W

Praise for *The Essentials of Clinical Reasoning for Nurses*

"This exciting new book presents a framework, the OPT Model of Clinical Reasoning, that nurses can use to guide their thinking about patient care. Case scenarios and patient stories demonstrate how to use the model in clinical practice, beginning with assessment and developing a patient-centered plan of care through deciding on interventions and outcomes. Nurse educators will find this book valuable. Effective learning strategies, such as Stop and Think questions and creating a Clinical Reasoning Web, are integrated in each chapter. These and other learning activities guide readers in reflection and using the clinical reasoning process in different patient situations—skills that are transferable to clinical practice. The OPT Model supports learning about and teaching clinical reasoning and care planning to students. With its many clinical examples, this book will be a valuable text for nursing students."

–Marilyn H. Oermann, PhD, RN, ANEF, FAAN
Thelma M. Ingles Professor of Nursing
Duke University School of Nursing
Editor, *Nurse Educator* and *Journal of Nursing Care Quality*

"This book brings clarity and depth to a complex nursing practice-based thinking process too often misrepresented as intuition or insufficiently described as the nursing process. The authors of this book reveal the underside of expert nursing judgment and decision making—systematic yet creative, and championing the patient's story and nursing knowledge and insights—through their eminently teachable OPT Model of Clinical Reasoning for entry-level professional nursing practice."

–Pamela G. Reed, PhD, RN, FAAN
Professor, The University of Arizona College of Nursing

"This book challenges nurses to deliberately integrate reflection and specific patient outcomes as they plan and provide care—and offers the OPT Model of Clinical Reasoning as a framework to do that. The model is explained clearly and applied brilliantly to the care of various patient populations, in community settings, and in clinical supervision. Using visuals that repeatedly illustrate application of the OPT Model to various case studies, the book clearly shows the reader how this approach promotes thinking skills of nurses and, ultimately, excellence in care. I highly recommend this book for educators, students, and nurses in practice."

–Theresa M. "Terry" Valiga, EdD, RN, CNE, ANEF, FAAN
Professor; Director, Institute for Educational Excellence; Chair, Division of Systems & Analytics
Duke University School of Nursing

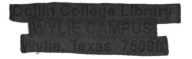

"The Essentials of Clinical Reasoning for Nurses *uses the widely acclaimed Outcome-Present State-Test (OPT) Model as a method for self-regulation in nursing and as a patient-centered clinical reasoning model to be used in the education of aspiring and practicing nurses. The book represents the seminal work that has been done on the model over the past 2 decades, including research that validates the model. I have used this model for over 20 years in my own teaching and highly recommend it for others who educate aspiring or practicing nurses.*"

–Deanna L. Reising, PhD, RN, ACNS-BC, FNAP, ANEF
Associate Professor, Indiana University School of Nursing

"*Nurse educators, nursing education students, and clinicians will find the strategies in this book to be invaluable in building clinical reasoning skills. The OPT Model of Clinical Reasoning builds on the traditional nursing process. The intuitiveness of the OPT Model makes it easy to teach, to learn, and to use. It helps users to identify the critical issue of care (keystone) for the client and to see how the keystone issue affects other issues for the client. In addition, the model guides the user in how to help clients move toward their desired outcome state. In times of scarce resources and challenges related to safety and quality in healthcare settings, the OPT Model can be a wonderful resource to aid in the timely, accurate, and efficient provision of care. I am glad to see a book where not only is the model well-explicated, but where examples of its use are provided to help the learner.*"

–Robin Bartlett, PhD, RN
Professor and Director of PhD in Nursing Program
University of North Carolina at Greensboro

"*The Outcome-Present State-Test (OPT) Model for reflective nursing practice is the most significant advance in clinical reasoning since the inception of the nursing process. When I teach students and present the OPT Model to practicing, experienced nurses and advanced practice nurses, the students and nurses tell me that the nonlinear, simultaneous processes in the OPT Model actually reflect the way they think and make clinical decisions in practice. The OPT Model advances clinical decision by combining narrative approaches to practice, including listening to patient-in-context stories; placing primary emphasis on outcomes; integrating standardized nursing languages (NANDA-NIC-NOC); framing the nursing situation within a nursing context; and using reflective nursing practice strategies—all integrated into one nursing practice model.*"

–Howard Karl Butcher, PhD, RN
Associate Professor, The University of Iowa
Editor, *Nursing Intervention Classification*

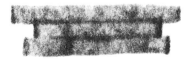

THE ESSENTIALS OF CLINICAL REASONING FOR NURSES

FOR NURSES

Using the Outcome-Present State-Test Model
for Reflective Practice

RUTHANNE KUIPER, PhD, RN, CNE, ANEF
SANDRA M. O'DONNELL, MSN, RN, CNE
DANIEL J. PESUT, PhD, RN, FAAN
STEPHANIE L. TURRISE, PhD, RN, BC, APRN, CNE

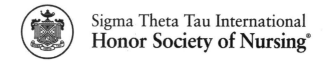

Sigma Theta Tau International
Honor Society of Nursing®

The Honor Society of Nursing, Sigma Theta Tau International (STTI) is a nonprofit organization founded in 1922 whose mission is to support the learning, knowledge, and professional development of nurses committed to making a difference in health worldwide. Members include practicing nurses, instructors, researchers, policymakers, entrepreneurs, and others. STTI has more than 500 chapters located at more than 700 institutions of higher education throughout Armenia, Australia, Botswana, Brazil, Canada, Colombia, England, Ghana, Hong Kong, Japan, Kenya, Lebanon, Malawi, Mexico, the Netherlands, Pakistan, Portugal, Singapore, South Africa, South Korea, Swaziland, Sweden, Taiwan, Tanzania, Thailand, the United Kingdom, and the United States of America. More information about STTI can be found online at www.nursingsociety.org.

Sigma Theta Tau International
550 West North Street
Indianapolis, IN, USA 46202

To order additional books, buy in bulk, or order for corporate use, contact Nursing Knowledge International at 888.NKI.4YOU (888.654.4968/US and Canada) or +1.317.634.8171 (outside US and Canada).

To request a review copy for course adoption, email solutions@nursingknowledge.org or call 888.NKI.4YOU (888.654.4968/US and Canada) or +1.317.634.8171 (outside US and Canada).

To request author information, or for speaker or other media requests, contact Marketing, Honor Society of Nursing, Sigma Theta Tau International at 888.634.7575 (US and Canada) or +1.317.634.8171 (outside US and Canada).

ISBN:	9781945157097
EPUB ISBN:	9781945157103
PDF ISBN:	9781945157110
MOBI ISBN:	9781945157127

Library of Congress Cataloging-in-Publication data

Names: Kuiper, RuthAnne, 1955- author. | O'Donnell, Sandra M., 1951- author.
  | Pesut, Daniel J., author. | Turrise, Stephanie L., author. | Sigma Theta
  Tau International, issuing body.
Title: The essentials of clinical reasoning for nurses : using the
  Outcome-Present State-Test model for reflective practice / RuthAnne
  Kuiper, Sandra M. O'Donnell, Daniel J. Pesut, Stephanie L. Turrise.
Description: Indianapolis, IN : Sigma Theta Tau International, 2017. |
  Includes bibliographical references.
Identifiers: LCCN 2017010413 (print) | LCCN 2017011431 (ebook) | ISBN
  9781945157097 (print : alk. paper) | ISBN 9781945157103 (EPUB) | ISBN
  9781945157110 (PDF) | ISBN 9781945157127 (MOBI) | ISBN 9781945157110 (Pdf) |
Subjects: | MESH: Nursing Assessment | Nursing Care--methods | Outcome
  Assessment (Health Care) | Educational Measurement
Classification: LCC RT48.6 (print) | LCC RT48.6 (ebook) | NLM WY 100.4 | DDC
  616.07/5--dc23
LC record available at https://lccn.loc.gov/2017010413

First Printing, 2017

Publisher: Dustin Sullivan	**Principal Book Editor:** Carla Hall
Acquisitions Editor: Emily Hatch	**Development and Project Editor:** Kezia Endsley
Editorial Coordinator: Paula Jeffers	**Copy Editor:** Charlotte Kughen
Cover Designer: Rebecca Batchelor	**Proofreader:** Todd Lothery
Interior Design/Page Layout: Rebecca Batchelor	**Indexer:** Joy Dean Lee

DEDICATION

To past, present, and future generations of nurses and nurse educators
who appreciate and value the creativity, complexity, and challenges
involved with learning and teaching clinical reasoning
for contemporary nursing practice.

ACKNOWLEDGMENTS

We admire and appreciate the clinical practice, insights, and wisdom of the following nurse educators who added to the development of the case study chapters in this book.

Angela Blake, BSN, RN-OB
Karen Monsen, PhD, RN, FAAN
Nancy Murdock, MSN, RN, CNS
Patricia H. White, MSN-Ed, RNC-NI, CNE

ABOUT THE AUTHORS

RUTHANNE KUIPER, PHD, RN, CNE, ANEF

RuthAnne Kuiper is a professor of nursing in the School of Nursing at the University of North Carolina, Wilmington. She earned a PhD in nursing from the University of South Carolina, Columbia; a master's of nursing degree as a clinical nurse specialist in cardio-pulmonary nursing from the University of California, Los Angeles; a BSN from Excelsior College, Albany, New York; and a diploma in nursing from Mountainside Hospital School of Nursing in Montclair, New Jersey. Kuiper's research interests include clinical reasoning, metacognition, self-regulated learning, and technologic innovation in nursing education. Kuiper has been the primary investigator for numerous studies related to nursing education and has many data-based publications from this work. She has been a grant reviewer for the National League for Nursing, Sigma Theta Tau International, INASCL, and the Department of Health and Human Services. She is on the editorial board for *Clinical Simulation in Nursing* and is a reviewer for multiple other professional journals. She is a member of Sigma Theta Tau International and has held multiple leadership positions in local chapters. She holds alumnus status from AACN for CCRN certification and has been a National League for Nursing Certified Nurse Educator since 2007.

In 2011, Kuiper was inducted into the Academy of Nursing Education Fellows. Kuiper was also included in the top 20 medical and nursing professors in North Carolina in 2013 based on being chosen as one of the top 100 nursing professors in the East by the Louise H. Batz Patient Safety Foundation. Kuiper's instructional and clinical expertise is in the area of adult health, specifically critical care nursing. She continues to teach nurse educator and nurse practitioner classes, supervises nurse educator practicums, and mentors graduate students across the country on master's and dissertation research projects. She has received a number of teaching awards in her professional career and is sought out by her colleagues for mentoring. Most recently, Kuiper has been faculty mentor in the Nurse Faculty Leadership Academy co-sponsored by Sigma Theta Tau International and Elsevier Foundation.

SANDRA M. O'DONNELL, MSN, RN, CNE

Sandra M. O'Donnell is a recently retired lecturer at the School of Nursing at the University of North Carolina, Wilmington. She earned her BSN and MSN, Nurse Educator from the School of Nursing at the University of North Carolina, Wilmington. She taught nursing for over 10 years. She received the graduate excellence award in 2006. She is currently a member of the Oncology Nursing Society, the National League for Nursing, the Nu Omega Chapter of Sigma Theta Tau International, and the Honor Society of Phi Kappa Phi. O'Donnell has taught clinical rotations in various clinical settings such as medical/surgical, oncology, cardiac step-down, renal, and progressive care units. She has taught undergraduate level health assessment, clinical reasoning, and scientific inquiry, pathophysiology, and the survey of professional nursing (an honors course). She also has experience in teaching online courses in the RN-BSN and the undergraduate clinical research programs. O'Donnell has been recognized numerous times by graduating seniors for her contributions to their learning experience, and she received the *Discere Aude* Award in 2008 for mentorship.

O'Donnell's research interests include the use of pedagogies in undergraduate classroom and clinical settings, and the development of increased self-efficacy among senior-level prelicensure students and new nurse graduates. O'Donnell has written several useful guidelines and handbooks currently used by prelicensure faculty in the nursing program. They include grading rubrics for written assignments, three clinical evaluation tools, a "Preceptor Handbook for Capstone" and "The Outcome-Present State-Test Handbook." For the past 10 years she has served as the editor of the quarterly UNCW School of Nursing newsletter, which is published on the School of Nursing website and distributed online to a large student, faculty, and alumni readership. Currently, O'Donnell serves in various volunteer roles in Wilmington, NC, which include the Lower Cape Fear Hospice board of directors and the New Hanover Regional Medical Center nurse volunteers.

DANIEL J. PESUT, PHD, RN, FAAN

Daniel Pesut is a professor of nursing in the Nursing Population Health and Systems Cooperative Unit of the School of Nursing at the University of Minnesota. He is director of the Katharine J. Densford International Center for Nursing Leadership and holds the Katherine R. and C. Walton Lillehei chair in nursing leadership. Pesut has worked in a number of settings. He was on active duty in the Army Nurse Corps from 1975–1978. He served on the faculty at the University of Michigan School of Nursing from 1978–1981 and completed his PhD in clinical nursing research at the University of Michigan in 1984. He served as the Director of Nursing Services at the William S. Hall Psychiatric Institute in Columbia, South Carolina (1984–1987), and was a faculty member at the University of South Carolina College of Nursing (1987–1997), Indiana University School of Nursing (1997–2012), and most recently at the University of Minnesota School of Nursing (2012–present). His work and scholarship in the areas of creativity, metacognition, and nursing education led to the creation and development of the Outcome-Present State-Test (OPT) Model of Reflective Clinical Reasoning.

Pesut is a fellow in the American Academy of Nursing. He served on the board of directors (1997–2005) and was president of the Honor Society of Nursing, Sigma Theta Tau International (2003–2005). He holds certificates in management development from the Harvard Institute for Higher Education and in integral studies from Fielding Graduate University. He is a certified Hudson Institute coach and member of the International Coach Federation. He is the recipient of a number of distinguished teaching and leadership awards. He has over 42 years of experience as a nurse clinician, educator, administrator, researcher, consultant, and coach who inspires and supports people as they create and design innovative practices with a desired future in mind.

STEPHANIE L. TURRISE, PHD, RN, BC, APRN, CNE

Stephanie L. Turrise is an assistant professor in the School of Nursing at the University of North Carolina, Wilmington. She earned a PhD and a master's of science in nursing, Adult Nurse Practitioner track, from Rutgers, The State University of New Jersey, Newark. She earned a post-master's certificate in nursing education from Indiana University-Purdue University Indianapolis and is a certified nurse educator. She earned her BSN from Bloomsburg University in Bloomsburg, Pennsylvania. Turrise's research interests include self-regulation both in nursing education and clinical research, specifically in individuals with chronic cardiovascular disease, and outcomes research surrounding transitions in care in chronic heart failure patients. She has been the principal investigator on internally funded grants with the most recent study being an interdisciplinary group examining the effects of mindfulness on outcomes in cardiac rehabilitation participants. She is an AACN board certified medical-surgical nurse and still practices in an outpatient cardiac rehab. She is a member of Sigma Theta Tau International and has held leadership positions in the local chapter.

TABLE OF CONTENTS

About the Authors vii
Foreword xvii
Introduction xix

I   MASTERING THE OPT MODEL OF CLINICAL
    REASONING. 1

1   THE DEVELOPMENT AND EVOLUTION OF
    CLINICAL REASONING IN NURSING 3
        Professional Nursing: Scope and Standards of Practice 4
        A Brief History of the Nursing Process 6
        The OPT Model of Clinical Reasoning 12
        Clinical Reasoning: Art and Science 15
        Summary 17
        Key Points 18
        Study Questions and Activities 19
        References 20

2   CLINICAL REASONING AND STANDARDIZED
    TERMINOLOGY 23
        Levels of Nursing Practice Data 24
        Standardized Terminologies: The Contributions of Nursing Informatics 29
        Harmonizing Nursing Language and Domains 37
        Future Evolution 42
        Summary 43
        Key Points 44
        Study Questions and Activities 45
        References 45

3   CLINICAL REASONING: THINKING ABOUT THINKING 47
        Thinking That Influences Clinical Reasoning 48
        The Kinds of Thinking That Support Clinical Reasoning 50
        Thinking Tactics That Support Mastery of Clinical Reasoning 58
        Summary 65
        Key Points 66
        Study Questions and Activities 67
        References 67

4   LEARNING THE OPT MODEL OF CLINICAL REASONING:
    PATIENT-IN-CONTEXT STORY AND THE CLINICAL
    REASONING WEB 71
        Sources of Health Data/Evidence 72
        Patient-in-Context 73
        The Clinical Reasoning Web: Strategy and Tool to Support
          Clinical Reasoning. 76
        Reflection on Clinical Reasoning. 83
        Key Points 88
        Study Questions and Activities 88
        References 89

5   LEARNING THE OPT MODEL OF CLINICAL REASONING:
    FRAMING, OUTCOME-PRESENT STATE-TEST 91
        Filtering, Framing, and Focusing. 92
        Reflection on Clinical Reasoning 105
        Key Points 109
        Study Questions and Activities 110
        References 110

6   LEARNING THE OPT MODEL OF CLINICAL REASONING:
    INTERVENTIONS, JUDGMENTS, AND REFRAMING 113
        Nursing Care Interventions 114
        Clinical Decisions. 116
        Judgments 118
        Reflection on Clinical Reasoning. 125
        Key Points 139
        Study Questions and Activities 140
        References 140

II APPLICATIONS OF THE OPT MODEL OF
    CLINICAL REASONING ACROSS THE LIFE SPAN 143

7   CLINICAL REASONING AND NEONATAL HEALTH ISSUES 145
        Case Study: Neonate with Jaundice. 146
        The Patient Story 148
        Patient-Centered Plan of Care Using the OPT Model of
          Clinical Reasoning. 150
        Patient Problems and Nursing Diagnoses Identification. 150
        Creating a Clinical Reasoning Web 155

Completing the OPT Model of Clinical Reasoning Worksheet 160
Summary 171
Key Points 172
Study Questions and Activities 172
References 173

8   CLINICAL REASONING AND ADOLESCENT HEALTH ISSUES . . 175
The Patient Story 177
Patient-Centered Plan of Care Using the OPT Model of
    Clinical Reasoning 179
Creating a Clinical Reasoning Web 181
Completing the OPT Model of Clinical Reasoning 190
Summary 201
Key Points 201
Study Questions and Activities 202
References 203

9   CLINICAL REASONING AND YOUNG ADULT
HEALTH ISSUES 205
The Patient Story 207
Patient-Centered Plan of Care Using the OPT Model of
    Clinical Reasoning 209
Patient Problems and Nursing Diagnoses Identification 209
Creating a Clinical Reasoning Web 211
Completing the OPT Clinical Reasoning Model 221
Summary 231
Key Points 232
Study Questions and Activities 233
References 233

10 CLINICAL REASONING AND WOMEN'S HEALTH ISSUES 235
The Patient Story 237
Patient-Centered Plan of Care Using the OPT Model of
    Clinical Reasoning 240
Patient Problems and Nursing Diagnoses Identification 240
Creating a Clinical Reasoning Web 248
Completing the OPT Model of Clinical Reasoning 253
Summary 263
Key Points 265
Study Questions and Activities 266
References 266

11   CLINICAL REASONING AND MEN'S HEALTH ISSUES......... 269
     The Patient Story 270
     Patient-Centered Plan of Care Using the OPT Model of
         Clinical Reasoning.. 272
     Patient Problems and Nursing Diagnoses Identification................. 273
     Creating a Clinical Reasoning Web 280
     Completing the OPT Model of Clinical Reasoning 285
     Summary... 296
     Key Points 298
     Study Questions and Activities 299
     References 299

12   CLINICAL REASONING AND GERIATRIC HEALTH ISSUES..... 303
     The Patient Story 306
     Patient-Centered Plan of Care Using the OPT Model of
         Clinical Reasoning.. 308
     Patient Problems and Nursing Diagnoses Identification................. 309
     Creating a Clinical Reasoning Web 314
     Completing the OPT Clinical Reasoning Model..................... 319
     Summary... 330
     Key Points 331
     Study Questions and Activities 331
     References 332

13   CLINICAL REASONING AND HOSPICE AND
     PALLIATIVE CARE 335
     The Patient Story 337
     Patient-Centered Plan of Care Using the OPT Model of
         Clinical Reasoning.. 338
     Patient Problems and Nursing Diagnoses Identification................. 339
     Creating a Clinical Reasoning Web 344
     Completing the OPT Clinical Reasoning Model..................... 349
     Summary... 359
     Key Points 360
     Study Questions and Activities 360
     References 361

III INNOVATIVE APPLICATIONS OF THE OPT MODEL OF CLINICAL REASONING. 363

14 USING THE OPT MODEL WITH THE OMAHA SYSTEM* 365
Community Care and Clinical Reasoning 366
Standardized Terminologies for Community Care: The Omaha System . . . 367
The Patient Story 375
Spinning and Weaving the Clinical Reasoning Web 376
Thinking Strategies That Support Clinical Reasoning 378
Summary. 389
Key Points 389
Study Questions and Activities 390
References 390

15 USING THE OPT MODEL FOR CLINICAL SUPERVISION. 391
Reflective Thinking Skills and Nursing Intelligence 392
Clinical Supervision and the Development of Successful Intelligence. 395
Using the OPT Model of Clinical Reasoning for Clinical Supervision 398
Summary. 403
Key Points 404
Study Questions and Activities 405
References 406

16 FUTURE TRENDS AND CHALLENGES 407
The OPT Model: Simulation Debriefing. 408
Curriculum Integration: Using the OPT Model of Clinical Reasoning
Across the Curriculum 410
The OPT Model and Interprofessional Education 415
Summary. 417
Key Points 418
Study Questions and Activities 418
References 419

GLOSSARY OF TERMS 423

INDEX. 435

FOREWORD

Have you ever encountered an idea or model that changed how you thought about your role as a nurse? That happened to me when I first learned about the Outcome-Present State-Test (OPT) Model.

I first encountered this way of "thinking about thinking" during a presentation by Daniel J. Pesut at some long-forgotten conference. As soon as I got home, I ordered the book he coauthored with JoAnne Herman—*Clinical Reasoning: The Art and Science of Critical and Creative Thinking*. Once in my hands, I read this small but powerful book cover to cover and was amazed by how well it fit with my passion for terminology development in my work on outcomes and interventions at the University of Iowa.

I immediately began using the OPT Model in my presentations on implementing standardized nursing terminologies into electronic health records. Many of these presentations were to international audiences, and I quickly learned to take a copy of the Pesut and Herman book with me to leave behind. I have given away at least 20 copies of the book in countries just starting to use the nursing process. I found the OPT Model very useful in helping nurses link nursing diagnoses, outcomes, and interventions. One idea I especially appreciate is the discussion about the generations of the nursing process. To me, this is critical in understanding where the nursing process began and where it is headed. Today, as we gather "big data," we are providing the foundation for moving our profession toward models of care for specific populations of patients, consistent with the generations of the nursing process.

Perhaps the OPT Model is most valuable when introducing beginning nursing students to ideas from *The Essentials of Clinical Reasoning for Nurses: Using the Outcome-Present State-Test Model for Reflective Practice*. They quickly learn to create web diagrams of case studies and start to think like nurses. My most rewarding experience in teaching happened after introducing clinical reasoning and the OPT Model. One of my students who participated in a home visit shortly after the OPT Model discussion wrote me an email describing how she had used what she had learned in class with her patient that night. The patient was not doing well following a cancer diagnosis and surgery. The student asked the patient to help her develop a web focused on the patient's problems. It became clear that the current care plan was not focused on the patient's priority issues. The student took her new web diagram back to the care team. They then generated a new plan of care to address the patient's needs, and the team complimented the student on her care of the patient. She was thrilled to have made a difference! I still have the email the student sent me that night. Her example shows the power of the OPT Model to help nurses meet the needs of patients based on individual patient stories.

I think that you, like me, will be greatly influenced by the content of *The Essentials of Clinical Reasoning for Nurses*. I warn you that the ideas may forever impact your clinical practice, how you teach, and even how you think about the problems you face in life. I know it did for me!

–Sue Moorhead, PhD, RN, FNI, FAAN
Director, Center for Nursing Classification and Clinical Effectiveness
Associate Professor
College of Nursing, University of Iowa

INTRODUCTION

In this book, we present and explain the Outcome-Present State-Test (OPT) Model of Clinical Reasoning. The OPT Model supports learning and teaching clinical reasoning, clinical supervision, and care planning. The structure and application of the model, definition of terms, and thinking strategies that support use of the model have education, practice, and research consequences for contemporary nursing. Students, clinicians, educators, managers, and administrators are invited to consider the OPT Model as an evolutionary development of traditional nursing process.

Based on our work with students in clinical reasoning courses, we have created, developed, and refined the OPT Model of Clinical Reasoning. OPT is a third-generation nursing process model that emphasizes reflection, outcome specification, testing, and the development of clinical judgment given the context of a client's or patient's story. The OPT Model supports the use and application of critical, creative, systems, and complexity thinking in clinical practice.

Application in Clinical Practice

Use and application of the OPT Model helps extract some of the covert thinking skills nurses use to reason about clinical care outcomes. By making the processes and thinking strategies and tactics more explicit, you can "unpack" the thinking used in reflective clinical reasoning. The OPT Model makes the invisible thinking of clinical reasoning clear and visible. Making these strategies more explicit has several benefits. Such analysis is likely to help teachers teach, students learn, and clinicians better reason. The focus on outcomes provides direction for care and benefits clients.

The OPT Model builds on the traditional nursing process and is different from the nursing process in several ways. First, the OPT Model organizes client needs and nursing care activities around a keystone issue. If keystone issues are resolved, then many of the more outlying problems will resolve themselves. Second, the OPT Model makes obvious the juxtaposition or gap analysis between a present state and a well-defined outcome state. The gap analysis creates a test. Test conditions activate clinical decisions, interventions, and evidenced-based judgments. Third, the model reinforces the concurrent, iterative characteristics of clinical reasoning. Fourth, the OPT Model is compatible with an outcome-driven healthcare system because it is built on a foundation of critical, creative, systems, and complexity thinking required for the development of reflective clinical judgments in practice.

Types of Thinking and Standardized Terminology

We have done our best to define the thinking strategies and tactics we believe are the essential ingredients of clinical reasoning. We outline the role of critical, creative, systems, and complexity thinking skills that support the reasoning core of the model. The OPT Model is a concurrent-iterative model of clinical reasoning. Reflection is an essential part of the reasoning process. The model uses the facts associated with a patient's or client's story and standardized nursing terminologies and systems thinking tactics to frame the context and content for clinical reasoning.

Clinical Decision-Making and Clinical Judgments

Clinical decision-making in this model is defined as choosing nursing actions. Clinical judgments are the conclusions drawn from tests that compare patient/client present state data to specified outcome state criteria. Concurrent judgments related to the match or mismatch of present state and outcome state data result in the need for clinical decisions. Clinical judgments result from the meaning one gives to tests created and outcome achieved. Reflections on judgments may indicate that outcomes were successfully achieved or may suggest the need for reframing the situation, creation of new tests, making additional clinical decisions, or alternative judgments about additional types of diagnoses, interventions, and outcomes needed to support quality care.

How the Book Is Organized

Part I, "Mastering the OPT Model of Clinical Reasoning," contains six chapters. In Chapter 1 we discuss the development and evolution of clinical reasoning in nursing. Chapter 2 describes and explains the importance and value of standardized terminologies for defining nursing knowledge and making nursing care visible. Chapter 3 provides a discussion and insights about the role of metacognition; critical, creative, systems, and complexity thinking; and ways that thinking strategies and tactics support the development of self-regulatory learning. Chapters 4, 5, and 6 provide a step-by-step approach to mastering the OPT Model that includes attention to the patient-in-context story and how to spin and weave a Clinical Reasoning Web to discern a keystone issue. Chapter 5 also describes and discusses the importance of filtering, framing, and defining the focus of care planning and reasoning efforts, and Chapter 6 details the elements associated with clinical decision-making, choice of interventions, and making clinical judgments.

Part II, "Applications of the OPT Model of Clinical Reasoning Across the Life Span," consists of seven chapters that illustrate the use of the OPT Model with specific clinical case studies. Readers will note that each of these chapters has a similar structure to support the teaching, learning, and application of the model with different clinical scenarios. The part begins with a neonatal health case and then focuses on application of the model with an adolescent and young adult. Chapters 10, 11, and 12 provide examples of how the model can be used with women's health-, men's health-, and older adult healthcare scenarios. Chapter 13 presents an end-of-life case and illustrates application of the model with a person receiving hospice and palliative care treatment.

Part III, "Innovative Applications of the OPT Model of Clinical Reasoning," consists of three chapters. Chapter 14 illustrates how the OPT Model can be used with the Omaha System, which is another standardized terminology that differs from the terminologies associated with the North American Nursing Diagnosis Association (NANDA-I), Nursing Intervention Classification (NIC), and Nursing Outcome Classification (NOC) systems. Chapter 15 describes and discusses how the structure, strategies, and tactics of the OPT Model can support clinical supervision and debriefing in simulation. Finally, Chapter 16 identifies and suggests how the OPT Model may evolve over and through time and support innovations in simulation debriefing, curriculum development, and interprofessional education. The glossary of terms assists the readers in defining new and familiar concepts that are used throughout the book.

As nursing science matures, the knowledge relevant to nursing practice expands. The OPT Model of Clinical Reasoning is a structure and process that builds on nursing's heritage and uses contemporary knowledge associated with the evolution and development of standardized terminologies to support the development and acquisition of critical, creative, systems, and complexity thinking skills necessary to reason into the future.

MASTERING THE OPT MODEL OF CLINICAL REASONING

1

THE DEVELOPMENT AND EVOLUTION OF CLINICAL REASONING IN NURSING

LEARNING OUTCOMES

- Review the current American Nurses Association Scope and Standards of Practice.

- Describe the development and evolution of the nursing process through time.

- Describe the role of standardized terminologies for clinical reasoning in the context of the nursing process.

- Describe the Outcome-Present State-Test (OPT) Model of Clinical Reasoning.

- Compare and contrast traditional nursing process models with the OPT Model of Clinical Reasoning.

The contributions of nurses are vital in meeting 21st century healthcare challenges. Advances in nursing knowledge work and the use of standardized terminologies support effective and efficient clinical reasoning and provide a foundation for the advancement of the profession (Pesut, 2006; Kuiper, Pesut, & Arms, 2016). The purpose of this chapter is to discuss the current scope and standards of practice for professional nurses as outlined by the American Nurses Association (2015). In addition, this chapter traces the history of nursing process over time and sets the context for learning about the Outcome-Present State-Test (OPT) Model of Clinical Reasoning.

PROFESSIONAL NURSING: SCOPE AND STANDARDS OF PRACTICE

Nursing as a profession has well-defined standards of professional practice and performance developed over time. Established professional standards guide practice and the education and socialization of the profession's members. The American Nurses Association (ANA) book *Nursing: Scope and Standards of Practice* 3rd edition (2015) provides a definition of nursing, explains the knowledge base for nursing practice, explains the differences between basic and advanced nursing practice, and discusses the professional, legal, and self-regulated governance of nursing practice for the benefit of society. The American Nurses Association (2015) provides several criteria by which a profession distinguishes itself from other occupations. Specifically, a profession has an orientation toward service within the context of a code of ethics. A profession uses a developed knowledge base and uses theory to guide actions. A profession is autonomous and self-regulating. Given the responsibilities of self-regulation, a profession is entrusted with the rights and responsibilities to regulate its own members and the services they provide. Professions are bound by a covenant and a social agreement to serve a greater good in the context of societal challenges and need.

To appreciate the development and evolution of professional nursing practice, it is important to learn about the history and evolution of the nursing process and the nature of thinking and reasoning that guides the assessment, diagnosis, outcome specification, planning, intervention, and evaluation of nursing care. The nursing process and the ways nurses think and reason about patient care situations have changed over time. The changes have been influenced by research and developments in nursing practice and education. Knowledge developed over time influences policy and practice standards. Nursing knowledge and concepts of professional duties have been influenced by legal, regulatory, and policy developments. Nursing education and teaching-learning principles linked with professional standards of practice have been informed by nursing education research. The current ANA Scope and Standards of Practice document (ANA, 2015) describes and explains the critical thinking model nurses use to provide a skilled level of nursing care. The model is commonly recognized as the nursing process. The model provides a structure for organizing thinking about nursing care for individuals, families, groups, and communities. This model is supported by a number of professional standards that guide practice.

Assessment as the first standard involves the collection of pertinent data and information related to the patient, family, or community's health. Assessment leads to a diagnosis. Diagnosis includes the analysis of data to determine actual or potential nursing problems or issues. From diagnoses, outcomes are derived. Outcomes identification is the process of determining desired results for the patient influenced by a nursing plan of care. Planning involves the design of strategies to achieve desired outcomes for the consumer or situation. Implementation or the execution of the developed plan also includes care coordination and activities related to health teaching and health promotion. Evaluation is the determination of progress toward outcome achievement. In addition to these standards of practice, there are standards related to professional performance that include:

- Ethical practice

- Attention to issues of cultural sensitivity

- Diversity and inclusivity

- Effective communication across all contexts

- Collaboration with all stakeholders including the healthcare consumer

Professional performance expectations include attention to leadership in practice settings and within the profession. The integration of research and evidence into practice positively impacts and promotes its quality. It mandates that one acquire knowledge and competence that reflect contemporary and futuristic thinking. There are professional performance standards related to practice evaluation of self and others, resource utilization, and environmental health. It is important to note that 2015 standards represent contemporary conceptions of nursing professional practice and build on the past development of standards and legal, educational, and political policies over time. The nature of the nursing process has changed over time. The authors believe it is important for students and clinicians to understand the history and development of the nursing process and how it has evolved over time.

Early nursing process models were organized around a problem-solving perspective. Over time, problem-solving models of the past have been replaced by contemporary developments related to an outcome orientation, with systems and complexity reasoning models that meet the demands of care planning and the clinical reasoning expected of today's nurses. Attention to contemporary nursing process models ought to include a discussion of standardized terminologies, systems thinking, outcome specification, and creative and complexity thinking. The following sections describe and trace the development and evolution of the nursing process through time.

A BRIEF HISTORY OF THE NURSING PROCESS

Since the 1950s, the nursing process provided the structure for clinical thinking in nursing. The traditional nursing process was designed to organize thinking to anticipate and quickly solve the problems patients encountered. Prior to the 1950s education in nursing was steeped in an apprenticeship model (Taylor & Care, 1999). Rituals, traditions, standard operating procedures, and apprenticeship models were replaced by an emphasis on developing problem-solving skills that supported clinical thinking. This first-generation nursing process (1950–1970) structured clinical thinking through a four-step problem-solving model of assessment, planning, intervention, and evaluation (APIE) (Pesut & Herman, 1998).

Bio-psycho-social and physical assessments revealed deviations from accepted norms and thus triggered problem identification, which was remedied by nursing actions, procedures, and interventions. Much of the nursing process and assessments were organized around framing issues from a body systems and pathophysiological approach. Filtering, framing, and focusing on specific problems were often directed by an assessment form or attention to deviations from a normal pathophysiological process. Over time, nurses began to differentiate nursing care perspectives from medical perspectives and set out to define and develop concepts, terms, and language to describe the scope and focus of nursing practice.

As problem-solution patterns emerged, a small group of nurses began to recognize redundancy of identified nursing concerns/problems. This attention to the pattern recognition and relationships between and among nursing care needs of specific client populations stimulated the development and self-organization of nurses who dedicated themselves to knowledge representation of nursing phenomena of concern. These nurses appreciated the complexity and self-similarity of patient care needs and nursing cures. They started to pay attention to patterns and relationships between and among behavioral cues, signs, and symptoms and defining characteristics associated with patient responses to their health and illness conditions. Nursing was defined as the diagnosis and treatment of human responses to actual or potential healthcare problems (ANA, 2015). This work evolved, and nurses systematically began to name, represent, and codify nursing phenomena into standardized knowledge taxonomies that have come to be known as nursing diagnoses, nursing interventions, and nursing outcomes.

Nursing diagnoses are standardized terminologies that represent, define, explain, and label patterns of behavior exhibited by patients within the domain of nursing practice. Pattern recognition and identification of relationships between and among cues, signs, and symptoms, and etiologies of these indicators evolved into a system of nursing diagnoses. The North American Nursing Diagnosis Association International (NANDA-I) continues to define the knowledge of nursing regarding problems and diagnoses (NANDA, n.d.). The nature and focus on understanding diagnosis and reasoning came to the foreground and informed the development of nursing knowledge for clinical practice.

The Evolution of the Nursing Process

As the issue of generating and developing nursing diagnoses moved to the foreground, the four-step problem-solving nursing process—assess, plan, implement, and evaluate (APIE)—changed and evolved. The knowledge representation, filtering, and framing work related to nursing diagnoses evolved to include interests in diagnostic reasoning. The four-step APIE model evolved into the five-step model of assess, diagnose, plan, intervene, and evaluate, or ADPIE. A second generation (1970–1990) of scholarship focused on defining and explaining the nature of diagnostic reasoning with a nursing filter and framework in mind (Pesut & Herman, 1998). Scholars began to explore how nurses were thinking about their practice and how caring, reasoning, and recognizing nurses as moral agents developed expertise and clinical wisdom. "Knowing the patient" and blending scientific knowing with the unique characteristics and context of a patient's story enabled nurses to practice the science and art of nursing (Tanner, 2006).

The work continues to support the creation of standardized terminologies that help define and explain nursing diagnoses, interventions, and outcomes. For example, a number of standardized terminologies used to filter, frame, and focus nursing care assessment and care planning emerged and have been recognized by the ANA. Some include the NANDA-I classifications, Nursing Intervention Classifications (NIC) system, Nursing Outcome Classification (NOC) system, the Omaha System, the International Classification for Nursing Practice (ICNP), the Clinical Care Classification (CCC) System, the Nursing Management Minimum Data Set (NMMDS), the Perioperative Nursing Data Set (PNDS), Systematized Nomenclature of Medicine—Clinical Terms (SNOMED CT), Alternative Billing Codes (ABC), and the Logical Observation Identifiers Names and Codes (LOINC) (ANA, 2012). The importance of these recognized standardized terminologies for clinical reasoning in nursing practice is discussed in the next chapter of this book.

The nature and nurture of clinical reasoning and clinical thinking became a focus for nursing education research and practice. Assessment and understanding of the "client-in-context" emerged as a priority regarding the development of expectations of nursing students and expert nurses (Tanner, 2006). Making the critical thinking in clinical reasoning explicit became an important topic and a major criterion for assessing students and accrediting nursing education programs (Facione & Facione, 1996; Bowles, 2000; Hicks, 2001; Scheffer & Rubenfeld, 2000; Kuiper & Pesut, 2004; NLN, 2006).

The Shift to Outcome Specification

As policies, rules, and regulations shifted in the healthcare industry, there was a shift from attention to problems to a concentration on the identification of desired outcomes or end results. Outcome specification, although implied, did not receive explicit attention in the first two generations of the nursing process—APIE and ADPIE. Scholars were busy creating standardized nursing classifications associated with nursing diagnoses and interventions and then later devoted time and attention to specifying outcomes (Butcher, Bulechek, Dochterman, & Wagner [in press]; Moorhead, 2013; Dochterman & Jones, 2003).

Enter the Outcome-Present State-Test (OPT) Model of Clinical Reasoning

As outcome specification assumed increased importance in nursing education programs, Pesut and Herman (1992, 1998, 1999) realized there was a need to help students master how they were thinking and reasoning about the complexity of patient care. So, Pesut and Herman (1999) created and developed the Outcome-Present State-Test (OPT) Model of Clinical Reasoning. These educators realized there was a need to create a model of clinical reasoning that embraced the unique complexity of the patient's story with attention to the complementary nature of the patient's identified problem with a specified outcome that could use the nursing terminologies that were being developed for the profession.

The OPT Model puts an emphasis on outcome specification given a presenting problem state that's derived from an analysis and evaluation of the competing issues clients may experience. The model suggests strategies that help clinicians gain insights into the juxtaposition between an identified present state and a desired outcome state. Problems and outcomes are two sides of the same coin, and when one is reasoning it is important to realize how the problems and outcomes are related and complementary in nature.

Kelso and Engstrøm (2006) observe nearly all problems and outcomes are complementary in nature. They suggest a new symbol to represent the complementary nature between a problem and an outcome and recommend use of the tilde (~) as a way to represent the complementary nature of problems ~ outcomes. Consider the complementary nature of nursing ~ negligence; pain ~ comfort; anxiety ~ anxiety control; suicidal ideation ~ will to live; self-care deficit ~ self-care. Every day nurses help people manage the dynamics of complementary needs and issues. Nurses help people transition from states of illness ~ health. A secret insight into the nature of clinical reasoning is the acknowledgment and recognition of the creative thinking that is required to appreciate the differences and complementary relationships between identified problems and desired outcomes.

The OPT Model was one of the first to make outcome specification an explicit part of the thinking and reasoning essential to the nursing process (Pesut & Herman, 1998, 1999). The OPT Model has been used in a number of schools of nursing and practice settings and has demonstrated effectiveness in helping students master the critical, creative, systems, and complexity clinical reasoning skills needed for contemporary nursing practice (Kautz, Kuiper, Pesut, Knight-Brown, & Daneker, 2005; Bartlett et al., 2008; Bland et al., 2009; Johnson et al., 2006; Kautz, Kuiper, Pesut, & Williams, 2006). The OPT Model foreshadowed the next iteration of the nursing process, which now includes attention to outcome specification. It is likely that in the future, additional generations of the nursing process will evolve (Pesut, 2006).

The Current Six-Step Nursing Process

The current standard of practice and description of nursing process offered by the ANA (2015) describes a six-step process with four additional subsets of steps under the implementation phase of the nursing process: assessment, diagnosis, outcome specification, planning, implementation (includes coordination of care, health teaching and promotion, consultation, and prescriptive authority and treatment), and evaluation (ANA, 2015). Figure 1.1 displays an adaptation of the ANA model of the nursing process.

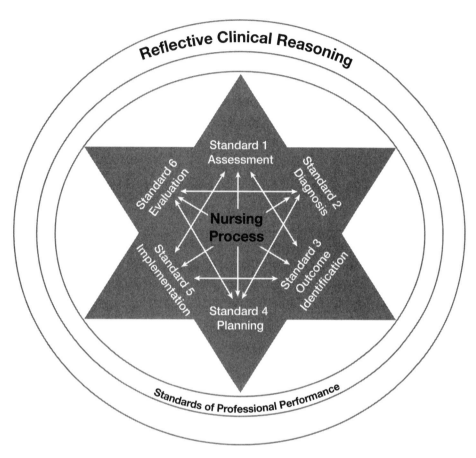

Figure 1.1 Nursing Process and Standards of Professional Nursing Practice.
*Adapted from the American Nurses Association (2015). *Nursing: Scope and standards of practice*, 3rd edition, ANA Publishing, Silver Spring, Maryland.

The current scope and standards embrace the essential elements of the OPT Model. As nurses monitor patients, they are always concurrently and iteratively "updating" the matrix of their thinking and reasoning about what is happening and how patients are responding. Nursing vigilance and attention are key skills that nurses need as they interact with patients. Nurses concurrently reason all the time about patient conditions and nursing care needs. The OPT Model of Clinical Reasoning provides structure—processes, strategies, and tactics that help students and clinicians master the complexities of clinical reasoning. The content of clinical reasoning or the clinical vocabulary one uses is based on the standardized terminologies. How one filters, frames, and focuses on clinical issues is often a function of philosophy and disciplinary perspective, structured from an electronic health record, or it's a policy associated with the use of standardized terminologies in an organization or practice context.

THE OPT MODEL OF CLINICAL REASONING

The OPT Model (see Figure 1.2) is a concurrent information-processing model that is iterative, recursive, and non-linear. This processing is in contrast to more traditional nursing process models, which are often presented as linear, step-wise, sequential information processing models. The OPT Model of Clinical Reasoning was developed to help students reason about the dynamics of patients' nursing care needs and master both the cognitive and metacognitive complexities of critical, creative, systems, and complexity thinking (Kuiper & Pesut, 2004). What follows is a brief discussion about the clinical reasoning that is supported by the OPT Model structure (Pesut & Herman, 1998, 1999; Pesut, 2001, 2004, 2006; Kuiper et al., 2016).

Clinical reasoning involves concurrent, creative, critical, systems, and complexity thinking. Clinical reasoning is supported by reflection and the intentional use of cognitive and metacognitive thinking skills and lower-order thinking strategies and tactics. The thinking tactics that enable one to perform clinical reasoning are gained through attention, practice, and conscious reflection about relationships among issues and the complexity of a client's story embedded given a specific context.

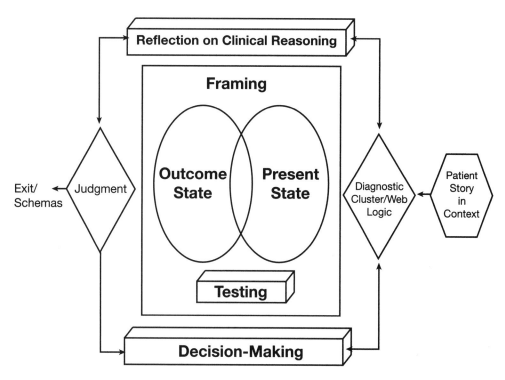

Figure 1.2   OPT Model of Clinical Reasoning (Pesut & Herman, 1998, 1999).

The OPT Model emphasizes reflection, outcome specification, decision-making, and tests of judgment within the context of individual patient stories and identified nursing care needs. The model advocates that clinicians simultaneously consider and understand relationships between and among competing nursing diagnoses and contemplate the interaction as well as balancing and reinforcing loops. It also advocates consideration of correlational as well as causal connections among the diagnoses. The OPT Model of Clinical Reasoning provides a structure, process, strategies, and tactics for considering patient stories in light of discipline-specific standardized terminologies. Relating elements of the story in a systemic way requires several kinds of thinking: critical, creative, systems, and complexity. Application of these different kinds of thinking leads a nurse to *frame, gain insight into competing issues, and understand the system dynamics and nursing care issues associated with a patient story.* Concurrent iterative thinking and reasoning leads to insight and understanding about the gaps that exist between a problem state and a desired outcome state. This *juxtaposition* of present states with desired outcome states reveals the complementary nature of problems ~ outcomes.

Once the gaps between a problem state and desired outcome state are defined, decision-making is activated and leads to simultaneous consideration of interventions that facilitate transitions from the present state to the desired outcome state. Judgments of outcome achievements are made by posing these questions:

- To what degree have outcomes been achieved?

- What else can be done to achieve the outcome?

- Is there a need to reconsider the filter, frame, name, and focus of the problem ~ outcome?

To help students and clinicians master the complexity thinking skills associated with the clinical reasoning in the OPT Model, relationships among diagnoses are represented in a visual way with a tool called a *Clinical Reasoning Web* (CRW). A CRW enables the clinician to "zoom out" and see the big picture and the complex nature of the client story and competing nursing diagnoses. As clinicians reflect, explain, and attend to interactive patterns and associations among the nursing diagnoses, what often emerges is complexity insight about the systemic dynamics of patient care needs.

After priority needs are identified, it becomes easier to "zoom in" and define outcomes associated with those present or problem state conclusions. Iterative reflection and expressed relationships between and among multiple nursing care needs leads to the identification of a keystone issue. The *keystone issue* is a central supporting element of the system dynamic and acts/serves as a *center of gravity* or leverage point in the system dynamic. Once this keystone issue is determined, efforts are put into specifying the problems ~ outcomes associated with the complementary nature of the "keystone problem ~ desired outcome." Evidence for outcome achievement is defined by criteria that are often included in standardized terminologies, for example Nursing Outcome Classification (NOC) (Moorhead,

2013). Nursing interventions are chosen and applied to help the client transition from the problem or presenting state to the desired or outcome state (Butcher et al. [in press]).

Clinical decision-making in the OPT Model is defined as the choice of nursing intervention or action that supports the transition from the present to desired outcome state. Clinical judgment in the OPT Model is an evaluation process about achievement of outcomes. To what degree was the gap between the present and desired outcome state achieved? Reflection on judgments might suggest the need for reframing situations or creating new gap analysis between problems and outcomes, making different intervention decisions or choices. Throughout the process, the nurse engages in iterative reflection and judgment about outcome achievement.

There are six logics embedded within the OPT Model. There is the logic of the patient story. The reasoning challenge begins with understanding the patient's story and reflecting on what the patient shares through the filtering of standardized knowledge representation. This logic leads to "framing" of a nursing care perspective. Every time nurses reason about a client story, they add to their repertoire of understanding and the resources they have to draw on for reasoning more effectively. These reasoning episodes help nurses develop schema that support pattern recognition in the future. There is the logic of the nursing diagnosis; the logic of relationships among competing diagnoses ~ outcomes; the logic of interventions that transition the client from present to desired outcome states; the logic of patterns and relationships among problems, outcomes, and interventions; and finally the logic of managing and self-regulating one's own thinking and reasoning efforts.

CLINICAL REASONING: ART AND SCIENCE

This book is devoted to helping students and clinicians understand how to reason more effectively about the nursing care needs of people. Understanding nursing in the larger context of society, what social forces are impinging on nursing, and what role nurses play in professional development and lifelong learning is a place to begin. The art and science of nursing is grounded in a social contract between nursing as a profession and society at large. As nurses strive to balance the art and science of nursing, the Scope and Standards of Practice (ANA, 2015) defines and outlines essential features of contemporary nursing practice. Essential features of contemporary nursing practice include:

- Attention to human responses to health and illness without restriction to a problem-focused orientation

- Integration of evidence and objective data with knowledge gained from an understanding of the client's story

- Application of scientific knowledge to the processes of thinking and reasoning about diagnosis and treatment

- Provision of a caring relationship that facilitates health and healing

As such, professional nurses are obligated to adhere to the 17 standards of practice and performance. Clinical reasoning presupposes you have certain skills and attitudes and have the knowledge you need to reason effectively. The prerequisite skills of clinical reasoning include activities associated with knowledge work: reading purposefully, memorizing, communicating ideas, understanding standardized terminologies, knowing the facts, putting facts together in meaningful ways, using facts, and deciding about the usefulness of facts for a particular situation. For example, in learning how the heart pumps blood, you needed to be able to read the text and memorize the information about the heart. Then you learned the vocabulary such as the right ventricle, aorta, contraction, and electrical innervations. This same kind of learning process takes place as you learn to use clinical reasoning in your nursing practice.

For example, to be a skilled nurse, you need to know the facts and use your knowledge. For example, normal blood pressure is 120/80 mmHg. Deviation from this indicates a problem. If you didn't know what was normal, it would be difficult to make decisions about deviations from the norm. Knowledge workers rely on standardized terminologies and the development of their critical, creative, systems, and complexity thinking skills. Reasoning is learned just as you learned how to use and work with knowledge to help yourself understand how the heart pumps blood. This book describes ways to think, reason, and reflect on patient stories. In the next few chapters, we describe and discuss essential ingredients of clinical reasoning and provide suggestions and strategies nurses and educators can use to develop clinical reasoning competencies.

SUMMARY

Professional nursing practice is influenced by developments in the discipline. Over and through time, the scope and standards associated with nursing practice have evolved. The nursing process is the thinking model associated with competent care. Since the 1950s, variations and versions of the nursing process have developed and evolved. Each subsequent development has been coupled with advances in nursing knowledge work. Early problem-solving models of the nursing process gave way to evolved models that focused more on diagnostic reasoning skills. As nursing knowledge classification systems developed and standardized terminologies were established, there was a need for nursing process models to incorporate standardized terminologies. As the complexity of nursing care increased, new models of clinical reasoning were needed to support systems and complexity thinking. The OPT Model of Clinical Reasoning provides the structure to help students and clinicians reason with critical, creative, systems, and complexity thinking skills in mind. The OPT Model is a *model of a model* or meta-model of clinical reasoning. It can be used by any of the health professions. What makes a difference with the use of the model is the clinical vocabulary or standardized terminologies that one uses to filter, frame, and focus the patient care issues at hand. Helping students and clinicians develop their thinking about thinking, or meta-cognitive skills, is one of the purposes of this text. The next chapter explores different levels of practice data and describes and discusses the importance of standardized terminologies for the clinical reasoning process.

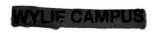

KEY POINTS

- Professional nursing practice is influenced by developments in the discipline. Over and through time, the scope and standards associated with nursing practice have evolved in response to contemporary political, legal, and educational developments.

- At least three generations of the nursing process have evolved over time. The first generation was focused on problems and process. The second generation focused on diagnosis and reasoning. The third generation is focused on the outcome specification with attention to the use and application of standardized terminologies.

- Standardized terminologies support filtering, framing, and focusing on issues relevant to patient care planning and nursing's contribution to the care planning process.

- The OPT Model of Clinical Reasoning is a third-generation nursing process that supports the development of cognitive and metacognitive aspects of clinical reasoning. The model taps into the critical, creative, systems, and complexity thinking skills that clinicians need to be successful.

- The OPT Model is a *model of a model* or meta-model of clinical reasoning. It can be used by any of the health professions. The difference with this model is the standardized terminologies one uses to filter, frame, and focus the patient care issues at hand. Helping students and clinicians develop their thinking about thinking, or metacognitive skills, is one of the purposes of this text.

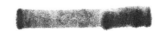

STUDY QUESTIONS AND ACTIVITIES

1. Read and study the third edition of the ANA (2015) *Nursing: Scope and Standards of Practice*. Pay particular attention to the appendices, which contain historical versions of the ANA Social Policy Statements over time. See http://www.nursingworld.org/nursingstandards.

2. Explore the North American Nursing Diagnosis Association website at http://www.nanda.org/.

3. Explore the Omaha System website at http://www.omahasystem.org/.

4. Explore the Center for Nursing Classification and Clinical Effectiveness at the University of Iowa website at http://www.nursing.uiowa.edu/center-for-nursing-classification-and-clinical-effectiveness.

5. Compare and contrast the work of the Center for Nursing Classification and Clinical Effectiveness with the work of the International Classification for Nursing Practice of the International Council of Nurses (ICNP) at http://www.icn.ch/what-we-do/international-classification-for-nursing-practice-icnpr/.

6. Develop a personal philosophy or position statement on the use of standardized terminology concerning professional nursing practice.

References

American Nurses Association (ANA). (2012). ANA recognized terminologies that support nursing practice. Retrieved from http://www.nursingworld.org/MainMenuCategories/ThePracticeofProfessionalNursing/ NursingStandards/Recognized-Nursing-Practice-Terminologies.aspx

American Nurses Association (ANA). (2015). *Nursing: Scope and standards of practice* (3rd ed.). Silver Spring, MD: ANA Publishing.

Bartlett, R., Bland, A. R., Rossen, E., Kautz, D. D., Benfield, S., & Carnevale, T. (2008). Evaluation of the Outcome-Present State-Test Model as a way to teach clinical reasoning. *Journal of Nursing Education, 47,* 337–344.

Bland, A., Rossen, E., Bartlett, R., Kautz, D., Carnevale, T., & Benfield, S. (2009). Implementation and testing of the OPT Model as a teaching strategy in an undergraduate psychiatric nursing course. *Nursing Education Perspectives, 30*(1), 14–21.

Bowles, K. (2000). Research briefs: The relationship of critical-thinking skills and the clinical-judgment skills of baccalaureate nursing students. *Journal of Nursing Education, 39*(8), 373–376.

Butcher, H. K., Bulechek, G. M., Dochterman, J. M., & Wagner, C. M. (in press). *Nursing Interventions Classification (NIC)* (7th ed.). St. Louis, MO: Mosby Elsevier.

Center for Nursing Classification and Clinical Effectiveness–University of Iowa. Retrieved from http://www. nursing.uiowa.edu/center-for-nursing-classification-and-clinical-effectiveness

Dochterman, J., & Jones, D. (2003). *Unifying nursing languages: The harmonization of NANDA, NIC, and NOC.* Washington, DC: American Nurses Association.

Facione, N. C., & Facione, P. A. (1996). Externalizing the critical thinking in knowledge development and clinical judgment. *Nursing Outlook, 44*(3), 129–136.

Herman, J., Pesut, D., & Conard, L. (1994). Using metacognitive skills: The quality audit tool. *Nursing Diagnosis, 5*(2), 56–64.

Hicks, F. D. (2001). Critical thinking: Toward a nursing science perspective. *Nursing Science Quarterly, 14*(1), 14–21.

International Council of Nurses (ICNP). (2016). Retrieved from http://www.icn.ch/what-we-do/ international-classification-for-nursing-practice-icnpr/

Johnson, M., Bulechek, G., Butcher, H., Dochterman, J. M., Maas, M., Moorhead, S., & Swanson, E. (2006). *NANDA, NOC, and NIC linkages* (2nd ed.). St. Louis, MO: Mosby.

Kautz, D., Kuiper, R., Pesut, D., Knight-Brown, P., & Daneker, D. (2005). Promoting clinical reasoning in undergraduate nursing students: Application and evaluation of the Outcome-Present State-Test (OPT) Model of Clinical Reasoning. *International Journal of Nursing Education Scholarship. 2*(1), Article 1. doi:10.2202/1548-923X.1052

Kautz, D. D., Kuiper, R. A., Pesut, D. J., & Williams, R. L. (2006). Unveiling the use of NANDA, NIC, and NOC (NNN) language with the Outcome-Present State-Test (OPT) Model of Clinical Reasoning. *International Journal of Nursing Terminologies and Classifications, 17,* 129–138.

Kelso, J. A., & Engstrøm, D. A. (2006). *The complementary nature.* Cambridge, MA: MIT Press.

Kuiper, R. A. (2002). Enhancing metacognition through the reflective use of self-regulated learning strategies. *Journal of Continuing Education in Nursing, 33*(2), 78–87.

Kuiper, R., & Pesut, D. (2004). Promoting cognitive and metacognitive reflective learning skills in nursing practice: Self-regulated learning theory. *Journal of Advanced Nursing, 45*(4), 381–391.

Kuiper, R., Pesut, D. J., & Arms, T. (2016). *Clinical reasoning and care coordination for advanced practice nursing.* New York, NY: Springer Publishing Company.

Martin, K. S. (2005). *The Omaha System: A key to practice, documentation, and information management* (reprinted 2nd ed.). Omaha, NE: Health Connections Press.

Moorhead, S., Johnson, M., Maas, M. O., & Swanson, E. (Eds.). (2013). *Nursing Outcomes Classification (NOC): Measurement of health outcomes* (5th ed.). St. Louis, MO: Elsevier.

NANDA-I. (n.d.). Retrieved from http://www.nanda.org/

National League for Nursing Accrediting Commission (NLN). (2006). *Accreditation manual with interpretive guidelines by program type: For post-secondary and higher degree programs in nursing.*

Omaha System. (2016). Solving the clinical data information puzzle. Retrieved from http://www. omahasystem.org/

Pesut, D. (2000). Knowledge work for 21st century nursing. *Nursing Outlook, 48*(2), 57.

Pesut, D. J. (2001). Clinical judgment: Foreground/background. *Journal of Professional Nursing, 17*(5), 215.

Pesut, D. (2004). Reflective clinical reasoning: The development of practical intelligence as a source of power. In L. Haynes, H. Butcher, & T. Boese (Eds.), *Nursing in contemporary society: Issues, trends, and transitions to practice* (pp. 146–162). Upper Saddle River, NJ: Prentice Hall.

Pesut, D. J. (2006). 21st century nursing knowledge work: Reasoning into the future. In C. Weaver, C. W. Delaney, P. Weber, & R. Carr (Eds.), *Nursing and informatics for the 21st century: An international look at practice, trends, and the future* (pp. 13–23). Chicago, IL: HIMSS.

Pesut, D. J., & Herman, J. (1992). Metacognitive skills in diagnostic reasoning: Making the implicit explicit. *Nursing Diagnosis, 3*(4), 148–154.

Pesut, D., & Herman, J. (1998). OPT: Transformation of the nursing process for contemporary practice. *Nursing Outlook, 46*(1), 29–36.

Pesut, D., & Herman, J. (1999). *Clinical reasoning: The art and science of critical and creative thinking.* New York, NY: Delmar Publishers.

Scheffer, B., & Rubenfeld, G. (2000). A consensus statement on critical thinking in nursing. *Journal of Nursing Education, 39*(8), 352–359.

Tanner, C. A. (2006). Thinking like a nurse: A research-based model of clinical judgment in nursing. *Journal of Nursing Education, 45*(6).

Taylor, L., & Care, W. (1999). Nursing education as cognitive apprenticeship: A framework for clinical education. *Nurse Educator, 24*(4), 31–36.

CLINICAL REASONING AND STANDARDIZED TERMINOLOGY

LEARNING OUTCOMES

- Describe three levels of nursing practice data.

- Discuss how each level of nursing practice data contributes to the generation and management of nursing knowledge.

- Explain why standardized terminologies are important for the organization of nursing knowledge, clinical reasoning, and care planning in professional nursing practice.

- Describe general features of recognized terminologies such as North American Nursing Diagnosis (NANDA-I), Nursing Interventions Classification (NIC), Nursing Outcomes Classification (NOC), the Omaha System, the International Classification of Nursing Practice (ICNP), the Clinical Care Classification (CCC) System, the Nursing Management Minimum Data Set (NMMDS), the Perioperative Nursing Data Set (PNDS), Systematized Nomenclature of Medicine–Clinical Terms (SNOMED CT), Alternative Billing Codes (ABC), and the Logical Observation Identifiers Names and Codes (LOINC).

- Discuss the harmonization of NANDA-I, NIC, and NOC with respect to a common unified nursing language and a framework for filtering, framing, and focusing nursing assessment and care planning.

- Explain how a common unified structure for nursing language supports the art and science of nursing and contributes to the generation and management of nursing knowledge.

Clinical reasoning presupposes an understanding of informatics and the role of standardized terminologies for the development of nursing knowledge work. Standardized terminologies are important for nursing practice at several levels of perspective. This chapter provides a brief orientation to the different levels of nursing practice data, and then the American Nurses Association (ANA)–recognized nursing knowledge classification systems are discussed. "A standardized terminology is one whose terms have agreed-upon definitions. It can be natural language, linear lists, taxonomic vocabularies, combinatorial vocabularies, or combinational vocabularies" (Sewell, 2015, p. 231; AMIA, 2015). Levels of nursing practice data influence the generation and management of nursing knowledge for care planning, organizational planning, evaluation, and nursing science development.

LEVELS OF NURSING PRACTICE DATA

Different levels of nursing practice data are used for different purposes regarding the allocation of resources and the generation and management of nursing knowledge that supports professional nursing practice. At the individual patient level, relationships between and among nursing diagnoses, interventions, and outcomes are important. As data and information about patients are aggregated, it becomes useful at the unit level for administrative and clinical decision-making. Data at the unit or organizational level is useful to support cost, quality, training, education, and effectiveness decisions. Finally, as organizations channel collected data to state and national entities, knowledge is generated and managed to support big data science and research. That, in turn, supports network-, state-, and country-level tracking of health outcomes and nursing care contributions.

The various levels of nursing practice data perspectives are illustrated in Figure 2.1. The Iowa Nursing Intervention project developed this model. It shows three levels of nursing practice data—the individual level, the unit/organization level, and the network/state/country level (Center for Nursing Classification and Clinical Effectiveness, 2015).

Standardized terminologies used in electronic health records that capture nursing data support the *filtering, framing, and focusing* plan that nurses use to reason about patient care needs, as well as interventions that produce desired nursing outcomes. Standardized terminologies are used to document the care that is delivered. Most students and clinicians are familiar with the individual level of practice because it is directly relevant to clinical reasoning. Managers and administrators are most interested in the organization- and unit-level data. Administrators and researchers are most interested in the network-, state-, and country-level data. Each level provides a different perspective about the nursing healthcare enterprise. All nurses need to be informed about these levels of practice data because data, once aggregated, defines, describes, and documents nursing's contribution to the healthcare enterprise. Appreciating the value of standardized terminology for the generation and management of nursing knowledge is a continuous professional responsibility and contributes to the metrics needed to monitor care, quality, and the effective use of resources.

Individual-Level Data

The level of immediate interest to most practicing nurses is the individual level. Information about the patient and the context is explained through the use of clinical knowledge that has been standardized in the form of classification systems or taxonomies. At this level, practice data is organized so that it is relevant and useful in explaining patient problems, nursing interventions, outcomes, and clinical choices and decisions that nurses can make. This data is often embedded into the electronic health record of an organization. If this information is collected and used according to a standardized system, it can be aggregated and used in a broader context at the unit or organizational level. Developments at this level are expanding as groups and organizations continue to focus on the development of nursing diagnoses, interventions, and outcomes and begin to aggregate nursing in the Nursing Management Minimum Data Set (NMMDS).

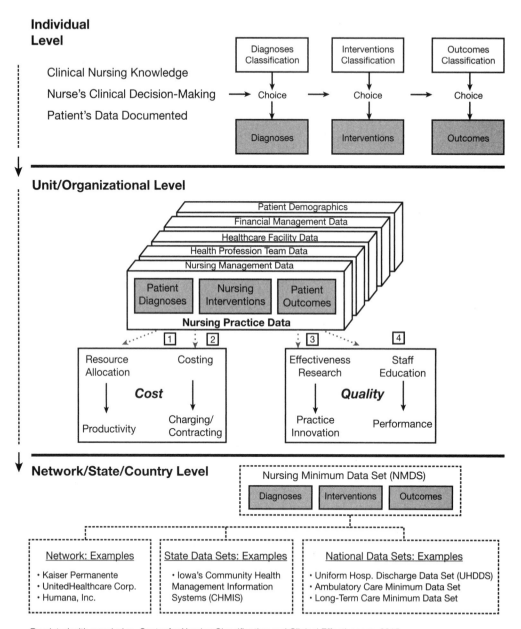

Figure 2.1 Nursing Practice Data: Three Levels.

Unit/Organization Level

At the unit or organizational level, data about individual patients is combined into one system. This system can be linked to other information systems, such as the medical care information system. At this level, analyses about common kinds of treatment can be performed according to four possible parameters: resources, costs, effectiveness, and education. Using data for resource allocation results in measures of productivity. Data related to costs provides information about charging and contracting. Data to support effectiveness research has consequences for practice innovations. Data about staff performance can be used for evaluation and planning. Each institution defines and specifies the type of information most useful for documenting patterns and trends for nursing service in the organization. If you have aspirations to become a nurse manager, this data will be important.

Network/State/Country Level

The network/state/country level represents the broadest scope of data about nursing activities. At this level, the Nursing Management Minimum Data Set (NMMDS) described next is an important contribution to the data management needs of many systems. What do you think are essential pieces of nursing information? A group of nurse researchers believes a nursing minimum data set is a good place to start. The NMMDS is a set of variables with uniform definitions and categories concerning the specific dimensions of nursing that meet the information needs of multiple data users in the macro healthcare system (Werley Devine, Zorn, Ryan, & Westra, 1991). The purpose of the NMMDS is to standardize information associated with nursing care that patients received in a variety of service settings. There are three elements in the data set: nursing care data, patient data, and service data.

Nursing care data elements consist of the following:

- Nursing diagnoses

- Nursing intervention

- Nursing outcome

- Intensity of nursing care

Patient data elements consist of personal identification, including date of birth, sex, ethnicity, and residence. Service data elements include the following:

- Unique facility or service agency number

- Unique health record of patient

- Unique number of principal registered nurse providers

- Episode admission or encounter date

- Discharge date

- Disposition of patient

- Expected payer

Benefits of this kind of data set include a uniform collection of data that can be compared across a variety of parameters, identification of trends related to patient problems and nursing care provided, and reliable data for quality assurance evaluation and cost of nursing service. Also, such a database promotes comparative research on nursing care, including research on nursing diagnoses, interventions, outcomes, and other clinical nursing research-based questions. Many organizations and projects are devoted to the development of the elements for the minimum data set. Consequences of this development include a data bank to research projects about nursing care. The Levels of Practice Data framework sets the stage and suggests distinctions between and among different levels of data collection, analysis, and evaluation. An important ingredient of each of these levels is the data itself. How specifically are data elements defined, coded, aggregated, and developed?

STANDARDIZED TERMINOLOGIES: THE CONTRIBUTIONS OF NURSING INFORMATICS

Nurse informaticists have a long history of scholarship and research related to the development of standardized terminologies and developing classification systems so that nursing knowledge can be represented, captured, and transformed into evidence-based practice guidelines. Nursing informatics scholars have spent many years representing and developing standardized terminologies to capture the *nursing framing* of client conditions. *Nursing informatics* is the "science and practice (that) integrates nursing, its information, and knowledge, with the management of information and communication technologies to promote the health of people, families, and communities worldwide" (AMIA, Special Interest Group on Nursing Informatics, 2009). Core areas of work include:

- Concept representation and standards to support evidence-based practice, research, and education

- Data and communication standards to build an interoperable national data infrastructure

- Research methodologies to disseminate new knowledge into practice

- Information presentation and retrieval approaches to support safe patient-centered care

- Information and communication technologies to address interprofessional workflow needs across all care venues

- Vision and management for the development, design, and implementation of communication and information technology

- Definition of healthcare policy to advance the public's health

The knowledge stored in these systems is useful for clinical reasoning, practice, and research purposes. The knowledge classification one uses in practice often serves as a *filter* for recording and ultimately thinking and reasoning about the management of problems, outcomes, and interventions. Filters help support *framing* and give specific meanings to a set of facts. Framing and meaning-making enable one to *focus* on a specific problem that, in turn, can be transformed into the desired outcome and influenced by the choice of an intervention. Capturing and organizing nursing knowledge in standardized ways supports the use of the data at several levels of practice and influences ongoing data mining and pattern recognition regarding the epidemiology of nursing diagnoses, interventions, and outcomes.

A useful standardized classification system is purpose-centric and has well-defined criteria for inclusion of items in categories—criteria that consistently and reliably assign items to categories and make sense to informed users. When classification systems meet these criteria, they provide the clinical vocabulary for clinical reasoning and assist the nurse in naming patient problems, communicating with peers concerning the patient, and communicating with other disciplines concerning the nature of nursing's contribution to care.

Why have classification systems? Mills (1991) argues that taxonomies provide language systems to identify relationships among essential elements and core nursing content. Such a systematic language system describes the culture of nursing. Taxonomies structure thinking and decision-making. Taxonomies facilitate memory and communication and promote consistency of care. Classification systems provide links to other classification systems. As you think about standardized terminologies, it is important to hold the following questions in mind:

- What is the purpose of this classification system?

- What criteria were used when classifying items? Criteria used to classify the content help define the meaning of the terms.

- How reliable are the classifications? To reliably classify content, you must have specific criteria for membership in a certain category.

- Is the classification system adequate?

- How specifically is the system evaluated regarding validity? Internal validity exists when the classification criteria can be used by anyone, and the same grouping will occur.

- Does the classification system make sense to the informed user?

As Kerr (1991) observes, the purposes of taxonomy are to understand one's world, communicate with others, provide information in a systematic manner, and identify gaps and relationships within knowledge. As our knowledge grows, taxonomies evolve and change.

Without standardized terminologies, it would be impossible to aggregate large amounts of data and information in a sensible way or use them consistently with the levels of practice data in mind. There are many classification systems used in the health professions. Classification systems organize and store knowledge. Classification systems systematically group ideas into categories based on shared characteristics or traits.

The knowledge that is used in the various levels of practice data is represented in a variety of resources. For example, nursing-specific knowledge developed over the last few years is stored in a variety of classification systems. Specifically, the work of the North American Nursing Diagnosis Association (NANDA-I) (n.d.), the Iowa Nursing Interventions Classification (NIC) project (Butcher, Bulechek, Dochterman, & Wagner [in press]), and the Iowa Nursing Outcomes Classification (NOC) project have made major contributions to the systematic development and classification of nursing knowledge (Moorhead, 2013). These internationally and nationally recognized resources are important because electronic health records are organized to map, translate, and capture the data in these knowledge representation systems to support the identification and tracking of essential health information at various levels of nursing practice.

Often it is the electronic health record (EHR) that is the vehicle through which nursing data derived from standardized terminologies is captured and stored. What is important regarding filtering, framing, and focus is that clinicians be conscious and purposeful about the way they frame the facts associated with a client's or patient's story. Standardized terminologies support disciplinary framing given the nature of the issues. For decades nurses have been defining and developing standardized terminologies that support nursing practice.

Nursing Documentation Organized by the ANA

For example, as far back as 1997, the ANA established the Nursing Information and Data Set Evaluation Center (NIDSEC). The purpose of this center was to develop and disseminate standards about information systems that support the documentation of nursing practice and to evaluate voluntarily submitted information systems against these standards. The target audience for these standards included consumers and vendors of clinical information systems. The need for an evaluation center emerged out of a long history of calls for standards about nursing data to information systems.

The workgroup established standards to evaluate the completeness, accuracy, and appropriateness of four dimensions of nursing data sets and the systems that contain them:

- Nomenclature

- Clinical content

- Clinical data repository

- General system characteristics

The Steering Committee on Classifications of Nursing Practice Data was organized to do the following:

- Support diversity in the development and testing of classification systems to describe nursing phenomena until stable systems evolve.

- Collaborate with multiple inter- and intra-disciplinary groups in identifying and developing classification systems for healthcare, as well as monitoring and studying the interrelationships of these systems to nursing classification systems.

- Promote or facilitate the classification of human responses that nurses diagnose and treat and for which they assume accountability.

- Ensure that classification systems developed or used by the nursing profession are adaptable to the various client/healthcare delivery situations in hospitals, nursing homes, and primary care.

- Promote consistent application of classification schemes that are selected, whether used for reimbursement, peer review, standards development, structuring practice, certification, or other purposes. Classification systems and integrated information systems are the building blocks for transforming data into nursing knowledge (Rutherford, 2008).

Today the ANA has recognized 12 standardized terminologies that support nursing practice, which are listed in Table 2.1. It is a professional responsibility and standard of practice to understand how standardized terminologies support professional nursing practice. Standardized terminologies provide the content knowledge and clinical vocabulary used in clinical reasoning. In this chapter, we introduce classification systems and standardized terminologies important for clinical reasoning in nursing practice. For most clinicians who work at the bedside, individual level of practice is most relevant. At this level clinicians make choices and decisions about the kind of patient problems they identify, the nursing diagnoses they make, the outcomes to establish, and the interventions they choose. The following chapters show how standardized terminologies are useful for thinking and reasoning about nursing care.

Given the context of practice or institutional policies, some of these classifications might be more familiar than others. It is important to realize that each standardized set of terminologies has contributed to the overall development of the profession and the healthcare enterprise (Sewell, 2015; Ackley & Ladwig, 2014). Understanding how to use and work with NANDA-I, NIC, and NOC is important clinical scholarship for the next few decades. NANDA-I diagnoses, NIC interventions, and NOC outcome classification provide the clinical vocabulary for clinical reasoning in nursing. The OPT Model of Clinical Reasoning provides the structure and some of the thinking strategies for combining, using, and integrating these classification systems in the service of care.

TABLE 2.1 ANA-RECOGNIZED STANDARDIZED TERMINOLOGIES FOR NURSING PRACTICE

Terminology	Description and Purpose	Link to More Information
Nursing Minimum Data Set (NMDS)	Defines and specifies categories of data needed to describe clinical practice. Includes patient demographics and unique patient number, unique nurse provider number, and nursing diagnoses, nursing intervention, nursing outcomes, and nursing intensity.	http://www.nursing.umn.edu/centers/center-nursing-informatics/center-projects http://www.nursing.umn.edu/sites/nursing.umn.edu/files/usa-nmds.pdf http://www.nursing.umn.edu/sites/nursing.umn.edu/files/nmds-monograph.pdf
Nursing Management Minimum Data Set (NMMDS)	Categories and terms useful to nurse managers and administrators for describing contextual factors necessary to plan, conduct, evaluate, and benchmark nursing services at local, regional, national, and international levels.	http://www.nursing.umn.edu/sites/nursing.umn.edu/files/nmds-implementation-guide.pdf http://www.nursing.umn.edu/sites/nursing.umn.edu/files/i-nmds.pdf
International Classification for Nursing Practice (ICNP)	Developed by the International Council of Nursing (ICN). Reference terminology containing nursing diagnosis, intervention, and outcomes that are combinational with parts of terms selected from seven specific axes: client, focus, judgment, means, action, time, and location.	http://www.icn.ch/what-we-do/international-classification-for-nursing-practice-icnpr/

Terminology	Description and Purpose	Link to More Information
North American Nursing Diagnosis Association International (NANDA-I)	Categories and definitions of nursing diagnoses. A nursing diagnosis is a clinical judgment about a human response to health conditions/life processes, or a vulnerability for that response, by an individual, family, group, or community. A nursing diagnosis offers the basis for selection of nursing interventions to achieve outcomes for which the nurse has accountability.	http://www.nanda.org http://kb.nanda.org/article/AA-00226/30/English-/Resources/Glossary-of-Terms.html
Nursing Interventions Classification (NIC)	Developed by the Center for Nursing Classification and Clinical Effectiveness at the University of Iowa College of Nursing. NIC categorizes and defines 554 nursing interventions grouped into 30 classes and 7 domains.	https://nursing.uiowa.edu/cncce/nursing-interventions-classification-overview
Nursing Outcomes Classification (NOC)	Developed by the Center for Nursing Classification and Clinical Effectiveness at the University of Iowa College of Nursing. NOC has 490 outcomes listed in alphabetical order. Each outcome has a definition and a list of indicators that can be used to evaluate patient status about the outcome on a five-point Likert scale.	https://nursing.uiowa.edu/cncce/nursing-outcomes-classification-overview
Omaha System	Classification of problems, interventions, and outcomes associated with patients, families, and communities in a home, public health, and community context.	www.omahasystem.com

continues

TABLE 2.1 ANA-RECOGNIZED STANDARDIZED TERMINOLOGIES FOR NURSING PRACTICE (CONTINUED)

Terminology	Description and Purpose	Link to More Information
Clinical Care Classification (CCC)	Developed to estimate home care expenses. The 21 Care Components provide the standardized framework for classifying each of the two interrelated CCC terminologies: CCC of Nursing Diagnoses and CCC of Nursing Interventions. They are used to code and classify the six steps of the nursing process: assessment, diagnosis, outcome identification, planning, implementation, and evaluation.	http://www.sabacare.com/
Perioperative Nursing Data Set (PNDS)	Provides standardized terminology and data related to the perioperative experience from preadmission to discharge. Developed as a means to generate and manage knowledge related to nursing contributions in an operative setting (Beyea, 2000).	http://www.aorn.org/aorn-org/education/individuals/continuing-education/online-courses/introduction-to-pnds
Alternative Billing Codes (ABC)	Developed to process alternative healthcare services not routinely included in traditional coding classification systems. Useful for documenting and billing for many alternative and complementary healthcare interventions. Includes many nursing procedures that are also referenced in NIC.	www.abccodes.com https://www.abccodes.com/faq/

Terminology	Description and Purpose	Link to More Information
Logical Observation Identifiers Names and Codes (LOINC)	A common language (set of identifiers, names, and codes) for clinical and laboratory observations. A catalog of measurements, including laboratory tests, clinical measures, standardized survey instruments, and more. Enables the exchange and aggregation of clinical results for care delivery, outcomes management, and research by providing a set of universal codes and structured names to unambiguously identify things you can measure or observe. Created to maximize interoperability and data exchange.	http://loinc.org/background http://loinc.org/downloads/files/LOINCManual.pdf
Systematized Nomenclature of Medicine–Clinical Terminology (SNOMED CT)	Comprehensive international healthcare reference terminology with subsets of nursing problems.	http://www.ihtsdo.org/snomed-ct/what-is-snomed-ct

From http://www.nursingworld.org/MainMenuCategories/Tools/Recognized-Nursing-Practice-Terminologies.pdf

HARMONIZING NURSING LANGUAGE AND DOMAINS

Table 2.2 represents an attempt to illustrate nursing domains of practice from the filtering and framing perspective. In this conceptualization, one sees the four domains of nursing practice and interest: functional, physiological, psychosocial, and environmental. Under these major domains are classes of diagnoses, outcomes, and interventions.

TABLE 2.2 HARMONIZING NURSING LANGUAGE AND DOMAINS: TAXONOMY OF NURSING PRACTICE: A COMMON UNIFIED STRUCTURE FOR NURSING LANGUAGE

Domains			
I. Functional Domain	**II. Physiological Domain**	**III. Psychosocial Domain**	**IV. Environmental Domain**
Includes diagnoses, outcomes, and interventions to promote basic needs.	Includes diagnoses, outcomes, and interventions to promote optimal biophysical health.	Includes diagnoses, outcomes, and interventions to promote optimal mental and emotional health and social functioning.	Includes diagnoses, outcomes, and interventions to promote basic needs.
Classes			
Includes diagnoses, class outcomes, and interventions that pertain to:			
Activity/Exercise: Physical activity, including energy conservation and expenditure.	**Cardiac Function:** Cardiac mechanisms used to maintain tissue profusion.	**Behavior:** Actions that promote, maintain, or restore health.	**Healthcare System:** Social, political, and economic structures and processes for the delivery of healthcare services.
Comfort: A sense of emotional, physical, and spiritual well-being and relative freedom from distress.	**Elimination:** Processes related to secretion and excretion of body wastes.	**Communication:** Receiving, interpreting, and expressing spoken, written, and nonverbal messages.	**Populations:** Aggregates of individuals, or communities having characteristics in common.
Growth and Development: Physical, emotional, and social growth and development milestones.	**Fluid and Electrolyte:** Regulation of fluid/electrolytes and acid-base balance.	**Coping:** Adjusting or adapting to stressful events.	**Risk Management:** Avoidance or control of identifiable health threats.
Nutrition: Processes related to taking in, assimilating, and using nutrients.	**Neurocognition:** Mechanisms related to the nervous system and neurocognitive functioning, including memory, thinking, and judgment.	**Emotional:** A mental state or feeling that may influence perceptions of the world.	

Classes Includes diagnoses, class outcomes, and interventions that pertain to:		
Self-Care: Ability to accomplish basic and instrumental activities of daily living.	**Pharmacological Function:** Effects (therapeutic and adverse) of medications or drugs and other pharmacologically active products.	**Knowledge:** Understanding and skill in applying information to promote, maintain, and restore health.
Sexuality: Maintenance of modification of sexual identity and patterns.	**Physical Regulation:** Body temperature, endocrine, and immune system responses to regulate cellular processes.	**Roles/Relationships:** Maintenance and modification of expected social behaviors and emotional connectedness with others.
Sleep/Rest: The quantity and quality of sleep, rest, and relaxation patterns.	**Reproduction:** Processes related to human procreation and birth.	**Self-Perception:** Awareness of one's body and personal identity.
Values/Beliefs: Ideas, goals, perceptions, and spiritual and other beliefs that influence choices of decisions.	**Respiratory Function:** Ventilation adequate to maintain arterial blood gasses within normal limits.	
	Sensation/Perception: Intake and interception of information through the senses, including seeing, hearing, touching, tasting, and smelling.	
	Tissues Integrity: Skin and mucous membrane protection to support secretion, excretion, and healing.	

The harmonization of language bridges the gaps among languages and supports the goal of standardization for health data analytic computations and projections. How one uses the knowledge stored in electronic health records depends on the context of one's practice, as well as one's knowledge, beliefs, values, and professional role. As nursing continues to evolve and data, information, and knowledge stored in electronic health records become an important *filter, frame, and focus,* the clinical scholarship will produce comparative, descriptive, prescriptive, and predictive health analytics (Ritt, 2014).

The purpose of NANDA-I is to provide a means to develop, organize, and test nursing diagnoses that are within the independent domain of nursing practice. Criteria are outlined in the procedures to develop and introduce diagnoses to the NANDA-I community. Reliability of NANDA-I diagnoses are supported by research literature, validation studies, and periodic refinement of labels and definitions. Labels and categories are tested to determine their adequacy. Diagnoses are accepted for clinical testing. As a result of use, diagnoses are tested and refined over time. Classifying nursing treatments is essential for the articulation and advancement of the knowledge base of nursing.

Nurses have been providing and documenting care for decades, but not in a uniform way. NIC provides a common language to communicate with ourselves and others the important work of nursing (Moorhead, 2013). A research team at the University of Iowa is doing important work regarding nursing-sensitive patient outcomes classification. Nursing-sensitive patient outcomes are variable patient or family states, behaviors, or perceptions responsive to nursing interventions and conceptualized at middle levels of abstraction. Nursing outcomes are one element needed to complete the nursing minimum data set.

The purpose of the Iowa NOC project is to:

- Identify, label, validate, and classify nursing-sensitive outcomes and indicators

- Evaluate the validity and usefulness of the outcomes classification through clinical field testing

- Define and test measurement procedures for the outcomes and indicators

The researchers developed outcomes as variable concepts so client states, in response to nursing interventions, could be documented over time and across contexts. Each outcome is associated with a group of indicators used to determine the outcome. For example, *fluid balance* as an outcome is defined as the balance of water in the intracellular and extracellular components of the body. Thinking of this on a continuum, five degrees of fluid balance are scaled. The range includes:

- Extremely compromised

- Substantially compromised

- Compromised

- Moderately compromised

- Not compromised

Use of a scaling method provides quantifiable information about outcome achievement. Indicators that fall under the fluid balance outcome definition include mean arterial and central venous pressure, pulmonary wedge pressure, 24-hour intake and output balance, body weight, presence or absence of sunken eyes, thirst, edema, or neck vein distention. NOC work is on the cutting edge and contributes a very important piece to the knowledge work needed in nursing.

The Omaha System was developed by integrating thoughts and ideas from a nursing theorist, researchers, community health nursing educators, and staff and supervisory nurses of the Visiting Nurses Association of Omaha (Martin & Sheet, 1992). The model is an approach to community health nursing. Three parts of the classification scheme are problem classification, intervention scheme, and problem rating scale for outcomes (Martin & Sheet, 1992).

In the Omaha System, four categories organize community health nursing practice. The categories or domains represent the first level of the problem classification scheme. These are environmental, psychosocial, physiological, and health-related behaviors. Within each defined domain, there are specified problems. Each problem is placed on a continuum that ranges from deficit to health promotion.

The second modifier identifies the focus of the problem as an individual or a family. Finally, associated signs and symptoms provide diagnostic clues to problem identification. The intervention scheme is a framework of nursing actions for use with nursing diagnoses.

There are four categories of nursing interventions: health teaching, treatment and procedures, case management, and surveillance. Health teaching involves such activities as giving information, anticipating client problems, responsibility for self-care, and coping. Treatments and procedures are actions directed toward prevention, identification, and alleviation of signs and symptoms. Case management includes nursing activities of coordination, advocacy, and referral. Surveillance includes detection, measurement, critical analysis, and monitoring to indicate client status about a given client condition.

The purpose of the Omaha System is to provide community health nurses with a systematic way to classify and code problems and interventions relevant to community and home healthcare nursing practice. Criteria were developed based on problems, interventions, and a problem rating scale for outcomes. The system is receiving increased attention regarding its reliability, adaptability, and cohesiveness to practitioners in the field (Martin, 2005).

FUTURE EVOLUTION

Members of the profession have an obligation and responsibility to stay informed and to use and refine the knowledge contained in standardized terminologies. The knowledge stored in these systems is the vocabulary of and for clinical reasoning. Imagine what the next 10 to 20 years will be like, as hospitals and healthcare agencies begin to incorporate standardized nursing language into the information systems and electronic records. Pesut (2008) suggests that over the next 10 years the fourth generation of nursing process (2020–2040) might be devoted to and organized around knowledge building. As databases and systems are linked with a common nursing language system, it becomes possible to discover and data-mine these repositories so that we can learn from the analysis of the patterns and relationships between and among nursing diagnoses, interventions, and outcomes.

As data accrues, it is likely that we will begin to develop the fifth generation of nursing process (2040–2050) archetypes derived from nursing analytic data that is empirically based and can inform best practices and provide new treatment options based on experience and clinical insights. As we refine these archetypes of care, we can learn the occurrence and epidemiology of nursing diagnoses, interventions, and outcomes for specific patient populations. We might also sort the data by type of institution or level of primary, secondary, or tertiary care needs. As we gain more experience and understanding of what patterns are occurring, nurses can plan more effectively and efficiently for the care patients need. We may in fact move to another generation of nursing process (2050–2060) whereby, given the data and prototypes of care that have been tested, we can develop predictive models of care based on the unique personal characteristics of the patient that can be compared with empirical data derived from data aggregated from several institutions or international databases of nursing knowledge. Simulations of patient care scenarios may, in fact, aid us in clinical reasoning, clinical decision-making, and better clinical judgments.

Evolution of these developments will focus nurses on the knowledge development and management strategies that support nursing care practices (Ritt, 2014). As explained in subsequent chapters, the OPT Model of Clinical Reasoning provides a structure that can use standardized nursing terminologies in a logical and artful way. The key to the success of this knowledge complexity work is appreciating and valuing the importance of nursing knowledge representation systems, the use of the electronic health record, and the evolving developments in nursing knowledge work supported by informatics and health analytic techniques and discoveries (Burke, 2013).

SUMMARY

There have been progressive developments in the area of nursing informatics and the development of standardized terminologies over the last 30 years. A series of projects resulted in the development of nursing classification systems, such as the NANDA-I, NIC, NOC, OMAHA System, ICNP, CCC System, PNDS, and

NMMDS. Additionally, nursing has been incorporated into interdisciplinary standardized terminologies such as ABC, LOINC, and SNOMED CT.

Through systematic research and peer review, these taxonomies developed labels, defined characteristics, and created structures that organize some of the most fundamental client problems, intervention, and outcomes that nurses deal with on a day-to-day basis. Standardized terminologies have several advantages. They provide a common language. Recognized standardized terminologies contribute to nursing's professional identity, role, and contribution to the healthcare enterprise. They provide a way to structure, generate, and manage knowledge. Taxonomies define the "what" and the nature of nursing care. Taxonomies are standardized so that it is possible to link payment to services and link nursing to other databases and healthcare classification systems. Standardized terminologies provide the content and vocabulary one uses for clinical reasoning. Accumulation of nursing knowledge at all levels of practice data provides the foundation for data science development and future types of nursing analytics.

KEY POINTS

- The development of standardized terminologies is important to build nursing knowledge at several levels of practice and perspectives.

- When examining classification systems, pay attention to the following issues: purpose, criteria used to create categories, classes, reliability, adaptability, and coherence or sense to the user.

- As of June 2012, the ANA has recognized 12 sets of standardized terminologies that support nursing practice: NANDA-I, NIC, NOC, Omaha System, NMDS, ICNP, CCC System, NMMDS, PNDS, SNOMED CT, ABC, and LOINC.

- Knowledge stored or classified in these systems becomes the clinical vocabulary and content for clinical reasoning.

- Harmonizing nursing language and domains provide a framework for assessment and evaluation of essential nursing care issues.

- Knowing the knowledge contained in these systems makes clinical reasoning easier, more effective, and efficient.

- Although there are a variety of recognized terminologies, the rest of this book relies on the use of NANDA-I, NIC, and NOC, as these standardized terminologies are most commonly embedded in electronic health records and used in clinical practice.

STUDY QUESTIONS AND ACTIVITIES

1. Which of the standardized terminologies described in this chapter are you most familiar with? Make a list of the advantages and disadvantages of each system described in this chapter.

2. Conduct a literature search on the system you know the least about. Find out what current information exists regarding this system.

3. One of the disadvantages of such systems is that they promote labeling of individuals given certain diagnoses. Discuss with a colleague the pros and cons of "labeling" clients using existing classification systems terminology.

4. Interview someone in another discipline and ask if the person uses standardized terminologies or specific knowledge classification systems in his or her work.

References

Ackley, B. J., & Ladwig, G. B. (2014). *Nursing diagnosis handbook: An evidence-based guide to planning care* (11th ed.). Maryland Heights, MO: Mosby.

American Medical Informatics Association (AMIA). (2015). Retrieved from http://www.amia.org/about-amia/mission-and-history

American Nurses Association (ANA). (2012). ANA recognized terminologies that support nursing practice. Retrieved from http://www.nursingworld.org/MainMenuCategories/ThePracticeofProfessionalNursing/NursingStandards/Recognized-Nursing-Practice-Terminologies.aspx

AMIA Nursing Special Interest Group. Retrieved from https://www.amia.org/programs/working-groups/nursing-informatics

Beyea, S. C. (2000). Perioperative data elements: Interventions and outcomes. *AORN Journal, 71*(2), 344–352.

Burke, J. (2013). *Health analytics: Gaining insight to transform health care.* Hoboken, NJ: John Wiley & Sons.

Butcher, H. K., Bulechek, G. M., Dochterman, J. M., & Wagner, C. M. (in press). *Nursing Interventions Classification (NIC)* (7th ed.). St. Louis, MO: Mosby.

Dochterman, J. M., & Jones, D. A. (Eds.). (2003). *Unifying nursing languages: The harmonization of NANDA, NIC, and NOC.* Washington, DC: American Nurses Association.

Kerr, M. (1991). Validation of taxonomies. In R. Carroll-Johnson (Ed.), *Classification of nursing diagnoses: Proceedings of the 9th conference* (pp. 6–13). Philadelphia, PA: Lippincott.

Martin, K. S. (2005). *The Omaha System: A key to practice, documentation, and information management* (2nd ed.). Omaha, NE: Health Connections Press.

Martin, K. S., & Scheet, N. J. (Eds.). (1992). *The Omaha System: Applications for community health nursing.* Omaha, NE: WB Saunders Company.

Mills, W. (1991). Why a classification system? In R. Carroll-Johnson (Ed.), *Classification of nursing diagnoses: Proceedings of the 9th conference* (pp. 3–6). Philadelphia, PA: Lippincott.

Moorhead, S. (2013). *Nursing Outcomes Classification (NOC): Measurement of health outcomes* (5th ed.). Philadelphia, PA: Elsevier Health Sciences.

NANDA-I. (n.d.). Nursing diagnoses: Definitions and classification. Retrieved from http://www.nanda.org/

Omaha System. (2016). Retrieved from http://www.omahasystem.org/

Pesut, D. (2008). Thoughts on thinking with complexity in mind. In C. Lindberg, S. Nash, & C. Lindberg (Eds.), *On the edge: Nursing in the age of complexity* (pp. 211–238). Bordentown, NJ: PlexusPress.

Ritt, E. (2014). Essential analytics in nursing education: Building capacity to improve clinical practice. *Journal of Nursing Education and Practice, 4*(12), 9–12.

Rutherford, M. (2008). Standardized nursing language: What does it mean for nursing practice. *OJIN: The Online Journal of Issues in Nursing, 13*(1), 243–250.

Sewell, J. (2015). *Informatics and nursing: Opportunities and challenges* (5th ed.). Philadelphia, PA: Wolters Kluwer.

Werley, H. H., Devine, E., Zorn, C. R., Ryan, P., & Westra, B. L. (1991). The Nursing Minimum Data Set: Abstraction tool for standardized, comparable, essential data. *American Journal of Public Health, 81*(4), 421–426.

3

CLINICAL REASONING: THINKING ABOUT THINKING

LEARNING OUTCOMES

- Identify five types of thinking that support the development and mastery of clinical reasoning.

- Describe relationships between and among critical thinking, self-regulatory thinking, creative thinking, systems thinking, and complexity thinking proposed to support clinical reasoning skill development.

- Describe the importance of reflection and self-regulation during the clinical reasoning process.

- Define 11 thinking tactics and strategies that support the development of clinical reasoning thinking skills.

THINKING THAT INFLUENCES CLINICAL REASONING

This chapter explores and describes different types of thinking required to support clinical reasoning. The importance of reflection and self-regulation is highlighted. It also discusses the influence of critical, creative, self-regulatory, systems, and complexity thinking. Finally, the chapter introduces several thinking tactics and strategies that facilitate and support the development of clinical reasoning skill sets.

Nursing practice has been influenced by trends and developments of technological advances. As noted in Chapter 1, the nursing process has evolved and transformed over time. What was once a four-phase problem-solving process has developed into a six-phase process that includes assessment, diagnosis, outcome specification, planning, implementation, and evaluation. Each phase of the process activates a different kind of thinking associated with the patient's story, history, care needs, and the healthcare issues being addressed. Different kinds of thinking influence how a nurse filters, frames, and focuses the data, knowledge, and evidence used to reason about a case. Knowledge and evidence management inform the nursing process and practice. Clinical reasoning activates many types of thinking. As nurses clinically reason with patients, families, and other providers within organizations and systems, they continuously develop critical, creative, systems, and complexity thinking skills. Mastery of clinical reasoning necessitates the development of *metacognitive* (thinking about thinking) self-regulation skills as well as cognitive thinking tactics and strategies (Kuiper & Pesut, 2004).

How is it that one develops the ability to think about one's thinking and *be aware of being aware?* One way is to make distinctions about the kinds of thinking that are involved in the clinical reasoning process. Another way is to make distinctions between the cognitive and metacognitive aspects of thinking. Metacognitive awareness requires the development of self-regulation skills. Self-regulation requires an attention to the processes of self-monitoring, self-evaluation, and self-reinforcement (Pesut & Herman, 1999; Kuiper & Pesut, 2004; Kuiper, Pesut, & Arms, 2016).

Metacognitive skills are important for determining the practice issues, interventions, and outcomes that support care plans in service of a quality outcome (Herman, Pesut, & Conard, 1994). Specific cognitive and metacognitive processes include the application of knowledge and experience to identify patient problems, make clinical judgments, and implement actions to support outcome achievement (Benner, Hughes, & Sutphen, 2008; Kuiper & Pesut, 2004; Kuiper et al., 2016).

Failure to develop one's thinking-about-thinking capacity is likely to lead to *hypocognition,* which has been defined as an inability to understand and think in a strategic way (Mariotto, 2010). In order to avoid hypocognition, nurses ought to consider the following strategies:

- Integrate basic science into clinical reasoning skills

- Practice translating evidence into practice from a pragmatic standpoint using the type of thinking that promotes it

- Be cautious about the use of algorithms created as an attempt to synthesize overwhelming amounts of clinical research data and deny and work against individuality of clinical decision-making (Mariotto, 2010)

Clinical expertise is needed to know when it is appropriate to deviate from evidence-based guidelines given the values and preferences of individual patients to deliver quality, patient-centered, safe care (Cronenwett et al., 2007). As nurses focus on different aspects of patient care needs, standardized terminologies and knowledge representations systems provide ways to help them filter, frame, and focus disciplinary contributions to care in a strategic and thoughtful way.

An essential part of the framing involves attention to patient and family needs, wishes, and preferences. Understanding the nature of a whole situation from different perspectives is embedded in a sense of salience and reasoning across time, through changes in the situation, or through one's understanding (frame) of the situation (Benner, Hooper-Kyriakidis, & Stannard, 2011; Bourdieu, 1990). This understanding brings to the forefront the importance of a nurse's ability to reflect and self-regulate using the appropriate thinking activities for the context and healthcare problem at hand.

THE KINDS OF THINKING THAT SUPPORT CLINICAL REASONING

The kinds of thinking essential to clinical reasoning are displayed in Figure 3.1. Cognitive (critical thinking) and metacognitive (reflective self-regulation, creative thinking, systems thinking, and complexity thinking) are listed to show the distinctions among these kinds of thinking. In practice, each of these types of thinking is used in a recursive, iterative way and is related to the others.

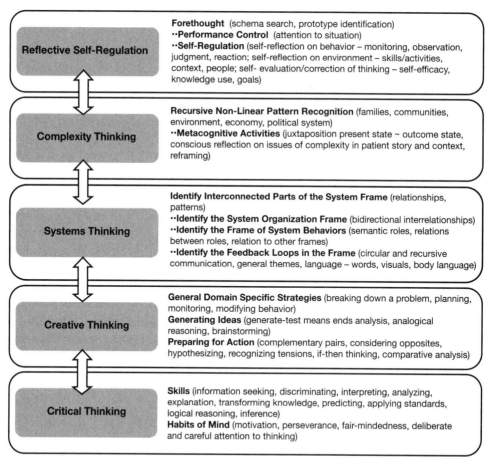

Reflective Self-Regulation

Forethought (schema search, prototype identification)
··**Performance Control** (attention to situation)
··**Self-Regulation** (self-reflection on behavior – monitoring, observation, judgment, reaction; self-reflection on environment – skills/activities, context, people; self- evaluation/correction of thinking – self-efficacy, knowledge use, goals)

Complexity Thinking

Recursive Non-Linear Pattern Recognition (families, communities, environment, economy, political system)
··**Metacognitive Activities** (juxtaposition present state ~ outcome state, conscious reflection on issues of complexity in patient story and context, reframing)

Systems Thinking

Identify Interconnected Parts of the System Frame (relationships, patterns)
··**Identify the System Organization Frame** (bidirectional interrelationships)
··**Identify the Frame of System Behaviors** (semantic roles, relations between roles, relation to other frames)
··**Identify the Feedback Loops in the Frame** (circular and recursive communication, general themes, language – words, visuals, body language)

Creative Thinking

General Domain Specific Strategies (breaking down a problem, planning, monitoring, modifying behavior)
Generating Ideas (generate-test means ends analysis, analogical reasoning, brainstorming)
Preparing for Action (complementary pairs, considering opposites, hypothesizing, recognizing tensions, if-then thinking, comparative analysis)

Critical Thinking

Skills (information seeking, discriminating, interpreting, analyzing, explanation, transforming knowledge, predicting, applying standards, logical reasoning, inference)
Habits of Mind (motivation, perseverance, fair-mindedness, deliberate and careful attention to thinking)

Figure 3.1 Kinds of Thinking That Support Clinical Reasoning.

Critical Thinking

For many years in nursing education programs, the curriculum was developed and organized around the value of critical thinking. In fact, the American Association of Colleges of Nursing (AACN, 2008) established critical thinking as a fundamental and essential part of baccalaureate nursing programs. Watson and Glaser (1964) suggest that *critical thinking* is a complex set of attitudes that support problem recognition, logic, and a search for evidence to support truths. Facione (1990) conducted an international Delphi study to determine a consensus statement on the essence of critical thinking and defined critical thinking as "purposeful, self-regulatory judgment." Critical thinking is a constellation of some skills that include interpretation, analysis, inference, explanation, evaluation, and self-regulation (Facione & Facione, 1996). Scheffer and Rubenfeld (2000) surveyed expert nurse educators and developed a definition of critical thinking that embraces deliberate and careful attention to thinking and the cognitive processes of information seeking, discriminating, analyzing, transforming knowledge, predicating, applying standards, and logical reasoning along with the characteristics of motivation, perseverance, and fair-mindedness.

According to Brookfield (2012), critical thinking happens when people attempt to discover assumptions that influence the way they think and act, check or appraise whether those assumptions are valid and reliable guides for action, look at these assumptions from multiple viewpoints or as others see them, and then take informed action.

Three types of assumptions are important for critical thinking:

- *Paradigmatic assumptions*—Ordering the world into fundamental categories

- *Prescriptive assumptions*—What we think ought to happen in a particular circumstance

- *Causal assumptions*—How the world works and the conditions under which these assumptions can be changed (Brookfield, 2012)

When critical thinking is linked to actions, the issue of "values" is raised because the next step in the process is to determine which actions are desirable and supported (Brookfield, 2012). Critical thinking is more than a mental process and is done with a greater purpose in mind, informed by the values of the situation and the context in which they occur. For example, a nurse using critical thinking skills will examine the assumptions and knowledge held by all parties concerned when decisions are made to vaccinate children. Knowing how to educate and present the best evidence to a parent will impact the values the parents place on preventative healthcare measures for their child.

Reflective Self-Regulation

Self-monitoring, a thinking activity used during self-regulation, leads to a change in an individual's strategies, cognitions, affects, and behaviors. When these thinking activities become habitual, as one repeats the processes in subsequent situations, the learner develops self-efficacy to attain goals and employ self-evaluation during reflection to make attributions for performance (Kuiper & Pesut, 2004; Schunk, 2012; Kuiper et al., 2016).

The self-regulation processes that coincide with learning are described by Zimmerman (1998, 2000) as forethought, performance control, and self-reflection. The forethought phase when applied to care planning precedes action and sets the stage for clinical reasoning. Performance control is the phase that coincides with clinical reasoning and affects the attention given to a situation and resulting actions. Self-reflection is the phase whereby people respond behaviorally and mentally to their actions. Social Cognitive Theory proposes that the interaction of the personal, behavioral, and environmental processes during self-regulated thinking is cyclic because the phases change as they are monitored during the process (Zimmerman, 1998, 2000).

When using the OPT Model of Clinical Reasoning, reflection is a component of executive thinking processes (Pesut & Herman, 1992, 1999). Reflection is the process of observing one's thinking while simultaneously thinking about patient situations. The goal of reflection is to achieve the best possible thought processes. The greater the reflection, the higher the quality of care delivered. Reflection involves the use of the skills of monitoring, analyzing, predicting, planning, evaluating, and revising (Herman et al., 1994). When effective clinical reasoning is employed, there is evidence of self-regulated learning and strategic thinking, as well as forethought and performance control for care planning that produces positive healthcare outcomes for patients, families, and communities (Kuiper, Pesut, & Kautz, 2009). Such strategic thinking builds on foundations of critical thinking but furthermore requires the development and application of creative, systems, and complexity thinking. The development of these thinking skills leads to clinical growth (Barkimer, 2016).

Creative Thinking

Creative thinking is a metacognitive process that supports clinical reasoning by generating associations, attributes, elements, images, and operations to solve problems or meet a need based on the complementary nature of a problem and outcome (Pesut, 1985, 2008, 2016). Creative thinking involves grappling with complementary pairs, tensions, and opposites (Pesut, 2008, 2016). Creative problem-solving, defined in a model by Treffinger (1985) and Treffinger and Isaksen (2005), consists of three stages: understanding a challenge, generating ideas, and preparing for action. It involves the metacognitive processes of planning, monitoring, and modifying behavior (Schunk, 2012). Consider how this model might apply to a clinical situation. Reflect on whether this process is evident in a clinical reasoning scenario.

First, as a problem is considered, general strategies—such as breaking down a problem into its components—are implemented that could be used across domains. These strategies are used early in creative thinking activities to understand the challenges in a problem. Second, generating ideas is accomplished by tactics such as generate-and-test, means-ends analysis, analogical reasoning, and brainstorming using domain-specific knowledge and experience (Schunk, 2012). The generate-and-test strategy uses knowledge to create a hierarchy of possible solutions and subsequent solution choice.

Second, fundamental to creative thinking is the means-ends analysis activity, which compares the situation at hand with the desired goal and compares and contrasts the differences between them. In the OPT Model of Clinical Reasoning, creative thinking is defined as juxtaposing a problem with an outcome. By identifying sub-goals and attaining each of them, one can move closer to a solution. *Analogical reasoning* is comparing a problem situation with one from experience, which requires good domain knowledge and previous exposure. *Brainstorming* requires defining a problem, generating solutions, determining criteria to judge solutions, and then selecting the best solution for the outcome. Brainstorming success is also determined by domain knowledge to be able to recognize the problem, generate workable solutions, and evaluate the outcome.

Third, preparing for action requires the use of production systems that are networks of condition-action sequences (Anderson, 1990, 1993, 2000). The conditions are the circumstances of the problem that activate the system, and the actions are the activities that occur. Proceeding through this stage of preparing for action requires the use of if-then comparisons synonymous with creative thinking. The "if" is the goal to be achieved and the "then" is the action. Problem-solving in care-planning situations that are not clearly defined and difficult require specific strategies, such as critical thinking and creative thinking, to maneuver through the healthcare systems of our day. Dealing with these systems requires additional strategies, such as systems and complexity thinking, to manage the multiple factors influencing the dynamics of the patient, contexts, and issues. Appreciating and attending to the whole ~ part relationships requires systems thinking.

Systems Thinking

Jennifer Mensik (2014) describes the importance of a systems-thinking mindset for systems-based leadership in healthcare and discusses the challenges of systems thinking from an individual trying to influence organizations from the bottom up and top down. *Systems thinking* is a framework that assists one to focus on relationships and patterns versus objects (Senge, 1990). Senge (1990) defines systems thinking as a way of thinking and a language for describing and understanding the actors, forces, elements, and interrelationships that shape the behavior of systems. Systems thinking spins around four key concepts:

- All systems are composed of interconnected parts, and a change to any part or connection affects the entire system.

- Structure and connections among the parts create patterns and reveal how a system is organized and behaves.

- System behavior is an emergent phenomenon because its parts and structure are constantly changing through iterative feedback loops.

- Feedback loops control a system's major dynamic behavior as each part influences the others in a circular pattern, creating complexity.

Barry Richmond (1993) defines systems thinking as the art and science of making reliable inferences about behavior through a deep understanding of the world's underlying structures with an appreciation that the world is a complex system in which dynamics are controlled via interactive feedback loops.

A more recent definition of systems thinking comes from Derek and Laura Cabrera (2015). They suggest systems thinking requires mastery and attention to distinctions (D), systems (S) rules, relationship (R) rules, and perspective (P) rules (DSRP). Systems thinking requires one to be able to make distinctions between and among ideas or things. Any idea or thing can be split into parts or lumped into a whole. Any idea can relate to other ideas or things. Finally, any thing or idea can be a point of view or perspective. For example, distinguishing standardized terminologies becomes important in clinical reasoning. How clinicians split terms or lump them together becomes important when considering disciplinary points of view or perspectives. Standardized terminologies can relate to other systems, and standardized terminologies provide a point of view or perspective regarding how one discipline over another filters, frames, and focuses on issues of interest.

The key to solving difficult, complex, social-system problems is to use systems thinking with a process that uniquely fits the problem at hand given the system dynamics. For example, thinking and reasoning about balancing and reinforcing causal loops in a system dynamic are done by taking in the whole picture. Relationships, whether they be visible or invisible, become obvious when systems-thinking interactions among all the elements that comprise the whole situation are considered (Senge, 1990).

Understanding the whole system of human activity in the environment in which it exists is one of the challenges for the nurse in care planning. Instead of the traditional, linear, cause-and-effect relationship among patient comorbidities, treatments, and outcomes, the whole complex and bidirectional interrelationships are considered concurrently to expose interconnectedness and relationships (Pesut, 2008; Kuiper et al., 2016). Another aspect of systems thinking is the consideration of the filter or frames one uses to interpret the facts of a situation. *Frames* or *schemas* as defined by Lakoff (2010) are unconscious structures that include semantic roles, relations between roles, and relations to other frames. Frames are strengthened and maintained by language, evoke emotion, and inform unconscious reasoning (thinking). So, developing a frame regarding the system in which one is working assists with interpreting and considering facts that must be communicated to others. The various frames brought to a care-planning situation by each healthcare provider may prohibit them from becoming involved in the system and understanding the real situation. For example, frames for care planning that all providers and patients understand equally well require practice with systems thinking. Lakoff (2010) asserts that a lack of frames results in hypocognition. Some strategies to help with new frame development include:

- Frame issues in terms of moral values

- Provide stories that emphasize values and evoke emotion

- Find general themes or narratives that incorporate important points

- Be aware of context and use words, visuals, and body language people can understand

Complexity Thinking

Complexity thinking transcends and includes systems thinking. Crowell (2015) notes that complexity science supports a new worldview that embraces the fact that situations are complex, uncertain, nonlinear, dynamic, and relationship-based. Complexity thinking strategies emerged from complexity theory, which is based on mathematics and quantum physics, in which "relationship is the key determiner of everything" (Wheatley, 1999, p. 11). The relationships of agents, actors, or components in a situation engage in a dynamic interaction that often reveals patterns and maps of relationships (Capra, 1996, p. 81). Complexity theory applied to nursing and healthcare proposes that a multitude of factors influence health, but it also acknowledges the uniqueness of each interaction with a patient resulting from creative thinking and innovation inherent in nursing activities (Burns, 2001).

Complexity thinking involves attention to the recursive nonlinear patterns that emerge between and among elements of patient care needs and nursing care concerns. This nonlinearity is a difficult idea to accept in a society that is constantly seeking specific causes and solutions for problems. The individual, whether it is the patient or healthcare provider, is in relationships embedded in larger structures like families and communities. Some broader patterns that affect people are the environment, the economy, and the political system.

Complexity theory studies the interactive relationships of multiple agents or components, in a system dynamic that often reveals complex forms in motion (Gleick, 1987). Lindberg, Nash, and Lindberg (2008) provide a primer on complexity science and make distinctions between and among problems that are simple, complicated, and complex. They apply complex adaptive systems theory to nursing and illustrate how nursing manages and leverages many of the characteristics of complex adaptive systems—i.e., order~disorder, diversity, self-organization, embeddedness, distributed control, adaptable elements, and non-linearity.

The knowledge representation and framing of nursing phenomena involving patient care needs are complex, and nurses have to adjust their thinking along with them. The specific complex thinking activities that enable one to perform clinical reasoning are gained through practice, conscious reflection, and attention to issues of complexity associated with a patient's story and context of practice. Complexity thinking defined in the OPT Model of Clinical Reasoning is derived from complexity principles and practices, which lead to filtering, framing, and focus with a concurrent understanding of system dynamics and ultimately the determination and juxtaposition of present states with desired outcome states.

With complexity thinking, one considers multiple interactions of various elements in a situation. Pesut (2008) notes complexity thinking involves attention to the recursive nonlinear pattern recognition associated with the identification and creation of Clinical Reasoning Webs, patient care needs, and nursing care responses. Many different kinds of thinking are involved in the clinical reasoning process. Making distinctions between and among the kinds of thinking offers insight into how thinking tactics might be applied. In the next section, suggested thinking tactics and strategies derived from the kinds of thinking are discussed.

THINKING TACTICS THAT SUPPORT MASTERY OF CLINICAL REASONING

Table 3.1 displays some specific tactics and strategies that support the development of clinical reasoning skills. Many of these strategies are metacognitive in nature. Each of the following strategies—attention to knowledge work, self-talk, prototype identification or pattern recognition (schema searches), hypothesizing, activation of if-then thinking, comparative analysis, juxtaposing to ascertain gaps between present and desired states, activating reflexive comparisons, reframing, and reflection checks—are discussed next.

Knowledge Work

Clinical reasoning presupposes that you have done the *knowledge work* of reading, memorizing, drilling, writing, and practicing. This knowledge work is necessary to gain the clinical vocabulary of standardized terminologies used to document and interpret data about the patient-in-context story. Often the information and knowledge one needs are available through the electronic healthcare record or the systems of care processes that are in place in an organization. It is very difficult to generate diagnostic hypotheses for a patient case if you do not know the definitions and classifications of disease states or domains of nursing care knowledge that provide the disciplinary knowledge base for the provider. Other fundamental knowledge needed to plan care for patients includes knowledge about physiological, psychological, and sociological functioning. Fundamental knowledge in these areas includes such things as normal and abnormal laboratory values and the psychodynamics of anxiety and fear. Fundamental knowledge in these areas helps you interpret, analyze, explain, and infer what is going on in a case to support clinical reasoning. The thinking strategies of self-talk, schema search, prototype identification, hypothesizing, if-then, how-so thinking, comparative analysis, juxtaposing, reflexive comparison, reframing, and reflection check are defined and described next.

Self-Talk

Self-talk is the process of expressing one's thoughts to one's self. Self-talk answers the question, "What are the nursing diagnostic possibilities associated with the medical conditions of disease states?" The answer to this question results in the identification of the diagnostic hypotheses relevant to the case. For example, the human responses to emphysema include such things as ineffective breathing pattern, impaired gas exchange, fatigue, anxiety, and fear. Self-talk or thinking out loud is useful when spinning and weaving Clinical Reasoning Webs. One has to think out loud and reason about the possible relationships and give voice to connections among diagnostic hypotheses and their relationships to one another.

Schema Search

Schema search is the process of accessing long-term memories that may explain or help identify and relate past experience to present/current situations. The reason students like a lot of clinical experiences are because the experiences help them build schema. Past clinical experiences are helpful in reasoning about a specific case. One way to develop expertise is to use self-talk as you build schema. Each experience nurses have with a patient creates a web in their minds. The more experiences one gains, the more complex the web, the greater number of patterns developed, and the easier it is to access those patterns or neural networks. Novices are in the process of spinning and weaving memory webs with each clinical experience. Experts have multiple webs superimposed on one another. The storage of information in memory is why experienced nurses can reason about situations effectively and quickly. The schema includes what this patient exhibited, what interventions were done, and what the outcomes were. These memories become the foundation for clinical reasoning expertise.

TABLE 3.1 THINKING TACTICS AND STRATEGIES DEFINITIONS

Thinking Strategy	Definition	Use Within the OPT Model of Clinical Reasoning
Knowledge Work	Active use of reading, memorizing, drilling, writing, reviewing, and practicing to learn clinical vocabulary	Patient-in-context story Nursing diagnoses terminology
Self-Talk	Expressing one's thoughts to one's self	Nursing diagnoses identification Reasoning web—spinning and weaving the web
Schema Search	Accessing general and/or specific patterns of past experiences that might apply to the current situation	Outcome-present state-test identification
Prototype Identification	Using a model case as a reference point for comparative analysis	Nursing diagnoses identification Outcome state Interventions
Hypothesizing	Determining an explanation that accounts for a set of facts that can be tested by further investigation	Reasoning web—spinning and weaving the web

Thinking Strategy	Definition	Use Within the OPT Model of Clinical Reasoning
If-Then, How-So Thinking	Linking ideas and consequences in a logical sequence with an explanation of how they are related	Reasoning web—spinning and weaving
Comparative Analysis	Considering the strengths and weaknesses of competing alternatives	Keystone identification
Juxtaposing	Putting the present state condition next to the outcome state in a side-by-side contrast	Present state-outcome state comparisons
Reflexive Comparison	A tactic that involves constant comparison of one state or situation to another	Compare the patient's state from one observation to the next
Reframing	Attributing different meaning to content or context given a set of cues, tests, decisions, or judgments	Reframe a keystone issue or change a plan of care for better patient/family management
Reflection Check	Reflecting and analyzing a patient scenario through the use of self-monitoring, self-correcting, and self-evaluating one's thinking about a task or situation	Pinpoint strategies and interventions to identify success or errors in patient care and determine how to correct them

Prototype Identification

Prototype identification is using a model case as a reference point for comparative analysis. A patient with a disease condition represents one instance of a person with that disease. Knowing what the prototypical patient in an acute crisis is likely to exhibit serves as a standard. With prototype identification, one uses textbook cases as the standard and a reference point for comparative analysis. Prototypes or simulations enable one to create the neural network connections that lead to the formation and development of patterns that can be recognized. A major part of clinical reasoning is the pattern recognition match between what one knows and has experienced and what one is observing and assessing. Patterns of experience through time help with the development of schemas. Prototype identification activates and reinforces schema development.

Hypothesizing

Hypothesizing is determining an explanation that accounts for a set of facts that can be tested by further investigation. Hypothesizing presupposes use and understanding of clinical vocabulary. Explanations for circumstances in a case are called *diagnostic hypotheses*. They are guesses about what might explain a situation and high-risk sequelae. Testing hypotheses one makes about patient cases has to be supported by data.

Diagnostic hypotheses become the origins and insertion points for making associations when one develops a Clinical Reasoning Web. Hypothesizing includes if-then, how-so thinking; however, it is a more formal statement or declaration about how specifically sets of facts are related. Hypothesis testing requires gathering of evidence under controlled conditions to affirm or negate the proposed relationship. Spinning and weaving the webs for individual case care planning results in some diagnostic hypotheses. Once diagnoses are identified, it is easier to see how these diagnoses might be related through hypothesizing.

If-Then, How-So Thinking

If-then, how-so thinking involves linking ideas and consequences in a logical sequence. This type of thinking is used in connecting diagnoses and care planning needs in the respective webs. The linking of ideas and consequences in a logical sequence is at the heart of clinical reasoning. It is also the place to start developing the plan of care and determining what resources are needed for care planning.

Comparative Analysis

Comparative analysis is a thinking strategy that involves considering the strengths and weaknesses of competing alternatives. Once diagnostic hypotheses and their relationships are made explicit using the webs, comparative analysis is used to determine which of these relationships is the keystone or the central supporting issue of a situation. Identifying the keystone issues enables the nurse to focus on care. Once a keystone issue is identified, it has a domino effect in that you can influence other problems and needs.

Juxtaposing

Juxtaposing is another essential tactic. Think of *juxtaposing* as the creation of a gap analysis. Juxtaposing involves putting the present state condition next to the outcome state. The side-by-side contrast of one state with the other illustrates the differences or gaps between the two states. The differences or gaps evident from the present to desired state help establish the conditions for the creation of a test in the OPT Model of Clinical Reasoning. A test is satisfied if the gap is closed.

As one determines the practice issues, interventions, and outcomes in the care planning model, the successive achievement of the desired outcome helps to close the gap and successfully pass the test(s). Juxtaposing enables one to set up essential elements between two states. Decisions that one makes and interventions one initiates help bridge the gap between juxtaposed conditions.

Reflexive Comparison

Reflexive comparison is a tactic that involves constant comparison of the patient's state from the time of observation to the next time of observation. For example, each time a laboratory test value is reviewed, the nurse or provider compares a patient's progress from one observation to the next. In this way, the nurse or provider is using the patient as his or her own standard regarding making progress toward the desired outcome state. This process represents an *ipsative* versus a normative model of comparison.

Reframing

Reframing is the strategy that attributes a different meaning to the content or context of a situation given a set of cues, tests, decisions, or judgments. Remember that clinical reasoning is reflective, concurrent, creative, critical, systems, and complexity thinking embedded in nursing practice that nurses use to frame, juxtapose, and test the match between a patient's present state and desired outcome state. It may be that one needs to reframe the keystone issue. The challenge now becomes how one assists a patient transition from one state to another. Another way to reframe the situation is to consider how, through care planning, the patient and family can more effectively manage their own therapeutic regime. Reframing is the thinking strategy that enables one to attribute different meaning given the story and context and reflection on the situation.

Reflection Check

A *reflection check* involves reflecting and analyzing the patient scenario. Reflection check is the process of intentionally using the self-regulation strategies of self-monitoring, self-correcting, self-reinforcing, and self-evaluating one's own thinking about a specific task or situation (Herman et al., 1994; Kuiper & Pesut, 2004; Kuiper et al., 2016; Pesut & Herman, 1992; Worrell, 1990). A reflection check pinpoints all that you have done correctly and identifies errors and provides an opportunity to understand how to correct them. A reflection check involves understanding how the thinking skills and strategies described thus far support clinical reasoning.

Thinking Tactics Applied to Clinical Decision-Making

The strategies described here and displayed in Table 3.1 come together during case analysis to make clinical decisions. Clinical decision-making involves the selection of interventions, actions, and issues that move patients from a present state to an outcome state. In other words, what actions and interventions coordinated by the nurse are necessary to bring the present state and outcome state closer together? Decision-making is supported through the use and application of schema searches and prototype identification. Comparative analysis is the process of considering the strengths and weaknesses of competing alternatives. If-then, how-so thinking also supports decision-making. During testing, the nurse determines how well the gap has been filled between the present and outcome state. Testing is accomplished through the use and application of comparative analysis and reflexive and ipsative comparison, which is the process of making a judgment about the state of a situation after gauging the presence or absence of some quality against a standard using the current case as a reference criterion. For example, how does a wound look one week after treatment? Conclusions related to tests are the bases of clinical judgments.

Judgments are made by drawing conclusions based on the findings from the tests of comparing the present state to a specified outcome state, and the result of organizational systems thinking. When judgments of present state closely match the desired outcomes (a wound is healed), the nurse can reason about other things. If a match or test is unsatisfactory (infection still present), reflection activates critical, creative, and concurrent thinking and decision-making. Regarding judgments, three conclusions are possible:

- A perfect match between outcome state and present state (e.g., a wound is healed)

- A partial match of outcome state with the present state (wound healing is progressing but not complete)

- No match between outcome and present state (not healed and looks worse)

Judgments result in reflection and clinical decision-making about achieving a satisfactory match between a patient's present state and the outcome state. Thinking strategies that support judgment are reframing or the process of attributing a different meaning to the facts or evidence at hand. Finally, a reflection about the entire process results in self-correction and adds to the expertise of the clinician.

Clinically, focusing on the present state or presenting problems does not provide explicit direction for action. After outcomes are specified, the path of action is clear, and the tests of achievement are explicit. Transforming problems into outcomes involves thinking beyond the present to the end results of action. This process must include care planning activities and reflection. One can appreciate how different kinds of thinking—both cognitive and metacognitive—support thinking strategies that provide a foundation for clinical reasoning.

SUMMARY

Understanding clinical reasoning begins with insight around the kinds of thinking that are involved in the clinical reasoning process. This chapter describes some distinctions between and among critical thinking (cognitive) aspects of the reasoning process and metacognitive kinds of thinking that support the development of reflection and self-regulation. The other kinds of thinking crucial to the clinical reasoning process include self-regulation of learning, creative thinking, systems thinking, and complexity thinking. Some specific thinking tactics and strategies were defined and described to support the development of clinical reasoning. Insight and mastery of the thinking tactics and strategies are important. The next few chapters illustrate the application of the different kinds of thinking, tactics, and strategies with the OPT Model of Clinical Reasoning. In Part II, each clinical case study illustrates how the thinking strategies support the use of the OPT Model of Clinical Reasoning across the life span.

KEY POINTS

- Clinical reasoning activates many types of thinking. As nurses clinically reason with patients, families, and other providers within organizations and systems, they need to develop critical, self-regulatory, creative, systems, and complexity thinking skills.

- Clinical reasoning is influenced by the cognitive and metacognitive thinking activities that permit the nurse to frame and consider the whole situation and associated relationships between and among problems, interventions, and outcomes in service of patient preferences for safe and effective care.

- Clinical reasoning challenges require nurses to think about their thinking and combine both cognitive and metacognitive skills in determining the practice issues, interventions, and outcomes that support care plans in service of quality outcomes.

- Specific thinking tactics and strategies that support the mastery of the OPT Model of Clinical Reasoning include intentional use of knowledge, self-talk, schema search, prototype identification and pattern recognition, hypothesizing, juxtaposing, if-then, how-so thinking, comparative analysis, reflexive comparison, reframing, and reflection checking.

STUDY QUESTIONS AND ACTIVITIES

1. Identify the differences and explain in your own words relationships among critical, creative, systems, and complexity thinking.

2. Describe the role of reflection and the different thinking tactics as they are applied to the OPT Model of Clinical Reasoning.

3. Try to recall some schema and prototypes you have become familiar with. Using critical reflection, analyze the clinical reasoning thinking strategies you will need to use in subsequent clinical situations.

4. Explore Diana Crowell's (2015) book *Complexity Leadership: Nursing's Role in Health Care Delivery*. Complete the Complexity Leadership Assessment profile, which can be found in Chapter 12 of her text. Relate your scores and assessments to the need for complexity thinking skills.

References

American Association of Colleges of Nursing (AACN). (2008). *The essentials of baccalaureate education for professional nursing practice*. Washington, DC: American Association of Colleges of Nursing.

American Nurses Association (ANA). (2015). *Nursing: Scope and standards of practice* (3rd ed.). Silver Spring, MD: ANA Publishing.

Anderson, J. R. (1990). *Cognitive psychology and its implications* (3rd ed.). New York, NY: W. H. Freeman and Company.

Anderson, J. R. (1993). Problem solving and learning. *American Psychologist, 48*(1), 35–44.

Anderson, J. R. (2000). *Learning and memory: An integrated approach* (2nd ed.). New York, NY: Wiley.

Bandura, A. (1997). *Self-efficacy: The exercise of control*. New York, NY: W. H. Freeman and Company.

Barkimer, J. (2016). Clinical growth: An evolutionary concept analysis. *Advances in Nursing Science, 39*(3), e28–e39.

Benner, P., Hooper-Kyriakidis, P., & Stannard, D. (2011). *Clinical wisdom and interventions in acute and critical care: A thinking-in-action approach*. New York, NY: Springer Publishing Company.

Benner, P., Hughes, R. G., & Sutphen, M. (2008). Clinical reasoning, decision making, and action: Thinking critically and clinically. In R. G. Hughes (Ed.), *Patient safety and quality: An evidence-based handbook for nurses* (pp. 1–23). Washington, DC: Agency for Healthcare Research and Quality.

Bourdieu, P. (1990). *The logic of practice*. Stanford, CA: Stanford University Press.

Brookfield, S. D. (2012). *Teaching for critical thinking: Tools and techniques to help students question their assumptions*. San Francisco, CA: Jossey-Bass.

Burns, J. P. (2001). Complexity science and leadership in healthcare. *Journal of Nursing Administration, 31*(10), 474–482.

Cabrera, D., & Cabrera, L. (2015). *Systems thinking made simple: New hope for solving wicked problems*. New York, NY: Odyssean Press.

Capra, F. (1996). *The web of life*. New York, NY: Doubleday.

Cronenwett, L., Sherwood, G., Barnsteiner, J., Disch, J., Johnson, J., Mitchell, P., . . . Warren, J. (2007). Quality and safety education for nurses. *Nursing Outlook, 55*(3), 122–131.

Crowell, D. M. (2015). *Complexity leadership: Nursing's role in health-care delivery*. Philadelphia, PA: F. A. Davis.

Facione, N. C., & Facione, P. A. (1996). Externalizing the critical thinking in knowledge development and clinical judgment. *Nursing Outlook, 44*(3), 129–136.

Facione, P. A. (1990). *The Delphi report executive summary* (pp. 1–22). Montclair, NJ: Montclair State University Center for Critical Thinking; and Millbrae, CA: The California Academic Press.

Gleick, J. (1987). *Chaos: Making a new science*. New York, NY: Penguin Books.

Herman, J., Pesut, D., & Conard, L. (1994). Using metacognitive skills: The quality audit tool. *Nursing Diagnosis, 5*(2), 56–64.

Institute of Medicine (IOM). (2001). *Crossing the quality chasm: A new health system for the 21st century*. Washington, DC: The National Academies Press.

Institute of Medicine (IOM). (2003). Greiner, A., & Knebel, E. (Eds). *Health professions education: A bridge to quality*. Washington, DC: The National Academies Press.

Kuiper, R. A., & Pesut, D. J. (2004). Promoting cognitive and metacognitive reflective clinical reasoning skills in nursing practice: Self-regulated learning theory. *Journal of Advanced Nursing, 45*(4), 381–391.

Kuiper, R. A., Pesut, D., & Arms, T. (2016). *Clinical reasoning and care coordination in advanced practice nursing*. New York, NY: Springer Publishing.

Kuiper, R., Pesut, D., & Kautz, D. (2009). Promoting the self-regulation of clinical reasoning skills in nursing students. *The Open Nursing Journal, 3*, 76–85.

Lakoff, G. (2010). Why it matters how we frame the environment. *Environmental Communication: A Journal of Nature and Culture, 4*(1), 70–81. doi:10.1080/17524030903529749

Lindberg, C., & Lindberg, C. (2008). Nurses take note: A primer on complexity science. In C. Lindberg, S. Nash, and C. Lindberg (Eds.), *On the edge: Nursing in the age of complexity* (pp. 23–48). Bordentown, NJ: PlexusPress.

Mariotto, A. (2010). Hypocognition and evidence-based medicine. *Internal Medicine Journal, 40*, 80–82. doi:10.111?j.1445-5994.2009.02086.x

Mensik, J. (2014). *Lead, drive & thrive in the system*. Silver Spring, MD: ANA Publishing.

Pesut, D. (1985). Toward a new definition of creativity. *Nurse Educator, 10*(1), 5.

Pesut, D. (2008). Thoughts on thinking with complexity in mind. In C. Lindberg, S. Nash, & C. Lindberg (Eds.), *On the edge: Nursing in the age of complexity* (pp. 211–238). Bordentown, NJ: PlexusPress.

Pesut, D. J. (2016) Transformed and in service: Creating the future through renewal . In W. Rossa (Ed.), *Nurses as leaders: Evolutionary visions of leadership* (pp. 165–178). New York, NY: Springer Publishing.

Pesut, D. J., & Herman, J. A. (1992). Reflection skills in diagnostic reasoning. *Nursing Diagnosis, 3*(4), 148–154.

Pesut, D., & Herman, J. (1999). *Clinical reasoning: The art and science of critical and creative thinking.* New York, NY: Delmar Publishers.

Richmond, B. (1993) Systems thinking: Critical thinking skills for the 1990s and beyond. *System Dynamics Review, 9*(2), 13–133.

Scheffer, B., & Rubenfeld, G. (2000). A consensus statement on critical thinking in nursing. *Journal of Nursing Education, 39*(8), 352–359.

Schraeder, C., & Shelton, P. (2013). Effective care planning models. In G. Lamb (Ed.), *Care coordination: The game changer: How nursing is revolutionizing quality care* (pp. 57–79). Silver Spring, MD: American Nurses Association Publishing.

Schunk, D. H. (2012). *Learning theories: An educational perspective* (6th ed.). Upper Saddle River, NJ: Pearson Prentice Hall.

Senge, P. (1990). *The fifth discipline: The art and practice of the learning organization.* New York, NY: Doubleday Currency.

Treffinger, D. J. (1985). Review of the Torrance Tests of Creative Thinking. In J. Mitchell (Ed.), *Ninth mental measurements yearbook* (pp. 1633–1634). Lincoln, NE: Burros Institute of Mental Measurement.

Treffinger, D. J., & Isaksen, S. G. (2005). Creative problem solving: The history, development, and implications for gifted education and talent development. *Gifted Child Quarterly, 49*(4), 342–353. doi:10.1177/001698620504900407

Waldrop, M. (1992). *Complexity: The emerging science at the edge of chaos.* New York, NY: Simon and Schuster.

Watson, G., & Glaser E. (1964). *Critical thinking appraisal manual.* New York, NY: Harcourt, Brace & World.

Wheatley, M. J. (1999). *Leadership and the new science* (2nd ed.). San Francisco, CA: Berrett-Koehler Publishers.

Worrell, P. (1990). Metacognition: Implications for instruction in nursing education. *Journal of Nursing Education, 29*, 170–175.

Zimmerman, B. (1998). Developing self-fulfilling cycles of academic regulation: An analysis of exemplary instructional models. In D. H. Schunk & B. J. Zimmerman (Eds.), *Self-regulated learning: From teaching to self-reflective practice* (pp. 1–19). New York, NY: Guilford Press.

Zimmerman, B. (2000). Attaining self-regulation: A social cognitive perspective. In M. Boekaerts, P. R. Pintrich, & M. Zeidner (Eds.), *Handbook of self-regulation* (pp. 13–39). San Diego, CA: Academic Press.

Zimmerman, B., & Schunk, D. S. (2001). *Self-regulated learning and academic thought.* Mahwah, NJ: Lawrence Erlbaum Associates.

4

LEARNING THE OPT MODEL OF CLINICAL REASONING: PATIENT-IN-CONTEXT STORY AND THE CLINICAL REASONING WEB

LEARNING OUTCOMES

- Explain the components of a patient-in-context story that are needed to create an OPT Model of Clinical Reasoning Web Worksheet.

- Describe the processes for spinning and weaving a Clinical Reasoning Web between and among key nursing diagnoses.

- Describe the different thinking skills that support clinical reasoning and the strategies and tactics for determining priorities from the Clinical Reasoning Web.

- Describe how data, knowledge, and evidence management is essential to address patient and family needs and nursing care responsibilities.

- Describe the critical meta-reflective processes that support the nurse's reflection, communication, and reasoning related to levels and perspectives associated with care planning for patients and families.

This chapter describes the processes of gathering data to create the patient-in-context story and the organization of that data using a Clinical Reasoning Web. Many different frameworks can be used to collect patient and family health data. It is important to acknowledge that the nurse filters, frames, and focuses data as a function of disciplinary perspective and professional standards. One might use a specific nursing or medical classification such as the North American Nursing Diagnosis Association (NANDA-I)/Nursing Interventions Classification (NIC)/Nursing Outcomes Classification (NOC)/Omaha Systems (Martin, 2005). Some nursing education programs or clinical nursing departments in an organization subscribe to a particular model, conceptual framework, or theory. Frequently, assessment is directed and influenced by these nursing structures or elements that are contained in an electronic health record. It is important to reflect on the nature and origins of the assessments that are used and understand how current organizational or institutional policies influence the way one thinks and reasons about the patient-in-context story. Electronic health record categories often vary in the way they guide assessment and the degree to which assessments are illness and problem focused or health strengths and wellness focused. The primary importance of the data gathering is to determine the present state of the patient care issues, as well as areas of strength and deviations from normal. Once a deviation or problem is identified, the focus and clinical reasoning are about how to transform the problem into desired outcomes to influence health promotion and health maintenance with the patients' preferences in mind.

SOURCES OF HEALTH DATA/EVIDENCE

Gathering data begins as soon as the nurse has contact with the patient and family. This process usually occurs when first hearing about the case, perhaps from a report from another healthcare provider, reading the history and physical from a medical record, or hearing the patient's chief complaint. Thinking processes are immediately activated by the nurse to determine what is known, what needs to be clarified, and what other data needs to be gathered. Documenting the data is very important so that all pieces of information can be considered to create and fully understand the patient story.

One also has to consider what standardized terminologies will be used to convey the story. Medical, pharmacological, psychological, and nursing languages and terms will all be used to filter, frame, and focus the data in the case and serve as communication devices so the healthcare for this patient and family can be managed between team members. The central issues in the story need to be identified to narrow the focus to essential healthcare problems. Some questions that could be used to reflect on the development of creating a patient-in-context story are displayed in Table 4.1.

TABLE 4.1 QUESTIONS FOR UNDERSTANDING THE PATIENT-IN-CONTEXT STORY

Patient-in-Context	Who is the patient?
	What is the patient story?
	How would I describe the patient and his or her story?
	How do I think about the patient situation?
	What are the contextual factors I need to consider?
	How do institutional policies and the assessment forms I am using influence my thinking and reasoning about the patient and his or her story?

PATIENT-IN-CONTEXT

Other sources of data for the patient-in-context story include the patient interview. The nurse gathers both verbal and nonverbal data during the history discussion when physical examination takes place. Significant others and family are also interviewed to verify information and obtain facts that the patient might not be able to share. Previous medical records, in whatever form they may be, are essential to understanding the past health problems, plans of care, interventions, and evaluation of outcomes. If the patient is a child or frail elderly, parents and caretakers might be the only source of information for the story.

With the increased use of electronic health records, there is an explosion of data and a greater volume of data that all healthcare providers must filter through (Goodwin, VanDyne, Lin, & Talbert, 2003). The enormity of this knowledge work, however, can interfere with decision-making and clinical judgment (Grier, 1985). The structure and process offered in the OPT Model of Clinical Reasoning assist novices in making decisions and judgments by bringing essential and significant data, information, and knowledge to the forefront and organizing it for planning patient care.

The specific nursing diagnoses and associated data used for the OPT Model of Clinical Reasoning Worksheet are nursing terminology labels that represent cues and concepts derived from the patient assessment. Cues are logically and deliberately structured from the patient-in-context story to discern the meaning for nursing care. Diagnostic cluster/cue logic can be inductive, deductive, or dialectic. *Induction* involves reasoning from specific cues toward a general judgment. For example, an elevated white blood cell (WBC) count and an increased temperature lead one to conclude that there is an infection, given a patient has an ulcer on the right heel. *Deduction* involves reasoning from a general premise toward a conclusion. For example, if the infection is present, then antibiotics are likely to be an effective treatment. *Dialectic thinking* considers both the deductive and inductive aspects of a situation regarding an open system subject to feedback and change. Once the patient with an infection has been on antibiotics for a while, the temperature should return to normal, and the WBC count should decrease.

Clinical evidence about the patient-in-context is processed according to the way the nurse filters, frames, and focuses the cues. Cue logic contributes information that helps structure and frame the patient situation. The thinking strategy of self-talk, which is expressing one's thoughts to one's self, supports the explanation and development of cue logic. Cue logic is influenced by experience and short- and long-term memory that is linked with the knowledge work from the past and combined with the learning of new information. Experiences are recorded in mental models or schemas. Based on an experience, a person may often retrieve memories from a schema to help explain and relate to a current situation.

The use of a model case or prototype is another way that helps people think and reason about a situation. *Prototypes* are model cases that serve as reference points that can be compared with the presenting situation to help discern similarities and differences with presenting cases. From the comparison, one can generate a hypothesis about what is going on given the conditions at hand. Hypothesizing involves determining an explanation that accounts for a set of facts and then testing them by further investigation. For example, consider the issue of the elevated white blood cell count. Identification of redness, drainage from an ulcer, and an increase in temperature leads one to ask (self-talk) the question about infection. Because experience influences thinking, perhaps previous experience with an infected ulcer influences reasoning? Textbook descriptions (prototypes) of ulcerative infections are helpful in using cue logic about this problem. Once treatment is initiated, one can compare the healing wound with a memory of what it looked like with the infection present. This reflexive comparison is a test. The differences between the infected and healing ulcer create a contrast and provide evidence to suggest the ulcer is healing or not healing. Figure 4.1 displays the Outcome-Present State-Test (OPT) Model of Clinical Reasoning Worksheet describing a particular patient story.

Diagnostic cluster/cue logic is useful in making sense of the patient's story and framing the nursing care needs given the story and context in which one is working. The nurse must ask, "Did I gather all the information about the patient? If so, did it include nursing-sensitive information as well as the pathophysiology of the patient's condition? Did I define the outcomes or did I first develop a problem list? If I have identified a problem, what might be a complementary positive outcome?"

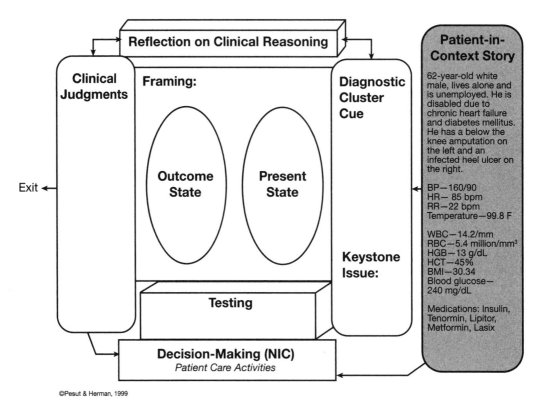

Figure 4.1   OPT Model of Clinical Reasoning Worksheet (Patient-in-Context Story).

THE CLINICAL REASONING WEB: STRATEGY AND TOOL TO SUPPORT CLINICAL REASONING

In the OPT Model, clinical reasoning is defined as the critical, reflective, concurrent, and creative thinking embedded in nursing practice that results in the juxtaposition of problems and outcomes that are subject to interventions and clinical judgments (Pesut & Herman, 1999). The OPT Model of Clinical Reasoning relies on critical thinking skills such as analysis, synthesis, evaluation, creativity, and judgment (Airasian et al., 2000). Creative thinking involves managing complementary pairs, tensions between choices, and opposites. Creative problem-solving requires three components: understanding a challenge, generating ideas, and preparing for action (Treffinger & Isaksen, 2005).

The OPT Clinical Reasoning Web Worksheet is a tool that supports clinical reasoning. Basically, the Clinical Reasoning Web is a visual-graphic representation of the relationships between and among the nursing diagnoses chosen from the analysis and synthesis of the data and cue logic associated with all possible resources. Consideration of each piece of data is related to the story as a whole and requires concurrent and iterative analysis, evaluation, and thinking.

The visual diagram that results illustrates dynamic relationships among issues as lines are drawn to connect the diagnoses. As the nurse thinks about a case and begins to spin and weave a Clinical Reasoning Web, relationships are identified among nursing diagnoses and are considered as concurrent consequences of medical conditions listed in the center circle of the web. By spinning and weaving the web, the nurse analyzes relationships among the diagnoses and a visual map evolves that ultimately converges on one specific keystone issue. The keystone issue represents the center of gravity of the system dynamics. Once the comprehensive process to draw all possible connections with arrows to connect the nursing diagnoses has been completed, often the keystone issue emerges as a central concern supporting the nursing diagnosis with the most connections. The example in Figure 4.2 and Table 4.3 shows a summary of connections for each nursing diagnosis to demonstrate the keystone priority. This keystone is then used as a focus to create the plan of care. Often, if the keystone diagnosis is identified and treated and the outcomes are achieved, the consequence is that other nursing diagnoses/problems often resolve. Even if the other nursing diagnoses are important, the issues may not represent the leverage point in the system to have maximum impact and influence.

The steps to create the OPT Model of Clinical Reasoning Web and Worksheet are as follows:

1. Place a general description of the patient and major medical diagnoses in the respective middle circle.

2. Determine which nursing domain and class is associated with the nursing diagnoses.

3. Choose the nursing diagnoses for each diagnostic cluster/cue logic of data. Nursing diagnoses are human responses to actual or potential health problems represented in standardized terminologies.

4. After the nursing diagnoses are identified, reflect on the total web worksheet and concurrently consider and explain how each of the diagnoses is or is not related to the other diagnoses. Draw lines of relationship to spin and weave the web connections or associations among diagnoses. As you draw the lines, think out loud, justify the reasons for the connections, and explain specifically how the diagnoses may or may not be connected or related. If there are functional relationships, connections are drawn until the process is exhausted and visually a web emerges. Some questions that could be used to reflect on the development of creating the diagnostic cluster/cue logic are displayed in Table 4.2.

TABLE 4.2   QUESTIONS FOR UNDERSTANDING THE DIAGNOSTIC CLUSTER/CUE LOGIC

Diagnostic	What diagnoses have I generated as a result of my thinking?
Cluster/Cue Logic	What is the complementary nature (~) of the problems and outcomes?
	What outcomes come to mind given the diagnoses?
	What data or evidence supports those diagnoses?
	How does a reasoning web reveal relationships among the identified problems (diagnoses)?
	How does the Clinical Reasoning Web relate ideas and thinking about the case?
	As themes emerge, what keystone issue(s) emerge?

5. When all connections are made, the lines leading to and from each oval with nursing diagnoses are counted and recorded. The numbers are recorded on the Clinical Reasoning Web Worksheet. For example, Table 4.3 shows the hierarchy of priorities for the patient in this example.

6. The nursing diagnosis with the most connecting lines radiating to and from that oval becomes the *keystone issue*. Figure 4.2 displays a completed Clinical Reasoning Web for this case.

7. Look once again at the sets of relationships and determine the theme or keystone that summarizes the patient-in-context or the patient's story.

8. Place the patient-in-context story, diagnostic cluster cue logic, and keystone issue on the OPT Model of Clinical Reasoning Worksheet.

TABLE 4.3 WEB CONNECTIONS AMONG NURSING DIAGNOSES

Nursing Domain	Class	Nursing Diagnoses	Web Connections
Psychosocial	Behavior	Ineffective Management of Therapeutic Regimen	8
Physiological	Tissues Integrity	Ineffective Tissue Perfusion	7
Functional	Nutrition	Imbalanced Nutrition More than Body Requirements	7
Psychosocial	Behavior	Ineffective Health Maintenance	7
Environmental	Risk Management	Ineffective Protection	6
Physiological	Physical Regulation	Risk for Infection	6
Psychosocial	Emotional	Risk for Loneliness	5
Environmental	Self-Perception	Disturbed Body Image	4

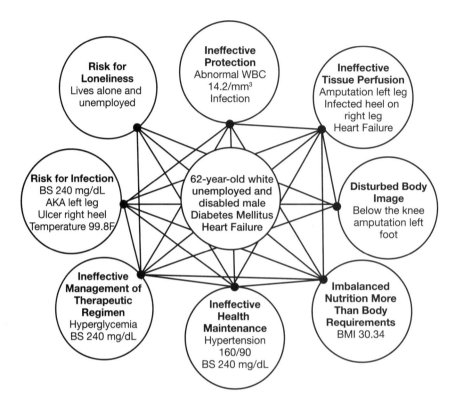

Figure 4.2 Clinical Reasoning Web.

Questions Frequently Asked About the Web

Students who have worked with the model often have questions about the cue logic and keystone issue. The most frequently asked questions are posed and answered here:

1. **Cue Logic:**

    a. *Question:* Is there a recommended number of nursing diagnoses to be inserted into the various ovals on the Reasoning Web?

    b. *Response:* The nursing diagnoses are chosen based on the nurse's analysis and synthesis of patient data gathered from all possible resources: patient history discussion, physical examination, interviews with significant others and family, and medical records (including past health problems, plans of care, interventions, and outcome evaluations). The data is patient-specific. Identification of problems and potential problems involves analysis and synthesis of the patient-specific data through various modes of thinking, and this process is described in Chapter 5.

c. A predetermined, across-the-board number of nursing diagnoses has not been established nor recommended. This clearly reinforces the value of the OPT Model and Clinical Reasoning Web in that these elements are individualized to the specific problems and risks of the patient or community. The number of diagnoses fluctuates according to identified problems, acuity levels, and clinical settings.

2. **Keystone:**

a. *Question:* What happens if there is a two-way or three-way tie in the number of connections between the nursing diagnoses in deciding which one becomes the keystone?

b. *Response:* As explained earlier in this chapter, the nurse begins to spin and weave a Clinical Reasoning Web through identification of relationships among the nursing diagnoses. These relationships are simultaneously considered with the medical condition listed in the center oval of the web. The keystone is the issue that emerges as the center of gravity or the central priority. It has the greatest impact and influence in planning care and becomes the focus from which to create the plan of care. As the keystone is treated and outcomes are achieved, other nursing diagnoses/problems often resolve.

c. *Response:* If more than one nursing diagnosis is assigned the highest number of connections, the nurse should reexamine relationships between the ovals. In doing so, the nurse should also consider and explain how each of the diagnoses is or is not related to the others. This process involves thinking out loud and justifying the reasons for the connections. It is essential that the nurse determine what theme of keystone *best* (italics added for emphasis) summarizes the patient-in-context story.

3. **Keystone:**

   a. *Question:* Can a "Risk for . . ." nursing diagnosis become the keystone issue?

   b. *Response:* No. NANDA-I defines a *risk nursing diagnosis* as "human responses to health conditions/life processes that may develop in a vulnerable individual, family, or community" (NANDA-I, 2017, p. 164). This is determined by risk factors that contribute to increased vulnerability. A risk nursing diagnosis differs from an actual diagnosis in which signs and symptoms validate the diagnosis, and a risk diagnosis depends on whether the filter, frame, or focus of the issue is primary, secondary, or tertiary preventive perspective. Risk factors validate a high-risk diagnosis (Carpenito, 2017). In other words, there are no signs or symptoms at present for a risk nursing diagnosis; instead, vulnerability exists that predisposes the *potential* for the patient to develop signs and symptoms.

Figure 4.3 displays the OPT Model of Clinical Reasoning Worksheet.

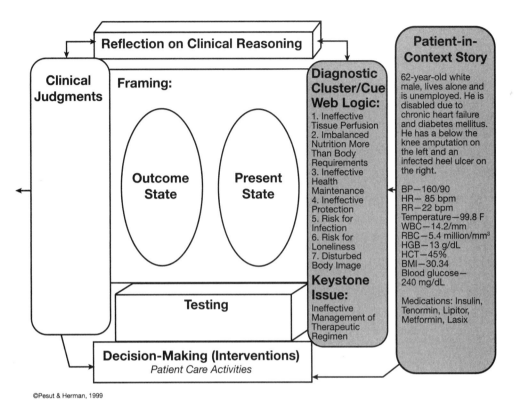

Figure 4.3   OPT Model of Clinical Reasoning Worksheet
(Diagnostic Cluster/Cue Logic).

REFLECTION ON CLINICAL REASONING

The clinical reasoning activities outlined previously are behaviors and skills that coincide with professional obligations, mandates, and responsibilities outlined by the American Nursing Association's *Nursing: Scope and Standards of Practice* (2015). Gathering and analyzing information and data in a clinical case is important to reinforce the need for nurses to develop competencies in care planning for patients and families using a clinical reasoning mindset that transcends and includes perspectives related to the contemporary healthcare arena. According to Hawkins, Elder, and Paul (2010), clinical reasoning has a purpose and is an attempt to figure something out, to settle some question, or solve a problem.

These critical thinking experts suggest that all clinical reasoning is based on assumptions and is done from a point of view, and based on data, information, and evidence. It is also influenced, informed, and expressed by concepts and theories. A clinical reasoning mindset also involves inference and interpretations that lead to conclusions that have consequences.

The clinical reasoning mindset filters information that is presented and is influenced by an individual perspective that includes the attitudes of a) intention, b) reflection, c) curiosity, d) tolerance for ambiguity, e) appreciation of perspectives, f) self-confidence, and g) professional motivation. The OPT Model of Clinical Reasoning provides a structure, process, and strategies for thinking about multiple competing patient care needs in the context of the patient's story.

Critical thinking skills are used to consider the patient-in-context story, and creative thinking is used to identify and reason about the most significant evidence that determines the keystone issue. Nursing students have found the OPT Model of Clinical Reasoning Worksheet and Web supportive structures helpful for organizing the content (data and evidence) in patient and family situations as they begin to develop plans of care (Kuiper, Pesut, & Kautz, 2009).

The thinking strategies in Table 4.4 describe the specific activities and outcomes used during this stage of the care planning with the OPT Model. Knowledge work and reflection through self-talk are important processes to recall prototypes and create schemas that organize information to reason about clinical cases. Developing cases create sensitivity to patterns and support the development of clinical confidence and competence. Table 4.4 describes several strategies and tactics that contribute to the development and mastery of clinical reasoning skills that are used in this case example.

TABLE 4.4 THINKING STRATEGIES THAT SUPPORT OPT MODEL CLINICAL REASONING

Thinking Strategy	Definition	Expected Outcomes
Knowledge Work	Active use of reading, memorizing, drilling, writing, reviewing, and using research to acquire content and clinical vocabulary with which to reason	• Knows common terms, specific facts, methods, procedures, basic concepts, and principles • Knows and values standardized terminologies • Has insight regarding the filtering, framing, and focus of knowledge work that supports clinical reasoning
Self-Talk	Expressing one's thoughts to one's self to support thinking and reasoning	• Think-out-loud explanation of relationships between and among cues, concepts, and hypotheses • Explanations about relationships among nursing diagnoses, interventions, and outcomes and associated and complementary medical standardized terms
Prototype Identification	A model clinical scenario or exemplar case study	• Comparative analysis of a given case with prototype • Identification of the similarities and differences with the exemplar case
Schema Search	Recall of experiences that support reasoning given the content and context of a patient story or clinical scenario	• Transfer of learning from the past to present case-based analysis

Knowledge Work

Clinical reasoning presupposes the knowledge work of reading, memorizing, drilling, writing, and practicing, which is necessary to gain the clinical vocabulary of the classification systems to interpret data about the patient-in-context story. The knowledge work that one needs is provided by clinical records, the electronic healthcare record, or the systems of care processes that are in place in an organization. It is very difficult to generate diagnostic hypotheses for a patient case if you do not know the definitions and classifications of disease states or domains of nursing care knowledge that provide the disciplinary knowledge base for the provider. The fundamental knowledge needed to plan care for this patient includes knowledge about physiological, psychological, and sociological functioning. The data gathered for this patient reveals that he lives alone and is unemployed. He is disabled due to chronic heart failure and diabetes mellitus. He has a below-the-knee amputation with an infected heel ulcer on the right. His vital signs include blood pressure (160/90 mmHg), heart rate (85 bpm), respiratory rate (22 bpm), and temperature (99.8° F). Laboratory values include a complete blood count, blood glucose, and body mass index. Other significant information includes his medication list (insulin, Tenormin, Lipitor, metformin, and Lasix). This knowledge helps the nurse to interpret, analyze, explain, and infer what is going on in the case to support clinical reasoning. Other thinking strategies are used next to reason through a possible plan of care: self-talk, schema search, prototype identification, hypothesizing, if-then, how-so thinking, comparative analysis, juxtaposing, and reflexive comparison.

Self-Talk

This strategy is the process of expressing one's thoughts to one's self. Self-talk answers the question, "What are the nursing diagnostic possibilities associated with the medical conditions of disease states?" The answer to this question results in the identification of the diagnostic hypotheses relevant to the case. For this case, the human responses to heart failure and diabetes include nursing diagnoses such as ineffective tissue perfusion; imbalanced nutrition, more than body requirements; ineffective health maintenance; ineffective protection; risk for infection; risk for loneliness; disturbed body image; and ineffective management of therapeutic regimen. Self-talk continues when spinning and weaving the Clinical Reasoning Web. Thinking out loud and reasoning about the relationships between these nursing diagnoses will emphasize the connections among diagnostic hypotheses and their relationships to one another.

Schema Search

Searching for schema is the process of accessing general and specific patterns of past experiences that might apply to the current situation. Past clinical experiences with patients who have heart failure and diabetes are helpful in reasoning about this specific case. Each experience with patients with these health problems creates a web in your mind. The schema includes what this patient exhibited, what interventions were implemented, and what the outcomes were. These memories become the foundation for clinical reasoning expertise.

Prototype Identification

Identifying prototypes is using a model case as a reference point for comparative analysis. A patient with heart failure and diabetes represents one instance of a person with that disease. Knowing what the prototypical patient with these conditions is likely to exhibit serves as a standard. With prototype identification, the textbook description of heart failure and diabetes serves as the standard and a reference point for comparative analysis. So, the nurse has to recall and reason about the pattern recognitions between prior cases and this case. Does the nurse have experience with heart failure and diabetes mellitus together? Does the nurse have experience with an adult male with these conditions who is also physically challenged and lives alone? Does the nurse have any experience with infected foot ulcers? Patterns of experience over time help with the development of schemas that could be recalled in this scenario. Determining if this schema aligns with the prototype reinforces schema development.

KEY POINTS

- Clinical reasoning for managing care begins with understanding and appreciating the story of the patient and family in context.

- Conscious attention to the way assessments are conducted and recorded influences the filtering, framing, and focus associated with the use of standardized terminologies.

- Creating a Clinical Reasoning Web is a scaffolding strategy for helping students think about patient problems and choosing priority care needs.

- Identification of significant cues, concepts, and principles and organizing them into a priority nursing diagnosis is the foundation for creating a plan of care that focuses on the present state, tests, interventions, outcomes, and clinical judgments.

- The process of creating and managing a plan of care through clinical reasoning involves critical, creative, systems, and complexity thinking skills that are supported by reflection and self-regulation of thinking.

STUDY QUESTIONS AND ACTIVITIES

1. Describe in your words the benefits and processes of describing a patient-in-context story to formulate a plan of care.

2. Create a list of all possible data sources for identifying patient and family healthcare needs. Categorize the problems by nursing domains and problem classifications.

3. Describe how the priority nursing diagnosis, once identified, could be incorporated into a plan of care and could impact other diagnoses identified in the Clinical Reasoning Web.

4. How could the information in a Clinical Reasoning Web be used to facilitate the communication between the members of a healthcare team during a report or placed in a healthcare record?

5. Identify all the possible standardized healthcare languages and communication strategies that are used in creating a patient-in-context story and a Clinical Reasoning Web. Do language differences impact communication and the development of a patient care plan?

6. Identify the relationship between reflection and critical and creative thinking strategies as applied to the patient-in-context story and the Clinical Reasoning Web.

References

Airasian, P. W., Cruikshank, K. A., Mayer, R. E., Pintrich, R., Raths, J., & Wittrock, M. C. (2000). The cognitive process dimension. In L. W. Anderson & D. R. Krathwohl (Eds.), *A taxonomy for learning, teaching, and assessing: A revision of Bloom's taxonomy of educational objectives*, pp. 63–92. Boston, MA: Allyn and Bacon.

American Nurses Association (ANA). (2015). *Nursing: Scope and standards of practice* (3rd ed.). Silver Spring, MD: ANA Publishing.

American Psychiatric Association. (2013). *DSM 5*. Arlington, VA: American Psychiatric Association Publishing.

Carpenito, L. J. (2017). *Nursing diagnosis: Application to clinical practice* (15th ed.). Philadelphia, PA: Wolters Kluwer Health.

Goodwin, L., VanDyne, M., Lin, S., & Talbert, S. (2003). Building nursing knowledge through informatics: From concept representation to data mining. *Journal of Biomedical Informatics, 36*(4–5), 379–388.

Grier, M. (1985). *Information processing in nursing practice: Annual review of nursing research* (pp. 265–287). New York, NY: Springer Publishing Company.

Hawkins, D., Elder, L., & Paul, R. (2010). *Clinical reasoning*. Tomales, CA: The Foundation for Critical Thinking.

Kuiper, R., Pesut, D., & Kautz, D. (2009). Promoting the self-regulation of clinical reasoning skills in nursing students. *The Open Nursing Journal, 3*, 76–85. Retrieved from http://www.ncbi.nlm.nih.gov/pmc/articles/PMC2771264/

Martin, K. S. (2005). *The Omaha System: A key to practice, documentation, and information management* (reprinted 2nd ed.). Omaha, NE: Health Connections Press.

NANDA-I. (2017). Defining the knowledge of nursing. Retrieved from http://www.nanda.org/nanda-international-glossary-of-terms.html

Pesut, D., & Herman, J. (1999). *Clinical reasoning: The art and science of critical and creative thinking*. New York, NY: Delmar Publishers.

Treffinger, D. J., & Isaksen, S. G. (2005). Creative problem solving: The history, development, and implications for gifted education and talent development. *Gifted Child Quarterly, 49*(4), 342–353. doi:10.1177/001698620504900407

LEARNING THE OPT MODEL OF CLINICAL REASONING: FRAMING, OUTCOME-PRESENT STATE-TEST

LEARNING OUTCOMES

- Explain the knowledge and data needed to frame a patient and family healthcare situation to present the most authentic circumstances for proceeding with a plan of care.

- Describe the processes of filtering, framing, and focusing to determine the present state issues that arise from the priority or keystone issue identified from the Clinical Reasoning Web.

- Describe the different clinical thinking processes that support the juxtaposing of the present and outcome states to determine the gaps in health and wellness.

- Describe how data and evidence management is essential to determine the outcome state to address patient and family needs.

- Describe the relationship between the frame and the present and outcome states, and how the reflection on these components of the OPT Model of Clinical Reasoning determines the tests and interventions selected for a plan of care.

This chapter describes the process of working with the data derived and organized from the using the Clinical Reasoning Web in Chapter 4. As the nurse reflects on the main health problems of a patient and family situation, priorities are determined, and the framing of the situation influences the identification of present-state issues that need attention to achieve identified outcomes. The patient's story is used to frame, or derive meaning, in the case. Significant issues that are identified help structure and guide thinking. Nurses filter health assessment and history information to create a frame for the issues associated with the patient care story. A focus on nursing-specific problems in the present state is managed and influences the creating of outcomes that are sensitive to nursing interventions. The OPT Model of Clinical Reasoning emphasizes filtering, framing, and focusing on patient/family assessments to identify gaps between present-state problems and the outcomes desired. The OPT Model identifies priorities in patient care scenarios, which help determine the outcomes desired for health and wellness. How the nurse applies clinical reasoning processes to determine outcomes for collaborative healthcare management is described in this chapter. Special emphasis is focused on the importance of filtering and framing, the complementary nature of a problem-outcome juxtaposition, and the definition of a test in the OPT Model.

FILTERING, FRAMING, AND FOCUSING

Intentional focus on the patient and family story enables the nurse to frame the relationships among the context, present state, and desired outcome state. The side-by-side comparisons that present themselves as a result of the OPT Model Worksheet promote concurrent and iterative thinking from the patient-in-context story and reveal the gaps that uncover the complementary nature of problems ~ outcomes. They can be influenced by interventions and are evaluated with tests. Nurses develop clinical reasoning skills with repeated practice as they analyze and understand individual patient stories and planning care for present ~ outcome states. Table 5.1 presents some reflection questions to use with the OPT Model of Clinical Reasoning to filter, frame, and focus on data given a particular patient case scenario.

TABLE 5.1 QUESTIONS THAT SUPPORT FILTERING, FRAMING, AND FOCUSING

Filtering and Framing	What are the background concerns operating in the patient story when I think about framing?
	What and how am I filtering the facts and data related to this story?
	How do the present state and outcome state relate, and what are the gaps between them?
	Considering a "frame" surrounding the patient's story, how best would I describe what is observed in this situation?
Outcome State	What are the primary healthcare problems related to the keystone issue?
Present State	What are the matching realistic and measurable goals or outcomes to be achieved through care management?
	How is the present state defined? How is the outcome state defined?
	What are the gaps or complementary pairs of outcomes and present states?
Tests	What are the clinical indicators from analysis and assessment of the patient regarding desired outcomes?
	On what scales will the desired outcomes be rated?
	How will I know when the desired outcomes are achieved?
	How am I defining the testing in this particular case?
	What tests are needed to analyze the interventions to achieve the goals of care management?

Filtering

Understanding nursing knowledge is essential to help filter information from the assessment and history of the patient and family. Nurses, as well as other healthcare professionals, filter information and use it to frame issues associated with patient care stories to then focus on a discipline-specific problem that is transformed into outcomes that are influenced by interventions. Filtering requires a clinical reasoning mindset to organize presented knowledge and data. The appreciation and consideration of such healthcare information has value regarding contemporary issues related to healthcare contexts, interprofessional team collaboration, informatics, and state-of-the-art therapies. The understanding, valuing, and insights gained through foundational professional preparation, use of clinical terminologies, practice with care plan development, reflective thinking, and guidance by faculty and staff help people "think like a nurse" (Tanner, 2006).

Novice nurses begin putting facts together in meaningful ways and recognizing patterns. They then decide about the usefulness of facts for current and future situations. Being conscious of how one filters information is important, as it reveals one's professional beliefs, values, and orientation to knowledge developed in the discipline. How one filters all the information that is presented in a case is influenced by a clinical reasoning mindset and individual perspective that includes the attitudes of a) intention, b) reflection, c) curiosity, d) tolerance for ambiguity, e) appreciation of perspectives, f) self-confidence, g) professional motivation, and h) strategic use of knowledge and standardized terminologies.

Filtering information involves the use of diagnostic cluster/cue logic, which is the deliberate structuring of patient-in-context story data to discern the meaning of nursing care. Clinical evidence influences filtering and framing about the patient-in-context story. Diagnostic cluster/cue logic and schemas stored in memory influence framing. Prototypes that are model cases that serve as reference points also influence filtering and framing. Consider the example of the infected foot ulcer. Identification of purulent drainage and an increase in temperature lead one to ask the question about infection. Because experience influences thinking, perhaps experience with an infected ulcer influences reasoning? Textbook descriptions of infected ulcers are helpful in using cue logic about this problem. After treatment is initiated and healing starts to take place, the nurse compares it with the memory of what it looked like with the infection present. This comparison is a test. The differences between the infected and healing ulcers create a contrast and provide evidence showing the ulcer is healing, or it is not healing.

Diagnostic cluster/cue logic from the knowledge work in assessment activities results in a list of nursing diagnoses. With the help of a Clinical Reasoning Web, a keystone priority issue is determined. This keystone then influences framing and nursing care needs. The diagnostic cluster/cue logic and framing are iterative and recursive. They shift like an optical illusion to oscillate between a foreground and background position. For example, the foreground would be the infected ulcer and the background would be living conditions of the patient. These two pieces of information are significant regarding the problem, but their significance moves back and forth in regard to the interventions.

Framing

A patient's story provides important information about the context and major issues for clinical reasoning. As the nurse listens to the patient and family, connects and communicates with them in meaningful ways, and gets the facts of the situation, meaning is attributed to the story. Note that at the top of the OPT Model Worksheet is a place to indicate the frame or theme that best represents the background context issues regarding the patient story (see Figure 5.1). The frame is the theme that often emerges after the creation of an OPT Model Clinical Reasoning Web. The frame helps organize the present state and outcome state, illustrates the gaps, and provides insights about what tests or interventions are needed to close the gaps. Frames depend on the nurse's filters and distinctions about obvious and not-so-obvious features of the story. Decision-making and reflection surround the framing process as the nurse thinks of all the patient-centered issues concurrently. Reflection is used to monitor and self-regulate one's thinking as a frame is created.

How you "frame" a story has implications for clinical reasoning. For example, consider the current case: George Appleton is a 62-year-old gentleman who lives alone and is unemployed. His medical history includes chronic heart failure and diabetes mellitus. In framing this situation, there is a need to manage the heart failure and diabetes so that he can be as independent as possible and prevent the complications of diabetes. How does such a frame guide and direct your thinking and doing? Would your thinking and doing be different if the "frame" or lens you used to view this situation involved "finding a caretaker for him"? How would your thinking and actions be different given these two different perspectives?

During the framing process, meaning is attributed to the connections in the case from the collected data, evidence, and cues. Previous schema or prototypes recalled from memory of previous experiences might apply to the current situation and influence framing. The result is establishing a structure for testing the achievement of outcomes, using the structure as a reference point for comparative analysis and hypothesizing, or determining an explanation that accounts for a set of facts that can be tested by further investigation.

If-then thinking is another strategy that involves future time projection that considers the consequences of specific actions. It makes a difference how one frames the facts about the right foot ulcer discussed in the earlier example. If the situation is framed as an infection, how does that guide one's thinking? If the situation is framed as ulcer management, how does that influence thinking? If the situation is framed as an ulcer that is healing, how does this influence thinking? If the situation is framed around elevated temperature, how does this influence thinking and doing? Considering the patient is a diabetic and the ulcer is on the right lower extremity, how does the framing of the problem shift? The fact is that one must consider all these possibilities at the same time. That process is concurrent, iterative, and recursive thinking, which supports clinical reasoning and describes the ideas about framing presented in Chapter 2.

Framing (Figure 5.2) is a process we use all the time as we create mental models or perceptual positions about issues, events, and meanings. Peter Senge (1990) discussed mental models in his book *The Fifth Discipline* and described them as how we make sense of the world and shape how we act. Senge (1990) describes mental models as simple generalizations, such as patients who engage in their healthcare, or complex theories, such as assumptions about why patients act as they do. If we believe patients are interested in their healthcare, we act differently than we would if we believed they were not. Becoming aware of frames or mental models regarding patient stories is an important aspect of clinical reasoning and guides perceptions and behaviors (Fairhurst & Sarr, 1996). As it applies to managing patient cases:

- Framing is a way to manage meaning and involves selecting and highlighting one or more aspects of a case while excluding others.

- Framing involves the use of language, thought, and forethought to focus, classify, remember, and understand one thing regarding another.

- Framing increases our chances of people's agreement because when the right frames are in place, the right behavior follows.

- Framing requires initiative with the clarity of purpose and a thorough understanding of the patient and family for whom we are managing meaning.

- Opportunities for framing occur with every communication we have in healthcare interactions.

- Our values play an important role in the kind of framing that we do and in the way that our frames are perceived (p. 22).

Framing involves thinking about the patient's story and distinguishes between the central issue or problem and peripheral problems. As the nurse uses clinical reasoning for framing, meaning in the story is created to establish a starting and stopping point for their efforts. A unique metaphor for framing is having different types of camera lenses. A wide-angle lens frames a scene much differently than a close-up zoom lens. Becoming aware of mental models and the frames we use for patient and family stories is important for successful clinical reasoning. We become aware of frames through stories patients share with us and the meanings we attribute to those stories. You could also think of framing as the backdrop or scenery of a stage play. As the scenery and contexts change, so do the actions and behavior of the actors. The background and context influence the action and events.

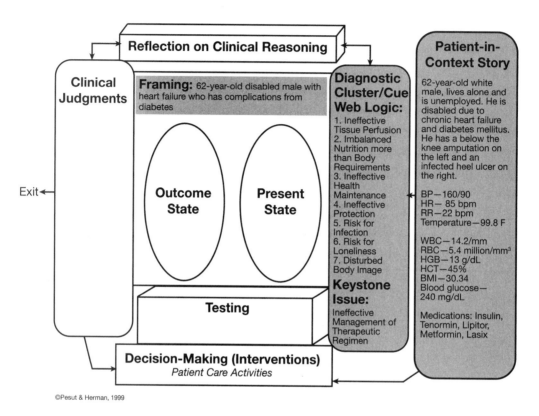

©Pesut & Herman, 1999

Figure 5.1   OPT Model of Clinical Reasoning Worksheet (Framing).

Framing is one of the unique aspects of the OPT Model that sets it apart from other care planning models. The frame interacts with and provides the organizing structure for establishing the present state and desired outcome state. The nurse must ask, "What are the central issues in the story?" then asks the questions, "What and how do I think about this story?" and "What lens have I used to view this situation?" Of course, how you frame or attribute meaning to the situation depends on how you organize the data or cues associated with the story. Hence, framing depends on the knowledge at hand and the diagnostic cluster/cue logic to make sense of what the nurse sees, hears, knows, and feels in a clinical situation.

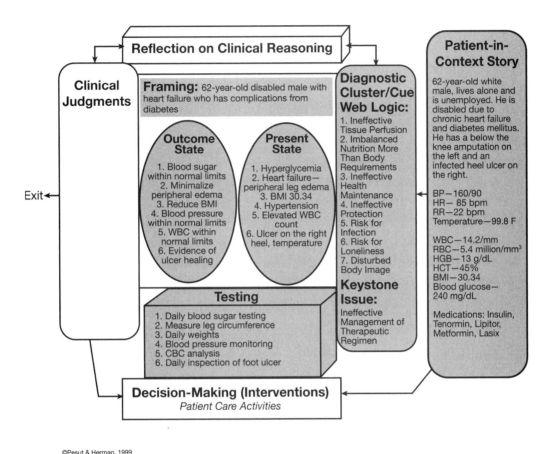

Reflection on Clinical Reasoning

Clinical Judgments

Framing: 62-year-old disabled male with heart failure who has complications from diabetes

Outcome State
1. Blood sugar within normal limits
2. Minimalize peripheral edema
3. Reduce BMI
4. Blood pressure within normal limits
5. WBC within normal limits
6. Evidence of ulcer healing

Present State
1. Hyperglycemia
2. Heart failure—peripheral leg edema
3. BMI 30.34
4. Hypertension
5. Elevated WBC count
6. Ulcer on the right heel, temperature

Diagnostic Cluster/Cue Web Logic:
1. Ineffective Tissue Perfusion
2. Imbalanced Nutrition More Than Body Requirements
3. Ineffective Health Maintenance
4. Ineffective Protection
5. Risk for Infection
6. Risk for Loneliness
7. Disturbed Body Image

Keystone Issue:
Ineffective Management of Therapeutic Regimen

Patient-in-Context Story
62-year-old white male, lives alone and is unemployed. He is disabled due to chronic heart failure and diabetes mellitus. He has a below the knee amputation on the left and an infected heel ulcer on the right.

BP—160/90
HR—85 bpm
RR—22 bpm
Temperature—99.8 F

WBC—14.2/mm
RBC—5.4 million/mm³
HGB—13 g/dL
HCT—45%
BMI—30.34
Blood glucose—240 mg/dL

Medications: Insulin, Tenormin, Lipitor, Metformin, Lasix

Exit◄

Testing
1. Daily blood sugar testing
2. Measure leg circumference
3. Daily weights
4. Blood pressure monitoring
5. CBC analysis
6. Daily inspection of foot ulcer

Decision-Making (Interventions)
Patient Care Activities

©Pesut & Herman, 1999

Figure 5.2   OPT Model of Clinical Reasoning Worksheet (Outcome-Present State-Test).

Focusing

With the frame as the background, what now comes to the foreground is the development of a present state and outcome state comparison. The *present state* (P) is a description of the client in context. Present state is the initial condition of the patient. The present state, which changes over time as a result of nursing actions, is derived from diagnostic cluster/cue logic and defined by standardized taxonomic terms. The foot ulcer example shows a present state of Impaired Skin Integrity. *Outcomes* (O) are desired or end states that result from nursing care.

Outcome states are the desired conditions of the client derived from the frame and initial present state data, as well as criteria that define the desired condition. In the foot ulcer example, an achievable outcome is healing, skin integrity, and resolved infection.

Given the frame of a situation, nurses use outcome-focused thinking (Pesut, 1989) to create outcomes derived from present state data. After an outcome is derived, a side-by-side comparison is made of present state ~ outcome state. *Juxtaposing* is the side-by-side comparison of specified outcome state criteria with present state data. Foreground issues of juxtaposed present and desired states emerge from background issues of "framing." The context is thus incorporated and supports the contrast of the juxtaposed present state ~ outcome state. The focus on this side-by-side comparison creates a test (T). A test is a process of juxtaposing the present state and outcome state and evaluating the gap between the two states. To perform a test one analyzes and compares data from the present state to the outcome state. Considering how the foot ulcer looked when infected and how it needs to look when healed is an example of the kind of side-by-side testing that comes from juxtaposing. Thus, the test, in this case, would be a complete assessment of the wound and surrounding skin. Other tests may include a white blood cell count and temperature assessment. Nursing care helps bridge the gap between present state and desired outcome state.

Once the keystone issue Ineffective Management of Therapeutic Regimen is identified, it is the basis for defining the patient's present state and contrasted with the desired outcome state. In this case, hyperglycemia, hypertension, peripheral edema, weight gain, and infected right foot ulcer would be the present state issues most in need of attention. The outcomes would be normalized blood sugars, normalized blood pressure, minimal peripheral edema, weight control, and evidence of ulcer healing. The evident gaps between the present state and outcome state are the focal point for analysis, implementation, and evaluation of nursing interventions. Therefore, the present and outcome states relate to the keystone issue, and the outcome state reflects improvement from the present state.

In one research study with generic undergraduate nursing students, it was found that with the OPT Model of Clinical Reasoning, framing was difficult for many students. OPT Model Worksheets analyzed over time revealed no differences overall ($p = .90$), but there were differences between and among students ($p < 0.01$) (Kautz et al., 2009). Attending to individual students' clinical work using the model is a way to assess, evaluate, and tailor instruction according to the individual's clinical reasoning abilities.

In another study with paramedic-to-bachelor degree students, there were significant positive differences in students' scores for capturing the patient-in-context story between weeks 1 and 6 ($p = .001$) and crafting judgment statements between weeks 1 and 6 ($p = .004$). Students also improved in retrieving the family history over time ($p = .000$) and the inclusion of judgment statements ($p = .000$) (Kautz, Kuiper, Pesut, Knight-Brown, & Daneker, 2005). Finally, in a study with fourth-year nursing students, it was found that knowledge level (i.e., skills, relationships with others, and understanding disease processes, treatments, and interventions) improved and enabled students to focus on priorities and participate effectively in the clinical environment (White, 2003). The OPT Model of Clinical Reasoning assists with forming these habits of mind and self-efficacy in practice. Framing is one of the most challenging concepts/aspects of the OPT Model. Following are some suggestions related to mastering this skill.

The steps to the creation of the frame, outcome-present state-test of the OPT Model Worksheet are as follows:

1. Carefully consider and filter all the information gathered for the patient-in-context story.

2. Frame the situation to select essential present-state issues using diagnostic cluster/cue logic and the deductive, inductive, and dialectic thinking processes about the priority issues of the case.

3. Reflect on the present-state issues to decide if resolving them would lead to positive outcomes for this patient and family.

4. Focus on the selected present-state issues and determine the complementary nature of problems with achievable outcomes.

5. Do a side-by-side comparison of present state and outcome state to identify and evaluate the gap between them.

6. Select the tests that would best analyze and provide evidence to conduct the gap analysis from the present state to the outcome state.

7. Reflect on the created plan and determine if the tests are appropriate, how the present and outcome states relate to the keystone issue, and whether the outcome state reflects an improvement from the present state.

Questions Frequently Asked About the Web

As with other parts of the OPT Model, students often have questions about issues related to framing, problem ~ outcome relationships, and the concept of testing. The most frequently asked questions are posed and answered here:

1. **Frame:**

   a. *Question:* What is unique about the framing statement that is not already written within the patient-in-context story?

   b. *Response:* The frame or theme represents the background issues in thinking about the patient story. It provides the structure for establishing the present state and desired outcome state. Think of framing as viewing a patient's story through the use of different types of camera lens. Consider framing as the backdrop or scenery of a stage play. As this scenery and context change, so do the actions and behavior of the actors.

   c. *Response:* Framing involves thinking about the patient's story and distinguishes between the central issue or problem and peripheral problems. When framing the patient's story, the nurse must consider the following: 1) the central issues of the story, 2) how and what to think about the story, and 3) the "lens" through which to view the situation. As a nurse, how would you "filter" and name, or give a headline to the patient story?

    d. *Response:* Conversely, the patient-in-context story is a description of information that is nursing-sensitive and information related to the pathophysiology of the patient's condition. It contains patient demographics, relevant diagnostic results, assessment data, family dynamics, and contextual factors that the nurse needs to consider for planning care. Given the facts, what are the nursing care consequences of the patient's medical condition?

2. **Present State:**

    a. *Question:* Do all present-state issues need to be related to the keystone issue?

    b. *Response:* Yes. The present state, which is the initial condition of the patient, must be related to the keystone issue. The keystone issue is the basis for defining the patient's present state and is contrasted with the desired outcome state. Over time the present state changes as a result of nursing actions.

3. **Outcome State:**

    a. *Question:* What are the recommended components of an outcome statement?

    b. *Response:* Outcomes are the goals of the patient's care or the desired results (Kuiper, Pesut, & Arms, 2016). They are derived from the frame and initial present-state data as well as criteria that define the desired condition. Outcome statements are specific to particular present-state data. They can be a state, behavior, or perception measured along a continuum in response to a nursing intervention (Butcher & Johnson, 2012). Outcomes are complementary to the present state and should be defined in positive terms rather than defined as negative to the present state. For example, pain/no pain is a negative definition. A better present ~ outcome state comparison would be pain/pain control.

4. **Outcome State:**

   a. *Question:* Is it necessary to include the NOC label for each outcome statement?

   b. *Response:* For clarification, outcome statements written for the case study
   examples in this book contain NOC labels, noted in bold type. Suggested
   outcomes depict the relationship between the patient's problems or current
   status and those aspects of the problems or status that are expected to be
   resolved or improved by nursing interventions.

5. **Tests:**

   a. *Question:* How does the nurse determine what tests should be considered
   for the patient's progression from present state to outcome state?

   b. *Response:* On the OPT Model of Clinical Reasoning, the nurse places each
   present-state condition next to the related outcome statement. This side-
   by-side contrast between one state and the other illustrates differences or
   gaps between the two states. The gap analysis is the test that needs to be
   satisfied. These differences or gaps establish conditions for the test (Kuiper
   et al., 2016). Evaluation of interventions are used to determine whether
   gaps have been closed or if partially so. In other words, the nurse must
   consider evidence to verify if the desired state has been achieved. Evidence
   may consist of laboratory study results, assessment data, patient
   verbalization, or written indications.

REFLECTION ON CLINICAL REASONING

Clinical reasoning practice is important to reinforce the need for nurses to develop competencies to filter, frame, and focus care planning. The OPT Model of Clinical Reasoning is a tool to support thinking by nurses as they makes concurrent and iterative side-by-side comparisons of outcomes with present state information from the patient story. The gap between a present state and desired state establishes a test that can be analyzed and evaluated after interventions are carried out. Judgments and conclusions result when evidence about their achievement are evaluated. There are some specific thinking strategies that support the development of clinical reasoning skills during this phase of the care planning.

The OPT Model of Clinical Reasoning relies on higher order critical thinking skills such as analysis, synthesis, evaluation, creativity, and judgment (Airasian et al., 2000). Many of these strategies are *metacognitive,* meaning thinking about your thinking. Each of the strategies—attention to knowledge work, self-talk, prototype identification or pattern recognition (schema searches), hypothesizing, activation of if-then thinking, comparative analysis, and juxtaposing—is used to ascertain gaps between present and desired states and activate reflexive comparisons.

Hypothesizing

This process determines an explanation that accounts for a set of facts that can be tested by further investigation. Hypothesizing presupposes use and understanding of clinical vocabulary. Explanations for circumstances in a case are called *diagnostic hypotheses*. They are guesses about what might explain a situation and high-risk sequelae. Our hypotheses we make about patient cases have to be supported by data, or we have to keep searching for the reality of a situation.

The diagnostic hypotheses become the origins and insertion points for making associations when one develops a Clinical Reasoning Web. Hypothesizing includes if-then, how-so thinking; however, it is a more formal statement or declaration about how specifically sets of facts are related. Hypothesis testing requires gathering evidence under controlled conditions to affirm or negate the proposed relationship. Spinning and weaving the webs for individual case management results in some diagnostic hypotheses. Once identified diagnoses are chosen, it is easier to see how these diagnoses relate by hypothesizing. For example, in the case of George Appleton, we could make the hypothesis that improving the self-management of the therapeutic regimen might improve health maintenance, reduce infection, and enhance tissue perfusion.

If-Then, How-So Thinking

This type of thinking involves linking ideas and consequences in a logical sequence, which is at the heart of clinical reasoning. If-then, how-so thinking is used in connecting diagnoses and care management needs in the respective webs. It is also the place to start developing the plan of care and determining what resources are needed for care management. In this case, *if* tissue perfusion improves with better management of the therapeutic regimen, *then* the infection would be resolved.

Comparative Analysis

This thinking strategy involves considering the strengths and weaknesses of competing alternatives. After diagnostic hypotheses and their relationships are made explicit using the webs, comparative analysis is used to determine which of these relationships is the keystone or the central supporting issues of a situation. Identifying the keystone issues enables the nurse to focus on care. Once a keystone issue is identified, a domino effect occurs in which other problems and needs are influenced. During the hypothesizing process, comparative analysis placed the nursing diagnoses in order of priority to gain the best impact and outcomes considering the multiple health issues at stake.

Juxtaposing

Think of juxtaposing as creating a gap analysis. Juxtaposing involves putting the present state condition next to the outcome state. The side-by-side contrast of one state with the other illustrates the differences or gaps between the two states. The differences or gaps evident from the present to desired state help establish the conditions for the creation of a test in the OPT Model. A test is satisfied if the gap is closed. As one determines the practice issues, interventions, and outcomes for managing care, the successive achievement of the desired outcome helps to close the gap and successfully pass the test(s). Juxtaposing enables one to set up essential elements between two states. For example, if the hyperglycemia in this patient improved with better health maintenance, the monitoring of blood sugar would determine if the gap closed and the outcome was achieved. Decisions that one makes and interventions one initiates help bridge the gap between juxtaposed conditions.

Reflexive Comparison

This strategy involves constant comparison of the patient's state from one time of observation to a later time of observation. For example, each time the size of an ulcer is measured, the nurse compares a patient's progress from one observation to the next. The patient serves as his/her own standard for making progress toward the desired outcome state.

The thinking strategies in Table 5.2 describe the specific activities and outcomes used during this phase of the care planning with the OPT Model. Framing the situation and then hypothesizing about the priority or keystone issue leads to some other strategies such as if-then, how-so thinking about tests, comparative analysis between present and outcome states, and juxtaposing outcomes with priority nursing diagnoses.

TABLE 5.2 THINKING STRATEGIES THAT SUPPORT THE OPT MODEL OF CLINICAL REASONING

Thinking Strategy	Definition	Expected Outcomes
Filtering	Filtering is the process of being conscious of the knowledge and perspectives one is using to gather data in a patient care scenario. The various healthcare disciplines filter patient data differently. The process of filtering is sifting through and choosing significant disciplinary knowledge and facts associated with a patient story.	• Identification of priority information related to nursing care planning. • Attention to the use of standardized terminologies. • Appreciation of interprofessional/disciplinary differences in scope of practice.
Framing	Frames are derived from filters and focus based on a particular conceptual-theoretical framework, or methods used to structure thinking and reasoning.	• Conscious identification of filtering, framing, and focusing based on models, theory, or practice conceptual framework used to structure and interpret the facts of a given situation. • Conscious choice of standardized terminologies.
Hypothesizing	Statements about how the facts or concepts in a given case are related to one another.	• Statement of integrated and associational relationships and directional, bidirectional, or multidirectional hypotheses.
If-Then, How-So Thinking	Linking ideas and consequences together in a logical sequence.	• Statement of specified relationships in an if-then, how-so format.
Comparative Analysis	Analysis of similarities and differences among facts in a given situation.	• Justification of plans and choices based on a compare-and-contrast process.
Juxtaposing	The process of contrasting present-state conditions with specified outcome states. Understanding the tension between opposites—for example, a nursing diagnosis and a corresponding nursing outcome.	• A side-by-side comparison of desired outcome and present-state data, which creates the test or gap analysis between the present and well-specified desired outcome states. (Note that an outcome is not the negative definition of the problem state.)

Thinking Strategy	Definition	Expected Outcomes
Testing	Concurrent thinking about the successive approximations of present-state transitions to outcome-state targets.	• Reflections and judgments related to transitional outcome achievements.
Reflexive Comparison	Use of the patient as the control for baseline and subsequent clinical observations.	• Identification of similarities and differences between time series observations.

KEY POINTS

- Filtering information and data from the patient-in-context story is used to frame the issues in healthcare scenarios.

- The frame is the theme about the background issues that lay the foundation for the plan of care that developed in a healthcare scenario.

- Clinical reasoning for managing care requires critical reflection to focus on the keystone and present-state issues that need attention for health promotion.

- Creative thinking, reflexive comparison, and juxtaposing are required to compare present-state issues with desired outcomes.

- After identified gaps are listed, hypothesizing and if-then, how-so thinking strategies are used to determine tests and scales that can determine whether outcomes are achievable.

STUDY QUESTIONS AND ACTIVITIES

1. Describe in your own words the information and data that has to be filtered to frame a healthcare situation.

2. When you examine a patient and family scenario, create a list of all the different frames that could emerge based on the type of healthcare provider managing particular problems.

3. Using an OPT Model Clinical Reasoning Worksheet, identify and match present state and outcome state for each nursing diagnosis in a completed Clinical Reasoning Web.

4. Describe how one keystone priority nursing diagnosis and present-state issues are most significant to choose in order to proceed to desired outcomes.

5. Complete a search for all possible tests that would monitor the progression from present to outcome states in a patient healthcare scenario and determine how you would pick the most practical ones for a particular case.

6. Reflect on the processes completed in the case discussed in this chapter and determine whether the filtering, framing, and focusing were correctly done. How you would change your thinking the next time you encountered this schema?

References

Airasian, P. W., Cruikshank, K. A., Mayer, R. E., Pintrich, R., Raths, J., & Wittrock, M. C. (2000). The cognitive process dimension. In L. W. Anderson & D. R. Krathwohl (Eds.), *A taxonomy for learning, teaching, and assessing: A revision of Bloom's taxonomy of educational objectives,* pp. 63–92. Boston, MA: Allyn and Bacon.

Butcher, H., & Johnson, M. (2012). Use of linkages for clinical reasoning and quality improvement. In M. Johnson, S. Moorhead, G. Bulechek, H. Butcher, M. Maas, & E. Swanson (Eds.), *NOC and NIC linkages to NANDA-I and clinical conditions* (3rd ed.), pp. 11–23. Maryland Heights, MO: Elsevier.

Fairhurst, G., & Sarr, R. (1996). *The art of framing: Managing the language of leadership.* San Francisco, CA: Jossey Bass.

Kautz, D., Kuiper, R., Bartlett, R., Buck, R., Williams, R., & Knight-Brown, P. (2009). Building evidence for the development of clinical reasoning using a rating tool with the Outcome-Present State-Test (OPT) Model. *Southern Online Journal of Nursing Research, 9*(1).

Kautz, D., Kuiper, R., Pesut, D., Knight-Brown, P., & Daneker, D. (2005). Promoting clinical reasoning in undergraduate nursing students: Application and evaluation of the Outcome-Present State-Test (OPT) Model of Clinical Reasoning. *International Journal of Nursing Education Scholarship, 2*(1), Article 1. Retrieved from http://www.bepress.com/ijnes/vol2/iss1/art1

Kuiper, R. A., Pesut, D. J., & Arms, T. (2016). *Clinical reasoning and care coordination in advanced practice nursing.* New York, NY: Springer Publishing Company.

Pesut, D. (1989). Aim versus blame: Using an outcome specification model. *Journal of Psychosocial Nursing and Mental Health Services, 27*(5), 26–30.

Pesut, D., & Herman, J. (1999). *Clinical reasoning: The art and science of critical and creative thinking.* New York, NY: Delmar Publishers.

Senge, P. (1990). *The fifth discipline.* New York, NY: Doubleday.

Tanner, C. A. (2006). Thinking like a nurse: A research-based model of clinical judgment in nursing. *Journal of Nursing Education, 45*(6), 204–211.

White, A. (2003). Clinical decision making among fourth-year nursing students: An interpretive study. *Journal of Nursing Education, 42*(3), 113–120.

C H A P T E R

6

LEARNING THE OPT MODEL OF CLINICAL REASONING: INTERVENTIONS, JUDGMENTS, AND REFRAMING

LEARNING OUTCOMES

- Explain how to choose evidence-based interventions that are most appropriate to achieve the desired healthcare outcomes for a patient and family scenario using the OPT Model of Clinical Reasoning.

- Describe the thinking processes used to evaluate tests and interventions to make judgments about their success in achieving the outcome state.

- Describe the thinking processes used to reframe a healthcare situation for determining a new set of present-state issues and desired outcomes.

- Explain how a new frame or keystone issue enhances patient and family health and well-being.

- Describe how the iterative and recursive process of reflective thinking and re-thinking is promoted by the OPT Model of Clinical Reasoning.

- Explain how the OPT Model of Clinical Reasoning supports the complexity thinking necessary to coordinate healthcare situations given current healthcare challenges and contexts.

Chapter 5 discusses choosing the appropriate tests to evaluate present-state ~ outcome-state gaps and whether or not the patient was moving closer to the desired outcomes. This chapter describes the process of choosing nursing interventions to assist the patient and family in reaching desired outcomes. This process requires making clinical judgments and decisions about changing tests and interventions, or reframing the situation to support a different focus or priority. As one set of problems is handled, others might arise that require a change in thinking. As the patient situation is reassessed, the nurse reflects on the remaining health problems in the situation. New health information and data are filtered to reframe the situation for a new set of present-state issues and desired outcomes. A focus on new nursing-specific problems in the present state is influenced by additional information, data, and results of interventions and transformed outcomes. As the nurse applies the clinical reasoning process during this section of the OPT Model of Clinical Reasoning, evidence-based interventions are chosen to achieve outcomes.

The nurse impacts the health and well-being of patients and families through the application and use of critical, creative, systems, and complexity thinking processes to manage patient problems with appropriate interventions in service of established patient-centered outcomes. It is important to reflect on the framing and complexity of patient issues to plan interventions to achieve desired outcomes. The decisions that one makes and interventions one initiates help bridge the gap between juxtaposed conditions of present ~ outcome states.

NURSING CARE INTERVENTIONS

As the nurse reflects on and analyzes how each of these current needs or issues impacts and influences all the other needs, patterns emerge that reveal focal points for intervention that can accelerate the achievement of outcomes by the use of effective and efficient evidence-based therapies. An important aspect of naming the interventions is classifying them according to a system that aligns with accepted knowledge and language for nursing. Nursing language is commonly understood by all nurses to describe care by providing them with a common means of communication about assessments, interventions, and outcomes

(Association of Perioperative Registered Nurses [AORN], n.d.; Keenan, 1999; Rutherford, 2008). The common language facilitates efficient documentation, particularly in electronic health records. The benefits of standardized languages are for better communication among nurses and other healthcare providers, increased visibility of nursing interventions, improved patient care, enhanced data collection to evaluate nursing care outcomes, greater adherence to standards of care, and facilitated assessment of nursing competency (Rutherford, 2008). Recall the information presented in Chapter 2 about clinical reasoning and standardized terminologies. Diagnoses, interventions, and outcomes are defined, described, and classified in all of the American Nurses Association (ANA)–recognized terminologies. Take a moment to review Table 2.1 in Chapter 2.

Development of the standardized terminologies was undertaken with a specific purpose in mind. Establishing criteria for a classification ensures reliability, adequacy, and usefulness for clinicians in practice. Each of the recognized classification systems represents standardized terminologies that are useful to clinicians as they reason about client problems, interventions, and outcomes. The examples in the OPT Model of Clinical Reasoning Worksheets used in Chapters 4, 5, and 6 are closely aligned with chronic physical and behavioral health problems. Based on the type of clinical case and the context of care, a specific type of standardized terminology may be required.

For teaching and learning purposes in this book, the authors have chosen to illustrate the use of the OPT Model of Clinical Reasoning with attention to the use of NANDA-I diagnoses, the Nursing Interventions Classification (NIC) (Butcher, Bulechek, Dochterman, & Wagner [in press]), and the Nursing Outcomes Classification (NOC) (Moorhead, 2013) systems. In Chapter 14, the authors illustrate how the OPT Model of Clinical Reasoning can incorporate the Omaha System (Martin, 2005).

How you use the knowledge stored in these classifications systems depends on the context of your practice, knowledge, beliefs, values, and professional identity. As nursing continues to evolve and classification systems become an important focus of clinical scholarship, members of the profession have an obligation and responsibility to stay informed and use and refine the knowledge contained in these systems. The knowledge stored in these systems is the vocabulary of and for clinical reasoning. As you will see in subsequent chapters, the OPT Model of Clinical Reasoning provides a structure that can use standardized terminologies in an artful way.

CLINICAL DECISIONS

Decisions are choices made about interventions that will help the patient transition from present state to the desired outcome state. One is constantly updating and "testing" the degree to which outcomes are being achieved or not based on the results of the interventions. Testing is concurrent and iterative as one gets closer and closer in successive increments toward goal or outcome achievement. Clinical decision-making is the selection of interventions and actions that move clients from a presenting state to a specified or desired outcome state. Decision-making is the process of selecting interventions from a repertoire of actions that facilitate the achievement of the desired outcome state.

In other words, what nursing actions and interventions are necessary to bring the present state and outcome state closer together in this case? You can use the prompts listed in Table 6.1 to support decisions about interventions for patient-centered care planning.

TABLE 6.1 QUESTIONS THAT SUPPORT DECISIONS IN THE OPT MODEL OF CLINICAL REASONING

Decision-Making (Interventions)	What clinical decisions or interventions help to achieve the outcomes?
	What specific intervention activities need implementation?
	Why consider these activities?

Decision-making in the OPT Model of Clinical Reasoning is the time to select interventions from a repertoire of actions that facilitate the achievement of the desired outcome state. Support for decision-making is aided with the use and application of schema searches and prototype identification from memory or resources. Comparative analysis is the process of considering the strengths and weaknesses of competing alternatives. If-then, how-so thinking also supports decision-making. Consideration for nursing interventions regarding treatment of the disease complications for patients is displayed in Table 6.2.

TABLE 6.2   INTERVENTIONS AND RATIONALES FOR INEFFECTIVE MANAGEMENT OF THERAPEUTIC REGIMEN*

Interventions	Rationales
Assess the patient's feelings, values, and reasons for not following the prescribed plan of care (e.g., monitoring blood sugar levels).	Assessment of individual's preferences for participation in decision-making will allow for enlisting involvement in decision-making at the preferred level (Florin, Ehrenberg, & Ehnfor, 2006).
Help the patient determine how to manage complex medication schedules.	Simplifying treatment regimens and tailoring them to individual lifestyles encourages adherence to treatment (Battaglioli-Denero, 2007).
Assess the patient's feelings, values, and reasons for not following the prescribed plan of care (e.g., dietary). Refer the patient to appropriate services as needed.	Assessment of individual's preferences for participation in decision-making will allow for enlisting involvement in decision-making at the preferred level (Florin et al., 2006). When appropriate referrals are missed, patients often experience poor outcomes, including complications, psychological distress, and hospital readmissions (Bowles, Foust, & Naylor, 2003).
Help the patient choose a healthy lifestyle and have appropriate diagnostic screening tests (e.g., complications of hypertension and monitoring strategies).	Healthy lifestyle measures, such as exercising regularly, maintaining a healthy weight, not smoking, and limiting alcohol intake, help reduce the risk of chronic illnesses (Holmes, 2006).

continues

TABLE 6.2   INTERVENTIONS AND RATIONALES FOR INEFFECTIVE MANAGEMENT OF THERAPEUTIC REGIMEN*   (CONTINUED)

Interventions	Rationales
Tailor both the information provided and the method of delivery of information to the specific patient and family (e.g., care of ulcers to prevent and treat infection).	Patient-centered educational interventions that support patient choice and self-management improve the quality of life, confidence in coping ability, and satisfaction, and they reduce the need for healthcare resources (Kennedy et al., 2004).
Tailor both the information provided and the method of delivery of information to the specific patient and family (e.g., signs and symptoms of infection and ulcer development, reporting them promptly).	Patient-centered educational interventions that support patient choice and self-management improve the quality of life, confidence in coping ability, and satisfaction, and they reduce the need for healthcare resources (Kennedy et al., 2004).

*Ackley, B., & Ladwig, G. (2014). *Nursing diagnosis handbook: An evidence-based guide to planning care.* St. Louis, MO: Mosby Elsevier.

JUDGMENTS

Making judgments is the process of drawing conclusions based on the findings from the test of comparing present state to a specified outcome state. Regarding judgments, there are three possible conclusions:

- A perfect match between outcome state and present state (e.g., fasting blood sugar is in acceptable range)

- A partial match of outcome state with present state (fasting blood sugar is lower than admission but not in acceptable range)

- No match between outcome and present state (fasting blood sugars are still out of range and high)

Judgments result from reflection and clinical decision-making about achieving a satisfactory match between the client's present state and the outcome state. Thinking strategies that support judgments include reflection checks, reframing the situation, and attributing a different meaning to the facts of the story. The prompts listed in Table 6.3 can be used to support judgments about interventions for patient-centered care planning.

TABLE 6.3 QUESTIONS THAT SUPPORT JUDGMENTS IN THE OPT MODEL OF CLINICAL REASONING

Judgments	1. What are the outcomes from the care management interventions for the essential needs of the patient?
	2. What is the meaning of the evidence collected from the testing of the gaps between the present and outcome states?
	3. What are the judgments of the successes or deficits from the plan of care?

During testing, the nurse determines how well the gap is closed. Nurses choose interventions to bring clients and families closer to the desired states based on present-state data. The thinking strategies of comparative analysis and reflexive comparison occur before and after testing instances and judgments. Judgments arise regarding the state of a situation after gauging the presence or absence of quality standards using the current case as a reference criterion (Fowler, 1994). Conclusions related to tests are the basis of clinical judgments. Research has shown that students improved in the use of goal-specific judgment statements over time ($p = .000$) (Kautz, Kuiper, Pesut, Knight-Brown, & Daneker, 2005).

A completed OPT Model of Clinical Reasoning (see Figure 6.1) uses the patient story, diagnostic cluster/cue logic, keystone priority, and present to outcome states to determine tests and scales and interventions for health and illness management that support the development and acquisition of clinical reasoning and judgment skills.

The steps to the creation of the interventions and judgments are as follows:

1. Carefully consider the gaps between the present and outcome states.

2. Select evidence-based interventions from a repertoire of actions that are necessary to bring the present state and outcome state closer together.

3. Use comparative analysis to consider the strengths and weaknesses of competing alternatives.

4. Make a decision if one or more interventions are appropriate for the situation.

5. Proceed with testing using comparative analysis and reflexive comparison to make a judgment about the state of the situation

6. Upon reflection, make conclusions or judgments about the efficacy of the interventions.

7. Based on results and outcomes of reflections, reframe the situation about the entire process, attributing new meanings to the gathered facts, if necessary.

8. Reflect on the plan and determine whether the tests are appropriate, the present and outcome states relate to the keystone issue, and the outcome state reflects on improvement from the present state.

9. Adjust or correct any part of the process to meet desired goals and outcomes for the health and well-being of the patient and family.

The example presented in Figure 6.1 shows the aspects of the OPT Model that are made explicit. The use of reflection, diagnostic cluster/cue logic, framing, and clinical decision-making will reveal a match and give judgment regarding the achievable outcome. The clinical reasoning used for completing the OPT Model Worksheet promotes critical, reflective, concurrent, creative, systems, and complexity thinking embedded in nursing practice that results in the juxtaposition of problems and outcomes that are subject to interventions and clinical judgments

(Kuiper, Pesut, & Arms, 2016; Pesut & Herman, 1999). The structure and process of the OPT Model promotes new ways to think about the role of interventions in achieving and making judgments about outcomes in complex patient care situations. Table 6.4 displays a side-by-side comparison of the outcome states, judgments, and rationales for the case depicted on the OPT Model Worksheet in Figure 6.1.

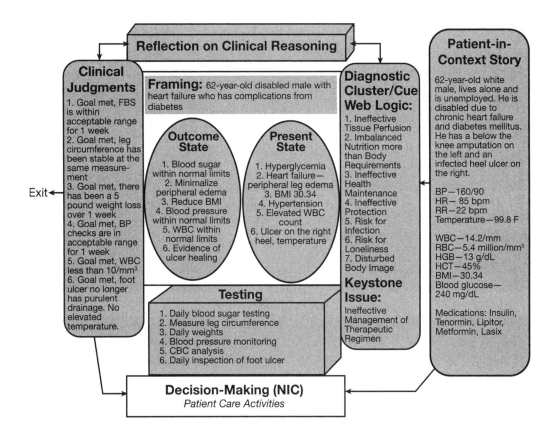

Reflection on Clinical Reasoning

Patient-in-Context Story

62-year-old white male, lives alone and is unemployed. He is disabled due to chronic heart failure and diabetes mellitus. He has a below the knee amputation on the left and an infected heel ulcer on the right.

BP—160/90
HR— 85 bpm
RR—22 bpm
Temperature—99.8 F

WBC—14.2/mm
RBC—5.4 million/mm³
HGB—13 g/dL
HCT—45%
BMI—30.34
Blood glucose—240 mg/dL

Medications: Insulin, Tenormin, Lipitor, Metformin, Lasix

Framing: 62-year-old disabled male with heart failure who has complications from diabetes

Outcome State
1. Blood sugar within normal limits
2. Minimalize peripheral edema
3. Reduce BMI
4. Blood pressure within normal limits
5. WBC within normal limits
6. Evidence of ulcer healing

Present State
1. Hyperglycemia
2. Heart failure—peripheral leg edema
3. BMI 30.34
4. Hypertension
5. Elevated WBC count
6. Ulcer on the right heel, temperature

Clinical Judgments
1. Goal met, FBS is within acceptable range for 1 week
2. Goal met, leg circumference has been stable at the same measurement
3. Goal met, there has been a 5 pound weight loss over 1 week
4. Goal met, BP checks are in acceptable range for 1 week
5. Goal met, WBC less than 10/mm³
6. Goal met, foot ulcer no longer has purulent drainage. No elevated temperature.

Diagnostic Cluster/Cue Web Logic:
1. Ineffective Tissue Perfusion
2. Imbalanced Nutrition more than Body Requirements
3. Ineffective Health Maintenance
4. Ineffective Protection
5. Risk for Infection
6. Risk for Loneliness
7. Disturbed Body Image

Keystone Issue:
Ineffective Management of Therapeutic Regimen

Testing
1. Daily blood sugar testing
2. Measure leg circumference
3. Daily weights
4. Blood pressure monitoring
5. CBC analysis
6. Daily inspection of foot ulcer

Exit

Decision-Making (NIC)
Patient Care Activities

©Pesut & Herman, 1999

Figure 6.1 OPT Model of Clinical Reasoning Worksheet (Judgments).

When all parts of the care planning are completed, and all the sections of the OPT Model Worksheet are filled in, the nurse can see the total picture of the patient care scenario. Table 6.5 displays the assessment domains, classes, patient cues/problems, NANDA-I nursing diagnoses, Nursing Outcomes Classifications (NOC), and Nursing Interventions Classifications (NIC) in a worksheet format that can be used to track and manage the care planning essentials for the specific case. This worksheet helps the nurse organize the information and the thinking during the evolution and development of the specific plan of care.

TABLE 6.4 TABLE OF OUTCOME STATES, JUDGMENTS, AND RATIONALES

Outcome State	Judgment	Rationale
Physiologic Health: Therapeutic Response. Blood sugar is within normal limits.	Fasting blood sugar is within the normal range for 1 week.	Patient is responding to diabetic education and is maintaining diet, medication regimen, and glucose monitoring.
Physiologic Health: Cardiopulmonary. Peripheral edema is minimized.	Leg circumference has been stable at the same measurement for 1 week.	While there remains some peripheral edema, the circumference of the leg has remained the same. This signifies adherence to the therapeutic regimen for diabetes and heart failure.
Physiologic Health: Metabolic Regulation. Body mass index (BMI) is reduced.	There has been a 5-pound weight loss over 1 week.	Patient has continued on the prescribed weight loss and diabetic diet for this care planning period. This is reflected in a weight reduction as calculated by his BMI.
Physiologic Health: Metabolic Regulation. Blood pressure is within normal limits.	Blood pressure checks are in acceptable range for 1 week.	The medical regimen for hypertension is being adhered to. In addition, the weight loss, infection, and blood sugar control have resulted in a decreased release of stress hormones that would be responsible for increasing the blood pressure.

Outcome State	Judgment	Rationale
Physiologic Health: Immune Response. White blood cell values are within normal limits.	White blood cells are less than 10/mm3.	The immune response has subsided, as the infection is being controlled and managed in this case.
Physiologic Health: Tissue Integrity. There is evidence of ulcer healing.	Foot ulcer no longer has purulent drainage. Temperature is not elevated.	There is improved tissue integrity as a result of the infection control. Signs of infection are abating.

Questions Frequently Asked About the Web

Students who have worked with the model often have questions about interventions, rationales, and judgments. The most frequently asked questions are posed and answered next.

1. **Interventions:**

   a. *Question:* Is more than one intervention required for each present state/outcome state?

   b. *Response:* The interventions are determined by the nurse in order to achieve the desired outcome state. The nurse or nursing instructor has the discretion to choose whether one or more interventions are chosen. In many of the case study examples provided in this book, more than one intervention has been offered.

2. **Rationales:**

   a. *Question:* Is it necessary to provide a rationale for each intervention listed?

   b. *Response:* Providing current evidenced-based rationales lends credence and strength to the chosen interventions, an aspect of nursing knowledge work that builds clinical expertise.

3. **Judgments:**

   a. *Question:* How does the nurse determine whether an outcome state-
       ment was achieved as described in judgments?

   b. *Response:* Judgment is the process of drawing conclusions based on the
       interventions (Butcher & Johnson, 2012). Based on the result of inter-
       ventions, the nurse must determine to what degree the patient's present
       state has changed. In doing so, the nurse relies on indicators, evidence,
       or tests for each outcome statement to make judgments. In turn, judg-
       ments result in reflection and conclusions as to the degree of match
       between the patient's present state and the outcome.

4. **Judgments:**

   a. *Question:* What if the patient does not achieve the desired outcome
       state?

   b. *Response:* Judgments result in reflection and clinical decision-making
       about achieving a satisfactory match between the patient's present state
       and the outcome state. Three conclusions are possible: 1) a perfect
       match between the outcome state and the present state, 2) a partial
       match of the outcome state with the present state, and 3) no match
       between the two states. If there was an unsatisfactory match, it may be
       that the nurse needs to reframe the keystone issue (Kuiper et al., 2016).
       This is a process of attributing a different meaning to the facts or evi-
       dence at hand. The entire process results in self-correction (Kuiper et
       al., 2016).

REFLECTION ON CLINICAL REASONING

The reflection box at the top of the worksheet is a reminder of the thinking strategies used for the patient situation. These strategies also make explicit many of the relationships among ideas and issues associated with the patient problems. When using the OPT Model of Clinical Reasoning Worksheets, the provider engages in reflection as a component of executive thinking processes that consist of critical, creative, and concurrent thinking. Reflection is the process of observing one's thinking while simultaneously thinking about patient situations. The goal of reflection is to achieve the best possible thought processes. The greater the reflection, the higher the quality of care delivered.

Reflection involves the use of the skills of monitoring, analyzing, predicting, planning, evaluating, and revising. Critical thinking consists of developing the following skills of interpretation: analysis, inference, explanation, evaluation, and self-regulation (Facione & Facione, 1996). These behaviors coincide with professional obligations, mandates, and responsibilities outlined by the ANA (2015) *Nursing: Scope and Standards of Practice* and the clinical reasoning mindset outlined in Chapter 4. Table 6.1 presents some reflection questions to use with the OPT Model of Clinical Reasoning when making decisions about nursing interventions and judgments regarding reaching desired outcomes.

As the nurse does concurrent and iterative as side-by-side comparisons of outcomes with present-state information from the patient story, gaps can be analyzed and evaluated as test conditions about judgments and conclusions given decisions and actions that fill the gaps. Table 6.6 presents the thinking strategies used by the nurse during this phase of the care planning process.

TABLE 6.5 ASSESSMENT DOMAINS, CLASSES (NANDA-I TAXONOMY II), PATIENT CUES/PROBLEMS, NURSING DIAGNOSES, NOC, AND NIC

Domain	Classes	Identified Patient Problems	NANDA-I Nursing Diagnoses	Nursing Outcomes Classifications (NOC)	Nursing Intervention Classifications (NIC)
Health Promotion: The awareness of well-being or normality of function and the strategies used to maintain control of and enhance well-being or normality of function	**Health Awareness:** Recognition of normal function and well-being				
	Health Management: Identifying, controlling, performing, and integrating activities to maintain health and well-being				
Nutrition: The activities of taking in, assimilating, and using nutrients for the purposes of tissue maintenance, tissue repair, and the production of energy	**Ingestion:** Taking food or nutrients into the body				
	Digestion: The physical and chemical activities that convert foodstuffs into substances suitable for absorption and assimilation				
	Absorption: The act of taking up nutrients through body tissues				

Domain	Classes	Identified Patient Problems	NANDA-I Nursing Diagnoses	Nursing Outcomes Classifications (NOC)	Nursing Intervention Classifications (NIC)
	Metabolism: The chemical and physical processes occurring in living organisms and cells for the development and use of protoplasm, the production of waste and energy, with the release of energy for all vital processes				
	Hydration: The taking in and absorption of fluids and electrolytes				
Elimination/Exchange: Secretion and excretion of waste products from the body	**Urinary Function:** The process of secretion, reabsorption, and excretion of urine				
	Gastrointestinal Function: The process of absorption and excretion of the end products of digestion				
	Integumentary Function: The process of secretion and excretion through the skin				
	Respiratory Function: The process of exchange of gases and removal of the end products of metabolism				
Activity/Rest: The production, conservation, expenditure, or balance of energy resources	**Sleep/Rest:** Slumber, repose, ease, relaxation, or inactivity				
	Activity/Exercise: Moving parts of the body (mobility), doing work, or performing actions often (but not always) against resistance				

continues

TABLE 6.5 ASSESSMENT DOMAINS, CLASSES (NANDA-I TAXONOMY II), PATIENT CUES/ PROBLEMS, NURSING DIAGNOSES, NOC, AND NIC   (CONTINUED)

Domain	Classes	Identified Patient Problems	NANDA-I Nursing Diagnoses	Nursing Outcomes Classifications (NOC)	Nursing Intervention Classifications (NIC)
	Energy Balance: A dynamic state of harmony between intake and expenditure of resources				
	Cardiovascular/Pulmonary Responses: Cardiopulmonary mechanisms that support activity/rest				
	Self-Care: Ability to perform activities to care for one's body and bodily functions				
Perception/Cognition: The human information-processing system including attention, orientation, sensation, perception, cognition, and communication	**Attention:** Mental readiness to notice or observe				
	Orientation: Awareness of time, place, and person				
	Sensation/Perception: Receiving information through the senses of touch, taste, smell, vision, hearing, and kinesthesia, and the comprehension of sensory data resulting in naming, associating, and/or pattern recognition				

continues

Domain	Classes	Identified Patient Problems	NANDA-I Nursing Diagnoses	Nursing Outcomes Classifications (NOC)	Nursing Intervention Classifications (NIC)
	Cognition: Use of memory, learning, thinking, problem-solving, abstraction, judgment, insight, intellectual capacity, calculation, and language				
	Communication: Sending and receiving verbal and nonverbal information				
Self-Perception: Awareness about the self	**Self-Concept:** The perception(s) about the total self				
	Self-Esteem: Assessment of one's own worth, capability, significance, and success				
	Body Image: A mental image of one's own body				
Role Relationship: The positive and negative connections or associations between people or groups of people and the means by which those connections are demonstrated	**Caregiving Roles:** Socially expected behavior patterns by people providing care who are not healthcare professionals				
	Family Relationships: Associations of people who are biologically related or related by choice				
	Role Performance: Quality of functioning in socially expected behavior patterns				

TABLE 6.5   ASSESSMENT DOMAINS, CLASSES (NANDA-I TAXONOMY II), PATIENT CUES/
PROBLEMS, NURSING DIAGNOSES, NOC, AND NIC   (CONTINUED)

Domain	Classes	Identified Patient Problems	NANDA-I Nursing Diagnoses	Nursing Outcomes Classifications (NOC)	Nursing Intervention Classifications (NIC)
Sexuality: Sexual identity, sexual function, and reproduction	**Sexual Identity:** The state of being a specific person in regard to sexuality and/or gender				
	Sexual Function: The capacity or ability to participate in sexual activities				
	Reproduction: Any process by which human beings are produced				
Coping/Stress Tolerance: Contending with life events/life processes	**Post-Trauma Responses:** Reactions occurring after physical or psychological trauma				
	Coping Responses: The process of managing environmental stress				
	Neuro-Behavioral Stress: Behavioral responses reflecting nerve and brain function				
Life Principles: Contending with life events/life processes	**Values:** The identification and ranking of preferred modes of conduct or end states				
	Beliefs: Opinions, expectations, or judgments about acts, customs, or institutions viewed as being true or having intrinsic worth				

Domain	Classes	Identified Patient Problems	NANDA-I Nursing Diagnoses	Nursing Outcomes Classifications (NOC)	Nursing Intervention Classifications (NIC)
	Value/Belief/Action Congruence: The correspondence or balance achieved among values, beliefs, and actions				
Safety/Protection: Principles underlying conduct, thought, and behavior about acts, customs, or institutions viewed as being true or having intrinsic worth	**Infection:** Host responses following pathogenic invasion				
	Physical Injury: Bodily harm or hurt				
	Violence: The exertion of excessive force or power so as to cause injury or abuse				
	Environmental Hazards: Sources of danger in the surroundings				
	Defensive Processes: The processes by which the self protects itself from the non-self				
	Thermoregulation: The physiological process of regulating heat and energy within the body for purposes of protecting the organism				
Comfort: Freedom from danger, physical injury, or immune system damage; preservation from loss; and protection of safety and security	**Physical Comfort:** Sense of well-being or ease and/or freedom from pain				

continues

TABLE 6.5 ASSESSMENT DOMAINS, CLASSES (NANDA-I TAXONOMY II), PATIENT CUES/ PROBLEMS, NURSING DIAGNOSES, NOC, AND NIC (CONTINUED)

Domain	Classes	Identified Patient Problems	NANDA-I Nursing Diagnoses	Nursing Outcomes Classifications (NOC)	Nursing Intervention Classifications (NIC)
	Environmental Comfort: Sense of well-being or ease in/with one's environment				
	Social Comfort: Sense of well-being or ease with one's social situation				
Growth/Development: Age-appropriate increases in physical dimensions, maturation of organ systems, and/or progression through the developmental milestones	**Growth:** Increases in physical dimensions or maturity of organ systems				

Butcher, H., Bulechek, G., Dochterman, J., & Wagner, C. M. (in press).;
Herdman, T. H., & Kamitsuru, S. (Eds.) (2014);
Moorhead, S., Johnson, M., Maas, M. O. & Swanson, E, (Eds.) (2013).

TABLE 6.6 THINKING STRATEGIES THAT SUPPORT THE OPT MODEL OF CLINICAL REASONING

Thinking Strategy	Definition	Expected Outcomes
Reflexive comparison	Use of the patient as their control for baseline and subsequent clinical observations	• Identification of similarities and differences between time series observations
Judgment	Conclusions are drawn from testing. Includes the 6 Cs: context, contrast, criterion, concurrent, consideration, and conclusion	• Statement about outcome achievement based on iterative concurrent reflections and judgments
Reframing	Consideration of different meanings regarding the context, facts, or change in the client's story based on filtering, framing, and post-judgment focus	• Reconsideration of clinical questions and reasoning related to diagnoses, interventions, and outcomes based on the new filter, frame, and focus
Reflection check	Self-observation, examination, and self-correction of thinking and reasoning based on testing and judgments	• Self-monitoring • Self-evaluation • Self-reinforcement • Self-correction of reasoning structures, process, and outcomes

Reflexive Comparison

Reflexive comparison is a strategy that involves constant comparison of the patient's state from one time of observation to another time of observation, on two occasions. For example, each time the blood sugar laboratory value is reviewed or the blood pressure is measured, the nurse compares a patient's progress from one observation to the next, so the patient serves as the standard regarding making progress toward the desired outcome state.

Reframing

Reframing is the strategy that attributes a different meaning to the content or context of a situation given a set of cues, tests, decisions, or judgments. Remember that clinical reasoning is reflective, concurrent, creative, critical, systems, and complexity thinking embedded in nursing practice that nurses use to frame, juxtapose, and test the match between a patient's present state and desired outcome state. It may be that one needs to reframe the keystone issue. The challenge now becomes how one assists a patient transition from one state to another. Another way to reframe the situation is to consider how, through care planning interventions, the patient and family can more effectively exercise self-care and manage the therapeutic regime. Reframing is the thinking strategy that enables one to attribute different meaning given the story and context and reflection on the situation.

Figure 6.2 shows how an OPT Model Worksheet is used to reframe the situation in this case and focus on the psychosocial issues that would directly affect the patient's psychological ability to manage self-care. The environment of living alone, a disturbed body image due to physical disabilities, and depression related to hypertensive medications will change the focus for testing and intervention.

Reflection Check

A reflection check involves reflecting and analyzing the patient-centered thinking using all the thinking strategies that support clinical reasoning. Reflection check is the process of intentionally using self-regulation strategies of monitoring, correcting, reinforcing, and evaluating one's thinking about a specific task or situation (Herman, Pesut, & Conard, 1994; Kuiper & Pesut, 2004; Pesut & Herman, 1992; Worrell, 1990). Research shows reflection promotes clinical reasoning development and skill (Kuiper, Pesut, & Kautz, 2009). A reflection check pinpoints efforts done correctly and identifies errors and provides an opportunity to understand how to correct them. For example, reframing this case changed the focus to psychosocial issues. The nurse might reflect whether the tests of evaluating companionship resources, monitoring attendance at counseling visits, weekly weights, and depression assessment were the best tests to use in this case. A reflection check involves understanding how the thinking skills and strategies described thus far support reflective clinical reasoning given the context in the patient story or framing. Table 6.7 can be used to support a reflection check about interventions for patient-centered care planning.

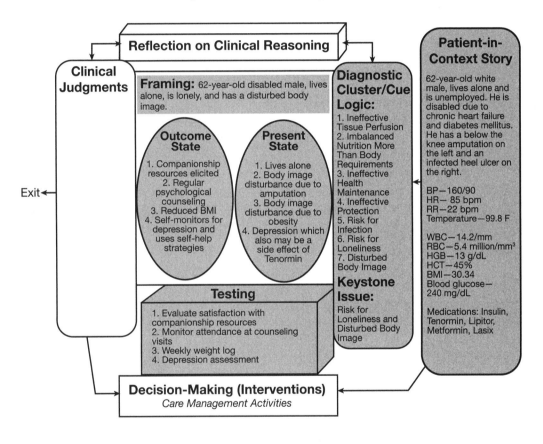

Reflection on Clinical Reasoning

Patient-in-Context Story

62-year-old white male, lives alone and is unemployed. He is disabled due to chronic heart failure and diabetes mellitus. He has a below the knee amputation on the left and an infected heel ulcer on the right.

BP—160/90
HR—85 bpm
RR—22 bpm
Temperature—99.8 F

WBC—14.2/mm
RBC—5.4 million/mm³
HGB—13 g/dL
HCT—45%
BMI—30.34
Blood glucose—240 mg/dL

Medications: Insulin, Tenormin, Lipitor, Metformin, Lasix

Clinical Judgments

Framing: 62-year-old disabled male, lives alone, is lonely, and has a disturbed body image.

Outcome State
1. Companionship resources elicited
2. Regular psychological counseling
3. Reduced BMI
4. Self-monitors for depression and uses self-help strategies

Present State
1. Lives alone
2. Body image disturbance due to amputation
3. Body image disturbance due to obesity
4. Depression which also may be a side effect of Tenormin

Diagnostic Cluster/Cue Logic:
1. Ineffective Tissue Perfusion
2. Imbalanced Nutrition More Than Body Requirements
3. Ineffective Health Maintenance
4. Ineffective Protection
5. Risk for Infection
6. Risk for Loneliness
7. Disturbed Body Image

Keystone Issue:
Risk for Loneliness and Disturbed Body Image

Testing
1. Evaluate satisfaction with companionship resources
2. Monitor attendance at counseling visits
3. Weekly weight log
4. Depression assessment

Exit

Decision-Making (Interventions)
Care Management Activities

©Pesut & Herman, 1999

Figure 6.2 OPT Model of Clinical Reasoning Worksheet (Reframing).

TABLE 6.7   QUESTIONS THAT SUPPORT A REFLECTION CHECK IN THE OPT MODEL OF CLINICAL REASONING

Reflection Check	1. Which clinical decision helps the patient transition from present state to outcome state?
	2. What abilities do I have to make clinical judgments for this situation?
	3. When I am considering the choices and decisions, what will I do if I need help?
	4. Is the environment conducive to making clinical judgments?
	5. What is my reaction to the clinical judgments made?
	6. What past experiences do I have that influenced my thinking in this situation?
	7. What were the consequences of the Reasoning Web for this situation?

Clinical Reasoning Outcomes

The strategies described in the previous sections and displayed in Table 6.6 come together during case analysis to help nurses make clinical decisions. Clinical decision-making involves the selection of interventions, actions, and issues that move patients from a presenting state to a specified or desired outcome state. In other words, what actions and interventions as coordinated by the nurse are necessary to bring the present state and outcome state closer together? Decision-making supports the use and application of schema searches and prototype identification. Comparative analysis is the process of considering the strengths and weaknesses of competing alternatives. If-then, how-so thinking also supports decision-making.

During testing, the nurse determines how well the gap is closed between the present and outcome states through the use and application of comparative analysis and reflexive comparison. Judgments are made about the situation after evaluating whether the present state is changed. Conclusions related to tests are the basis of clinical judgments.

Judgments are conclusions drawn based on the findings from the tests of comparing the present state to a specified outcome state, and the result of systems thinking. Once judgments of present state closely match the desired outcomes (e.g., healed ulcer), the nurse can reason about other things. If a match or test is unsatisfactory (e.g., infection still present), reflection activates critical, creative, concurrent thinking and decision-making. Regarding judgments, three conclusions are possible:

- A perfect match between outcome state and present state (e.g., healed ulcer)

- A partial match of outcome state with present state (ulcer healing is progressing but not complete)

- No match between outcome and present state (not healed and looks worse)

Judgments result in reflection and clinical decision-making about achieving a satisfactory match between the patient's present state and the outcome state. Thinking strategies that support judgment are reframing or the process of attributing a different meaning to the facts or evidence at hand. Finally, a reflection about the entire process results in self-correction.

Clinically, focusing on the present state or presenting problems does not provide explicit direction for action. Once outcomes are specified, the path of action is clear, and the tests of achievement are explicit. Transforming problems into outcomes involves thinking beyond the present to the end results of action. This process includes care management activities and reflection by the healthcare team to achieve success. One can appreciate how thinking strategies and critical thinking skills are embedded in reflective clinical reasoning. Table 6.8 compares some thinking strategies, critical thinking skills, and reflective clinical reasoning, which are used during the process of care planning for a patient and family.

TABLE 6.8 COMPARISON OF THINKING STRATEGIES, CRITICAL THINKING SKILLS, AND REFLECTIVE CLINICAL REASONING

Thinking Strategies	Critical Thinking Skills	Reflective Clinical Reasoning
Reading	Interpreting	Knowledge work
Memorizing	Categorizing	Clinical vocabulary
Drilling	Decoding sentences	Standardized terminologies
Writing	Clarifying meaning	
Reviewing		
Practicing		
Self-talk	Analyzing	Cue logic
Schema search	Examining ideas	Cue connection
Prototype identification	Identifying arguments	Induction
Hypothesizing	Analyzing arguments	Deduction
		Retroduction
Schema search	Making inferences	Framing
Prototype identification	Querying evidence	Cue connection
Hypothesizing	Conjecturing alternatives	Scenario development
If-then, how-so thinking	Drawing conclusions	Outcome specification
		Test creation
Schema search	Explaining	Decision-making
Prototype identification	Stating results	Interventions
Comparative analysis	Justifying procedures	Alternatives
If-then, how-so thinking	Presenting arguments	Consequences
Juxtaposing	Evaluating	Testing
Comparative analysis	Assessing claims	Conducting test
Reflexive comparison	Assessing arguments	Evaluating
Reframing	Self-regulation	Judgment
Reflection check	Self-examination	Attributing meaning to the test outcome
	Self-correction	Framing the new situation
		Creating a new test

Evidence suggests students who used the OPT Model and methods strengthened thinking skills and realized differences in how they thought about patient care problems (Kuiper et al., 2009). The structure and process of OPT guarantee that nursing care outcomes were well defined and promote new ways to think about the role of interventions in achieving and making judgments about outcomes in complex patient care situations. Also, strengthening clinical reasoning self-efficacy is the goal as the nurse practices the thinking skills and strategies in each subsequent clinical situation.

KEY POINTS

- The development of classification systems is important to standardize language about nursing diagnoses, interventions, and outcomes.

- NANDA-I diagnoses, NIC interventions, and NOC outcomes provide the clinical vocabulary for clinical reasoning in nursing. The OPT Model provides the structure and some of the cognitive processes for integrating these classification systems in the service of care.

- Knowing the knowledge contained in these systems makes clinical reasoning easier, more effective, and efficient. Knowledge stored or classified in these systems is the content for clinical reasoning.

- Analyzing and evaluating tests and interventions are key to making judgments about the plan of care using the OPT Model Worksheet.

- Reflection checks and reframing are significant steps in the clinical reasoning process to work with an iterative care planning process.

- Clinical schema and prototypes are developed with the OPT Model of Clinical Reasoning for the nurse in future care situations.

STUDY QUESTIONS AND ACTIVITIES

1. Describe in your own words the significance of standard nursing language and classification systems as they relate to effective and efficient clinical reasoning.

2. When you examine a keystone issue in a clinical scenario, create a list of all the different interventions that could emerge based on the needs of the patient and family.

3. Using an OPT Model Clinical Reasoning Worksheet, identify tests and interventions using a particular classification system for each nursing diagnosis in a completed Clinical Reasoning Web.

4. Describe how the keystone priority nursing diagnosis could change during the reframing process.

5. Complete a search for all possible interventions for a particular keystone issue that would influence present-state circumstances, and choose the most practical ones for a particular case.

6. Reflect on the thinking strategies you used with an OPT Model Worksheet and make judgments about the outcomes achieved and schema that was created. Could you use this schema again?

References

Ackley, B., & Ladwig, G. (2014). *Nursing diagnosis handbook: An evidence-based guide to planning care.* St. Louis, MO: Mosby Elsevier.

American Nurses Association (ANA). (2006). Recognized terminologies and data element sets. Retrieved from http://www.nursingworld.org/MainMenuCategories/Tools/Recognized-Nursing-Practice-Terminologies.pdf

American Nurses Association (ANA). (2015). *Nursing: Scope and standards of practice* (3rd ed.). Silver Spring, MD: ANA Publishing.

Association of Perioperative Registered Nurses (AORN). (n.d.). Perioperative nursing data set. Retrieved from www.aorn.org

Battaglioli-Denero, A. M. (2007). Strategies for improving patient adherence to therapy and long-term patient outcomes. *Journal of the Association of Nurses in AIDS Care, 18*(suppl 1), S17–S22.

Bowles, K. H., Foust, J. B., & Naylor, M. D. (2003). Hospital discharge referral decision making: A multidisciplinary perspective. *Applied Nursing Research, 16*(3), 134–143.

Butcher, H. K., Bulechek, G. M., Dochterman, J. M., & Wagner, C. M. (in press). *Nursing Interventions Classification (NIC)* (7th ed.). St. Louis, MO: Mosby Elsevier.

Butcher, H. K., Bulechek, G. M., Dochterman, J. M. M., & Wagner, C. (2013). *Nursing Interventions Classification (NIC)*. Philadelphia, PA: Elsevier Health Sciences.

Butcher, H., & Johnson, M. (2012). Use of linkages for clinical reasoning and quality improvement. In M. Johnson, S. Moorhead, G. Bulechek, H. Butcher, M. Maas, & E. Swanson (Eds.), *NOC and NIC linkages to NANDA-I and clinical conditions* (3rd ed.), pp. 11–23. Maryland Heights, MO: Elsevier.

Facione, N. C., & Facione, P. A. (1996). Externalizing the critical thinking in knowledge development and clinical judgment. *Nursing Outlook, 44*(3), 129–136.

Florin, J., Ehrenberg, A., & Ehnfor, M. (2006). Patient participation in clinical decision-making in nursing: A comparative study of nurses' and patients' perceptions. *Journal of Clinical Nursing, 15*(12), 1498–1508.

Fowler, L. (1994). *Clinical reasoning of home health nurses: A verbal protocol analysis* (Unpublished doctoral dissertation). University of South Carolina, College of Nursing, Columbia, SC.

Herdman, T. H., & Kamitsuru, S. (Eds.). (2014). *NANDA International nursing diagnoses: Definitions & classification, 2015–2017*. Oxford, England: Wiley Blackwell.

Herman, J., Pesut, D., & Conard, L. (1994). Using metacognitive skills: The quality audit tool. *Nursing Diagnosis, 5*(2), 56–64.

Holmes, S. (2006). Nutrition and the prevention of cancer. *Journal of Family Health Care, 16*(2), 43–46.

Kautz, D., Kuiper, R., Pesut, D., Knight-Brown, P., & Daneker, D. (2005). Promoting clinical reasoning in undergraduate nursing students: Application and evaluation of the Outcome-Present State-Test (OPT) Model of Clinical Reasoning. *International Journal of Nursing Education Scholarship, 2*(1), Article 1. Retrieved from http://www.bepress.com/ijnes/vol2/iss1/art1

Keenan, G. (1999). Use of standardized nursing language will make nursing visible. *Michigan Nurse, 72*(2), 12–13.

Kennedy, R. (2003). The nursing shortage and the role of technology. *Nursing Outlook, 51*(3), S33–S34.

Kennedy, A. P., Nelson, E., Reeves, D., Richardson, G., Roberts, C., Robinson, A., . . . Thompson, D. G. (2004). A randomised controlled trial to assess the effectiveness of cost of a patient orientated self-management approach to chronic inflammatory bowel disease. *Gut, 53*(11), 1639–1645.

Kuiper, R. A., & Pesut, D. J. (2004). Promoting cognitive and metacognitive reflective clinical reasoning skills in nursing practice: Self-regulated learning theory. *Journal of Advanced Nursing, 45*(4), 381–391.

Kuiper, R. A., Pesut, D., & Arms, T. (2016). *Clinical reasoning and care coordination in advanced practice nursing*. New York, NY: Springer Publishing.

Kuiper, R., Pesut, D., & Kautz, D. (2009). Promoting the self-regulation of clinical reasoning skills in nursing students. *The Open Nursing Journal, 3*, 76–85. Retrieved from http://www.ncbi.nlm.nih.gov/pmc/articles/PMC2771264/

Martin, K. S. (2005). *The Omaha System: A key to practice, documentation, and information management* (reprinted 2nd ed.). Omaha, NE: Health Connections Press.

Moorhead, S., Johnson, M., Maas, M. O., & Swanson, E. (Eds.). (2013). *Nursing Outcomes Classification (NOC): Measurement of health outcomes* (5th ed.). St. Louis, MO: Elsevier.

NANDA-I. (n.d.). *Nursing diagnoses: Definitions and classification*. (2016). Retrieved from http://www.nanda.org/

Omaha System. (2016). Retrieved from http://www.omahasystem.org/

Pesut, D. (1989). Aim versus blame: Using an outcome specification model. *Journal of Psychosocial Nursing and Mental Health Services, 27*(5), 26–30.

Pesut, D. J., & Herman, J. A. (1992). Reflection skills in diagnostic reasoning. *Nursing Diagnosis, 3*(4), 148–154.

Pesut, D., & Herman, J. (1999). *Clinical reasoning: The art and science of critical and creative thinking.* New York, NY: Delmar Publishers.

Robb, M. K. (2016). Self-regulated learning: Examining the baccalaureate millennial nursing student's approach. *Nursing Education Perspectives, 37*(3), 162–164.

Rutherford, M. (2008). Standardized nursing language: What does it mean for nursing practice? *OJIN: The Online Journal of Issues in Nursing, 13*(1). doi:10.3912/OJIN.Vol13No01PPT05

Worrell, P. (1990). Metacognition: Implications for instruction in nursing education. *Journal of Nursing Education, 29*(4), 170–175.

APPLICATIONS OF THE OPT MODEL OF CLINICAL REASONING ACROSS THE LIFE SPAN

7

CLINICAL REASONING AND NEONATAL HEALTH ISSUES

The authors would like to acknowledge Mrs. Patty White and Mrs. Nancy Murdock for their consultation on the material for this chapter.

LEARNING OUTCOMES

- Explain the components of the OPT Model of Clinical Reasoning that are essential to clinical reasoning to manage the problems, interventions, and outcomes of a newborn patient who has elevated levels of bilirubin and is jaundiced.

- Identify relevant nursing diagnoses specific to the health issues of the neonatal patient with hyperbilirubinemia.

- Identify outcomes appropriate for the health problems assessed in a neonatal scenario.

- Describe relevant tests and clinical judgments used to reason about present-state to outcome-state changes for an infant who has hyperbilirubinemia.

- Describe the different thinking processes that support clinical reasoning skills and strategies to determine priorities and desired outcomes for an infant with neonatal jaundice.

CASE STUDY: NEONATE WITH JAUNDICE

This chapter presents a case study involving a 37-week-old neonate with jaundice, a yellow discoloration of the skin and sclera. Neonatal jaundice is caused by deposition of a yellowish orange pigment from bilirubin in the skin and mucus membranes (Porter & Dennis, 2002). After birth, converting the unconjugated bilirubin into the water-soluble conjugated form becomes a function of the liver. When high levels of bilirubin have accumulated in the blood serum, a condition termed *neonatal hyperbilirubinemia* occurs (Blackburn, 2013; Porter & Dennis, 2002).

The high incidence of jaundice in newborns is the result of normal physiological processes or "physiological jaundice," and its occurrence is usually harmless (Clark, 2013). An explanation for jaundice includes an excess of red cells after birth are broken down, causing more bilirubin to be produced. However, due to immature functioning of the newborn's liver, the unconjugated bilirubin can build up in the blood, tissues, and body fluids, resulting in hyperbilirubinemia (Lantzy, 2016). Other contributing factors include infant prematurity, bruising resulting from the birthing process, delayed passage of meconium (the first stool), cephalohematoma (an accumulation of blood under the scalp), gestational diabetes, and delayed breastfeeding (Shortland & Hussey, 2008). Another type of jaundice is "pathological jaundice," which is caused by other disease factors (i.e., sepsis, hypothyroidism, immune and nonimmune hemolytic anemia, and a deficiency of G6PD, a condition in which red blood cells are damaged or destroyed) that are superimposed on physiological jaundice (Lantzy, 2016).

Most hyperbilirubinemia is benign. However, the most serious pathological consequence of hyperbilirubinemia is permanent neurological damage: athetosis (slow, writhing movements observed in the extremities), deafness, cerebral palsy, neurological developmental issues, and/or cognitive problems (American Academy of Pediatrics [AAP], 2004). *Kernicterus* is the term for the most devastating condition in which unconjugated bilirubin has passed through the blood brain barrier and has attached to neural membranes. The result is encephalopathy.

A bilirubin level is routinely conducted on newborns. Other tests may be recommended if the bilirubin level is elevated and these include: 1) a complete blood count (CBC); 2) the Coombs Test, which looks for antibodies present on red blood cells causing premature cell death; and 3) a reticulocyte (immature red blood cells) count to check for possible hemolytic anemia (MedlinePlus, 2016).

In this case study, one risk factor for developing neonatal jaundice is "breastfed jaundice," a term that suggests the infant is not receiving sufficient breast milk. Because there is a decrease in milk intake, low calorie intake, and possible dehydration, the circulation of bilirubin is increased. When the newborn does not receive enough breast milk, the meconium stool output is decreased and the reabsorption of bilirubin can result, thereby raising the levels of unconjugated bilirubin. Also, contributing to "breastfed jaundice" is infant lethargy resulting in a decreased likelihood of the newborn receiving nourishment, thereby repeating the cycle (Preer & Philipp, 2011).

Another contributing factor in this case study is ABO incompatibility resulting in red blood cell hemolysis. In this situation, the mother's blood type does not match that of the fetus, and the mother's immune system creates antibodies against the fetus's blood type (Shortland & Hussey, 2008). These antibodies are able to travel across the placenta to the fetus. After birth, some of the baby's red blood cells may be coated with the maternal antibodies that lead to destruction (hemolysis) of some of the red blood cells by the newborn's immune system. This condition is also referred to as "hemolytic disease of the newborn," and its earliest signs are high bilirubin levels and jaundice (MedlinePlus, 2015).

The mainstay of treatment is phototherapy, which involves the use of fluorescent white light (Lantzy, 2016). This treatment uses light to change the shape and structure of unconjugated bilirubin to convert it to molecules that can be excreted by the liver and kidney (Maisels & McDonagh, 2008). Two types of treatment used for severe hyperbilirubinemia are: 1) exchange transfusion, and 2) intravenous administration of immunoglobulin (IVIG). An exchange transfusion can rapidly remove bilirubin from circulation that occurs with immune-mediated hemolysis (the "hemolytic disease of the newborn"). The second treatment, IVIG, is used to help counteract the potential adverse effects of any antibodies acquired from the mother during gestation by infusing donor blood plasma with Immunoglobulin G (IgG). This process blocks the maternal antibodies circulating in the newborn's bloodstream from destroying the baby's red blood cells, thereby halting the progression of hemolytic anemia (Martin, Jerome, Epelbaum, Williams, & Walsh, 2008).

The chart "Bilirubin Levels and Risk of Significant Hyperbilirubinemia" illustrates the risk for significant hyperbilirubinemia in healthy-term and near-term, well newborns. The risks, based on age-specific total serum bilirubin levels, can be classified as high (above 95%), intermediate (40 to 95%), or low (below 40%) (Bhutani, Johnson, & Sivieri, 1999). For neonates born at 35 weeks gestation or later, phototherapy is an option when unconjugated bilirubin is greater than 12 mg/dL and may be indicated when unconjugated bilirubin is greater than 15 mg/dL at 25 to 48 hours, 18 mg/dL at 49 to 72 hours, and 20 mg/dL for a period at 72 hours or more (AAP, 2004; Porter & Dennis, 2002).

THE PATIENT STORY

Meet Jason Smith, a newborn Caucasian male who is currently 24 hours old. Jason was born at 37 weeks gestation to a 27-year-old gravida 4, para 4. His mother received routine prenatal care. Laboratory testing included blood type (O +), group B streptococcus screening, rubella immune antibodies, human immunodeficiency virus, Hepatitis B antibodies, and syphilis antibodies. All the laboratory test results were negative. Spontaneous rupture of membranes with clear fluid was followed by Pitocin® augmentation. Active labor lasted 8 hours with 20 minutes of pushing. Jason was delivered via vaginal delivery and had Apgar Scores of 8 at 1 minute and 9 at 5 minutes. Jason's birth weight was 3300 grams (7.26 pounds). He received Erythromycin ophthalmic ointment and Vitamin K injection mandated by institutional policy. The newborn physical exam and vital signs were within normal limits. After birth, he was swaddled and placed on his mother's chest for bonding and initiation of breastfeeding.

Physical Assessment

Vital signs at birth include temperature was 98.6° Fahrenheit, pulse was 152 beats per minute, respiratory rate was 48 breaths per minute (even and unlabored), and blood pressure was 64/48 mm Hg. Blood glucose levels remained stable with values of 50 to 65 mg/dL. The physical exam was unremarkable except for skin assessment, where he exhibited jaundice on his face, in his sclera, and on his chest. The elimination record shows one medium meconium stool since delivery and one urine void. The initial breastfeeding went very well after delivery. However, as time progressed since delivery, the neonate has required encouragement to feed. His mother is performing skin-to-skin stimulation and has attempted to breastfeed five times since delivery, with little success.

Psychosocial Assessment

Jason's mother has expressed her concern and appears anxious over the nature and cause of the jaundice. According to his mother, Jason's older siblings (ages 6, 4, and 2 years) were "never a problem" as far as feeding was concerned and did not have "skin turning yellow."

Treatment Plans

Jason was admitted to the Neonatal Intensive Care Unit (NICU) at 18 hours of age with a diagnosis of hemolytic jaundice due to ABO incompatibility. Intravenous fluids and intensive phototherapy were initiated. At 24 hours of age, with a bilirubin of 20 mg/dL, he received one dose of 500 mg/kg of intravenous Immunoglobulin G (IVIG). With continued aggressive fluid management to treat the hyperbilirubinemia, his bilirubin peaked at 22 mg/dL on day of life (DOL) 3. On day of life (DOL) 5, Jason's bilirubin was 8.9 mg/dL and phototherapy was discontinued, as the bilirubin levels continued to decline. Rebound bilirubin was 9.2 mg/dL at 24 hours after phototherapy was discontinued. The intravenous fluids were discontinued on DOL 5 as breastfeeding was well established and blood glucose levels were stable. Jason was discharged on DOL 7 with an appointment scheduled with his pediatrician at 48 hours after discharge.

PATIENT-CENTERED PLAN OF CARE USING THE OPT MODEL OF CLINICAL REASONING

The patient story in this case study has been obtained from all possible sources, including a physical examination, a current list of medications, and care conferences. The lists of patient problems and relevant nursing diagnoses support the creation of the Clinical Reasoning Web Worksheet that helps the nurse begin to filter the assessment data and information, frame the context of the story, and focus on the priority care needs and outcomes (Butcher & Johnson, 2012).

PATIENT PROBLEMS AND NURSING DIAGNOSES IDENTIFICATION

The first step of care planning is to identify the various problems and cues presented by the patient and select the nursing diagnoses whose defining characteristics capture these cues and problems. The medical diagnosis for this patient is hemolytic anemia with resulting hyperbilirubinemia, causing jaundice.

Nursing Care Priority Identification

The nurse identifies the cues and problems collected from the history, physiological, psychosocial assessment, and the medical record. Similar problems and cues are clustered for interpretation and meaning. Then relevant nursing diagnoses that "fit" the cluster of cues and problems are identified based on definitions and defining characteristics of each nursing diagnosis.

An assessment worksheet listing the major taxonomy domains, classes of each domain, patient cues and problems, relevant NANDA-I diagnoses with definitions (Herdman & Kamitsuru, 2014), Nursing Outcomes Classification (NOC) (Moorhead, Johnson, Maas, & Swanson, 2013), and Nursing Interventions Classification (NIC) (Butcher, Bulechek, Dochterman, & Wagner [in press]) labels has been created. This worksheet is designed to assist the nurse in organizing patient care issues and to generate appropriate nursing diagnoses. An example of a completed table of the taxonomy domains, classes, patient cues and problems, relevant nursing diagnoses, and suggested NOC and NIC labels for this case study is presented in Table 7.1.

STOP AND THINK

1. What taxonomy domains are affected, and which diagnoses have I generated?

2. Which cues/evidence/data from the patient and evidence from the patient assessment support the diagnoses?

TABLE 7.1 DOMAINS, CLASSES (NANDA-I TAXONOMY II), PATIENT CUES/PROBLEMS, NURSING DIAGNOSES, NOC AND NIC LABELS

Domain	Classes	Identified Patient Problems	NANDA-I Nursing Diagnoses	Nursing Outcomes Classifications (NOC)	Nursing Intervention Classifications (NIC)
Functional	Nutrition	• Inability of infant to sustain an effective suck • Lethargy of infant	**Ineffective Infant Feeding Pattern:** Impaired ability of an infant to suck or coordinate the suck/swallow response, resulting in inadequate oral nutrition for metabolic needs	• Breastfeeding Establishment • Swallowing Status: Oral Phase	• Breastfeeding Assistance • Lactation Counseling • Nonnutritive Sucking
Physiologic	Fluid and Electrolytes	• Breastfeeding pattern not well established • Minimal voids • Phototherapy with insensible water loss • Lethargy of infant	**Deficient Fluid Volume:** Decreased intravascular, interstitial, and/or intracellular fluid. This refers to dehydration, water loss alone without change in sodium.	Nutritional Status: Food & Fluid Intake	Fluid Monitoring Breastfeeding Assistance

continues

TABLE 7.1 DOMAINS, CLASSES (NANDA-I TAXONOMY II), PATIENT CUES/PROBLEMS, NURSING DIAGNOSES, NOC AND NIC LABELS (CONTINUED)

Domain	Classes	Identified Patient Problems	NANDA-I Nursing Diagnoses	Nursing Outcomes Classifications (NOC)	Nursing Intervention Classifications (NIC)
	Tissues Integrity	• Yellow skin and mucous membranes • Breastfeeding not established • ABO incompatibility • Dehydration • Bilirubin: 17.5 mg/dL • Hematocrit: 35.8% • Reticulocyte count: 19%	**Neonatal Jaundice:** The yellow orange tint of the neonate's skin and mucous membranes that occurs after 24 hours of life as a result of unconjugated bilirubin in the circulation	• Newborn Adaptation	• Phototherapy: Neonate • Newborn Monitoring
Psychosocial	Coping	• Mother is anxious over yellow skin and verbalizes that "my older children did not have this yellow skin" • Mother is anxious about neonate's lack of breastfeeding • Mother is anxious about the infant's admission to the Neonatal Intensive Care Unit	**Anxiety (parents):** Vague uneasy feeling of discomfort or dread accompanied by an autonomic response (the source often nonspecific or unknown to the individual); a feeling of apprehension caused by anticipation of danger. It is an alerting signal that warns of impending danger and enables the individual to take measures to deal with threat	• Coping	• Anxiety Reduction • Coping Enhancement

Domain	Classes	Identified Patient Problems	NANDA-I Nursing Diagnoses	Nursing Outcomes Classifications (NOC)	Nursing Intervention Classifications (NIC)
	Knowledge	• Mother indicates a lack of knowledge relating to hyperbilirubinemia • Mother expresses a lack of knowledge as to how to initiate a better feeding pattern with infant	**Deficient Knowledge:** Absence of deficiency of cognitive information related to a specific topic	• Client Satisfaction: Teaching • Knowledge: Breastfeeding	• Breastfeeding Assistance • Lactation Counseling • Teaching: Procedure/Treatment
		• Mother expresses desire to manage treatment after discharge: • When to call the physician • Possible preventative measures	**Readiness for Enhanced Health Management (Parents):** A pattern of regulating and integrating into daily living a therapeutic regimen for treatment of illness and its sequelae, which can be strengthened	• Knowledge: Treatment Regimen	• Health Education
Environmental	Risk Management	• Ineffective thermoregulation • Electrolyte imbalance • Elevated bilirubin • Intravenous fluids (invasive) • Blood glucose levels fluctuate	**Risk for Injury:** At risk of injury as a result of environmental conditions interacting with the individual's adaptive and defensive resources	• Risk Control • Risk Detection	• Nutritional Monitoring • Infection Control • Parent Education: Infant

continues

TABLE 7.1 DOMAINS, CLASSES (NANDA-I TAXONOMY II), PATIENT CUES/PROBLEMS, NURSING DIAGNOSES, NOC AND NIC LABELS   (CONTINUED)

Domain	Classes	Identified Patient Problems	NANDA-I Nursing Diagnoses	Nursing Outcomes Classifications (NOC)	Nursing Intervention Classifications (NIC)
		• Anticipated interruption of attachment process due to phototherapy • Parental anxiety related to admission to the Neonatal Intensive Care Unit and IV therapy	Risk for Impaired Parent Infant Attachment: Vulnerable to disruption of the interactive process between parent/significant other and child that fosters the development of a protective and nurturing reciprocal relationship	• Parent-Infant Attachment	• Attachment Promotion
		• ABO incompatibility • Ineffective breastfeeding • Elevated bilirubin level • Decreased hematocrit and elevated reticulocyte count	Risk for Complications of Hyperbilirubinemia: A newborn with or at high risk for development of an abnormally high concentration (give the age in hours of the infant) of the bile pigment bilirubin in the blood	• Restoration of Physiologic Stability	• Infant Monitoring

*Butcher, H., Bulechek, G., Dochterman, J., & Wagner, C. M. (in press).
Herdman, T. H., & Kamitsuru, S. (Eds.). (2014).
Moorhead, S., Johnson, M., Maas, M. O., & Swanson, E. (Eds.). (2013).

CREATING A CLINICAL REASONING WEB

The *Clinical Reasoning Web* is a means by which the nurse analyzes and reasons through complex patient stories for the purpose of finding and prioritizing key healthcare issues. Using the web, the nurse defines problems based on patient cues in the data, identifies nursing diagnoses to address and define the various problems, and determines relationships among these diagnoses (Kuiper, Pesut, & Kautz, 2009). The web is a visual representation and iterative analysis of the functional relationships among diagnostic hypotheses and results in a *keystone issue* that requires nursing care. In other words, the Clinical Reasoning Web represents a graphic illustration of how the elements of the patient's story and issues relate to one another and is depicted by sketching lines of association among the nursing diagnoses (Kuiper, Pesut, & Arms, 2016). Whereas medical diagnoses are consistent labels for a cluster of symptoms, patient stories vary, and each Clinical Reasoning Web is written to reflect the patient's unique story and the human response to actual or potential health problems best represented in nursing diagnoses. For example, given two patients with identical medical diagnoses, the nurse might determine that different nursing diagnoses and keystone issues are the priority for each based on thinking strategies and diagnostic hypotheses associated with each case.

Constructing the Clinical Reasoning Web

After the problems are identified from the assessment data, evidence, and cues and the nursing diagnoses are chosen, the Clinical Reasoning Web is constructed using the following steps.

1. Place a general description of the patient in the central oval with the primary medical diagnoses. In this case study it is a 24-hour-old newborn with hemolytic anemia, hyperbilirubinemia, and jaundice. He has recently undergone treatment to decrease the bilirubin level and to increase the amount of intake during breastfeeding.

2. Place each NANDA-I nursing diagnosis generated from the patient cues in the ovals surrounding the middle circle.

3. Under each nursing diagnosis, list supporting data that was gathered from the patient's story and assessment.

4. Because each nursing diagnosis is directly related to the center oval containing a brief description of the patient's situation, the nurse draws a line from the central oval to each of the outlying nursing diagnosis ovals. Figure 7.1 displays the beginning steps of constructing the Clinical Reasoning Web for this case study.

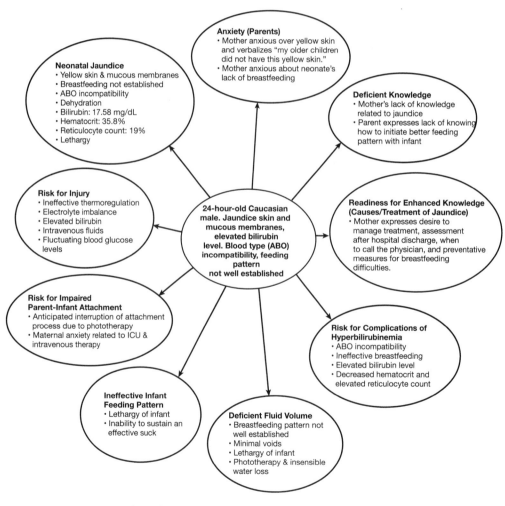

Figure 7.1   Clinical Reasoning Web: Neonatal Jaundice: Connections from Medical Diagnosis to Nursing Diagnoses.

Spinning and Weaving the Reasoning Web

In spinning and weaving the Clinical Reasoning Web, the nurse must relate, analyze, and explain the relationships between and among the nursing diagnoses. This process involves thinking out loud, using self-talk, using schema search, hypothesizing, if-then, how-so thinking, and using comparative analysis, as described in Chapter 3 of this book. In doing so, the nurse determines possible connections and relationships among the nursing diagnoses contained in the outlying ovals.

The nurse continues to spin and weave using the following steps:

1. Consider how each of the nursing diagnoses and the healthcare issues it defines relates to all the other diagnoses. If there is a functional relationship between two diagnoses, then a line with a one-directional arrow is drawn to indicate a one-way connection; a line with two-directional arrows is drawn to indicate a two-way connection. For example, what is the relationship between Neonatal Jaundice and Anxiety (on the part of the parents)? How are these two diagnoses related? How do they influence one another? In the case of Jason Smith, the nurse would consider whether Neonatal Jaundice would cause Anxiety with the parents, or in a reciprocal fashion, whether feeling anxious would cause Neonatal Jaundice. In this case, there is only a one-way connection leading from Neonatal Jaundice to Anxiety and not the reverse. Another example would be to consider how the nursing diagnosis Readiness for Enhanced Knowledge (parents) relates to the issue of Risk for Complications of Hyperbilirubinemia. In this case, there
is no relationship. Therefore, no connection is made between these two diagnoses.

2. The first step is iterative, recursive, and repeated with each of the other ovals to determine relationships for connections. If there are functional relationships, connections are drawn until the process is exhausted; visually, the web emerges.

3. When all connections are made, the lines leading to and from each oval with nursing diagnoses are counted and recorded. The numbers can be recorded on the Clinical Reasoning Web Worksheet. A table showing the hierarchy of priorities of Jason Smith's problems based on the number of connections is displayed in Table 7.2.

4. The nursing diagnosis with the most connecting lines radiating to and from that oval becomes the *keystone* issue. Figure 7.2 displays a completed Clinical Reasoning Web for this case.

TABLE 7.2   NURSING DOMAINS, NURSING DIAGNOSES, AND CONNECTIONS

Nursing Domain	Class	Nursing Diagnoses	Web Connections
Physiological	Tissue Integrity	Neonatal Jaundice	9
Psychosocial	Knowledge	Deficient Knowledge	7
Environmental	Risk Management	Risk for Complications of Hyperbilirubinemia	5
Functional	Nutrition	Ineffective Infant Feeding Pattern	4
Psychosocial	Coping	Anxiety (Parents)	4
	Knowledge	Readiness for Enhanced Knowledge (Parents)	3
Environmental	Risk Management	Risk for Injury	3
Physiological	Fluids and Electro-lytes	Deficient Fluid Volume	2
Environmental	Risk Management	Risk for Impaired Parent Infant Attachment	2

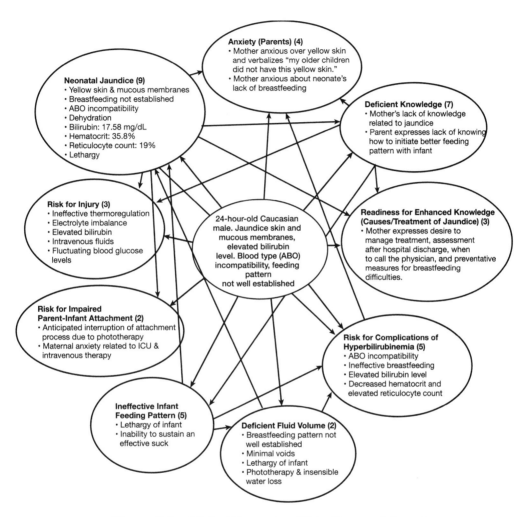

Figure 7.2   Clinical Reasoning Web: Neonatal Jaundice:
Connections Among Nursing Diagnoses.

The keystone issue, the nursing diagnosis with the most connections, emerges as a priority problem. It is the basis for defining the patient's present state, and this in turn is contrasted with a desired outcome state (Kuiper et al., 2009). Identifying the keystone issue guides clinical reasoning by identifying the central NANDA-I diagnosis that needs to be addressed first and enables the nurse to focus on subsequent care planning (Butcher & Johnson, 2012). After a keystone issue is identified, knowledge work continues to identify the complementary nature of the problems ~ outcomes using the juxtaposing thinking strategy. The keystone issue in this case is Neonatal Jaundice.

Interventions are chosen to assist baby Jason with resolving his elevated levels of bilirubin and neonatal jaundice. In doing so, these interventions are likely to influence other issues that are identified on the web.

STOP AND THINK

1. What are the relationships between and among the identified problems (diagnoses)?

2. What keystone issue(s) emerge?

COMPLETING THE OPT MODEL OF CLINICAL REASONING WORKSHEET

After the Reasoning Web has been completed with identification of the keystone and cue logic, the OPT Model of Clinical Reasoning can be completed. All sections of the OPT Model are completed with the case study described in this chapter.

Patient-in-Context Story

Exhibit 7.1 displays the patient-in-context story for the newborn Jason Smith. On the far right side of the OPT Model in Figure 7.3, the patient-in-context story is recorded. This story underscores the patient demographics, medical diagnoses, and current situation. The information placed in this box is presented in a brief format with some relevant facts that support the rest of the model.

EXHIBIT 7.1

Patient-in-Context Story

Jason Smith, a 24-hour-old Caucasian male baby born at 37 weeks gestation to a 27-year-old gravida 4, para 4 mother. Routine prenatal care and laboratory tests all negative. Labor uneventful with spontaneous rupture of membranes and clear fluid, Pitocin® augmentation. Active labor lasted 8 hours with 20 minutes of pushing. Vaginal delivery, Apgar Scores 8 at 1 minute and 9 at 5 minutes. Birth weight 3300 grams (7.26 lb). Newborn physical exam within normal limits. Infant swaddled and placed on mother's chest for bonding initiation of breastfeeding.

Physical Exam: Vital Signs: Temperature - 98.6° F, pulse - 152 beats per minute, respiratory rate - 48 breaths per minute (even and unlabored), blood pressure - 64/48 mmHg. Blood glucose: levels remained stable at 50–65 mg/dL. Skin: skin assessment, jaundice noted on face, sclera, and chest. Elimination: one medium meconium stool since delivery and one urine void.

Feeding: Initial breastfeeding normal but neonate needed encouragement to feed over time. Mother attempted breastfeeding five times since delivery.

Psychosocial: Mother is concerned and anxious about baby jaundice color. The older siblings (ages 6, 4, and 2 years) were "never a problem" as far as feeding or "skin turning yellow."

Labs at 24 hours of life: hematocrit - 35.8%, reticulocytes - 19%, bilirubin (initial) - 175 mg/dL (high risk).

Diagnostic Cluster/Cue Logic

The next step in the care planning process is completing the *diagnostic cluster/cue logic*. The keystone issue is placed at the bottom of the column with all the other identified nursing diagnoses and listed above it in priority order. At this point, the nurse reflects on this list to ask if there is evidence to support these nursing diagnoses and whether the keystone issue is correctly identified. Diagnostic cluster/cue logic is the deliberate structuring of patient-in-context data to discern the meaning for nursing care (Butcher & Johnson, 2012). In this case study, the nursing diagnoses depicted in the outlying ovals on the Reasoning Web are recorded under diagnostic cluster/cue logic on the OPT Model Clinical Reasoning Worksheet along with the number of arrows radiating to and from each diagnosis. Exhibit 7.2 displays the identified keystone issue, in this case as Neonatal Jaundice, and it is listed directly below the other nursing diagnoses.

EXHIBIT 7.2

Diagnostic Cluster/Cue Logic

1. Deficient Knowledge (7)

2. Risks for Complications of Hyperbilirubinemia (5)

3. Ineffective Infant Feeding Pattern (5)

4. Anxiety (parents) (4)

5. Risk for Injury (4)

6. Readiness for Enhanced Knowledge (3)

7. Risk for Injury (3)

8. Deficient Fluid Volume (3)

9. Risk for Impaired Parent-Infant Attachment (2)

Keystone Issue/Theme
Neonatal Jaundice (9)

EXHIBIT 7.3

Frame

A 24-hour-old Caucasian male with jaundice of skin and mucous membranes, and an elevated bilirubin level. There is blood type (ABO) incompatibility, and the feeding pattern has not been well established. The mother is anxious over infant's lack of feeding and the upcoming treatment for hyperbilirubinemia.

Framing

In the center and top of the worksheet is a box to indicate the *frame* or theme that best represents the background issue(s) regarding the patient-in-context story. The frame of this case is a 24-hour-old Caucasian male with jaundice of skin and mucous membranes and an elevated bilirubin level. There is blood type (ABO) incompatibility, and the feeding pattern has not been well established. Jason's mother is anxious over the infant's lack of feeding and the upcoming treatment for hyperbilirubinemia. This frame helps to organize the present state and outcome state and to illustrate the gaps between them to provide insights about essential care needs. The frame is the lens or background view to help the nurse differentiate this patient schema and prototype from others the nurse may have dealt with in the past. The interventions and tests that will be used in this care plan are specific to the frame that is identified. Exhibit 7.3 displays the frame in the case of the newborn Jason Smith.

Present State

The *present state* is a description of the patient-in-context story or the initial condition of the patient (Butcher & Johnson, 2012). The items listed in this section change over time as a result of nursing actions and the patient's situation. The cues and problems identified for the patient listed under the keystone capture the present state of the patient. These are the problems in which the care of the patient will be planned, implemented, and evaluated. The present-state items are listed in the oval of the identified keystone and, in this case, there are five primary issues related to the keystone issue: 1) bilirubin level of 17.5 mg/dL; 2) maternal anxiety regarding ineffective breastfeeding; 3) neonatal weight loss since birth (231 grams or 0.5 lb); 4) dehydration; and 5) maternal anxiety over upcoming treatments (phototherapy and infusion of Immunoglobin G). Exhibit 7.4 displays the list of present-state issues related to the keystone issue that will be subjected to tests to determine whether the identified outcomes are achieved.

Outcome State

Given a defined present state, consideration must be given to desired outcomes that will be achieved to resolve the keystone issue. In other words, one *outcome state* or goal is listed for each present-state item, and each can be tested and achieved through nursing and collaborative interventions. In this case study, the outcome states with NOC labels (in bold) aim to assist the newborn Jason Smith and his mother in the following ways: 1) Jason will receive appropriate therapy to enhance indirect biliriubin excretion; 2) his mother will manifest positive self-esteem in relation to the infant feeding process; 3) Jason will not experience further weight loss while hospitalized; 4) Jason will maintain hydration as evidenced by moist buccal membranes, four to six wet diapers in a 24-hour period, and weight loss not greater than 10% of his birth weight; and 5) both parents will receive information on neonatal jaundice prior to the infant's discharge. Exhibit 7.5 displays the outcome states for this case study.

EXHIBIT 7.4

Present State

Bilirubin: 17.5 mg/dL

Maternal anxiety regarding ineffective breastfeeding

Neonatal weight loss since birth (231 grams or 0.5 lb)

Dehydration

Maternal anxiety over upcoming treatments: phototherapy and infusion of Immunoglobin G

EXHIBIT 7.5

Outcome State

Newborn Adaptation: Appropriate therapy to enhance indirect bilirubin excretion.

Anxiety Level: Mother will manifest positive self-esteem in relation to the infant feeding process.

Breastfeeding Maintenance: No further infant weight loss while hospitalized.

Fluid Balance: Infant will maintain hydration (moist buccal membranes, four to six wet diapers in 24 hours, and weight loss no greater than 10% birth weight).

Patient Satisfaction: Parents will receive information on neonatal jaundice prior to discharge.

Because each present state and its corresponding outcome state directly relate to each other, they are placed next to each other for juxtaposition. This placement will assist the nurse with comparative analysis and reflection while the nurse exercises clinical reasoning in this care situation.

Tests

The differences or gaps between the present state and outcome state become the foci of concern in the next step of care planning. The nurse must consider what tests and related interventions are most appropriate to fill the gap between the present state and the desired outcomes. Based on these clinical decisions, the nurse considers evidence that may indicate whether the gaps have been filled. In collaboration with other healthcare providers and the patient, tests are conducted to measure changes and gather data. The nurse asks what and if clinical indicators are available for each desired outcome state—that is, what to consider as to whether the desired outcome is achieved. The tests chosen in this case include 1) the bilirubin, hematocrit, and reticulocyte assessments; 2) verbalization of relaxed feelings during feedings; 3) daily weights; 4) wet diaper count, skin and mucous membrane assessment for dryness, daily weights; and 5) parental expression of satisfaction with planned treatment. The tests for newborn Jason are displayed in Exhibit 7.6.

EXHIBIT 7.6

Tests

Bilirubin level, hematocrit, and reticulocyte assessments

Verbalization of relaxed feelings during feedings

Daily weights

Wet diaper count; skin and mucous membrane assessment for dryness; daily weights

Parental expression of satisfaction with planned treatment

STOP AND THINK

1. Is the patient-in-context story complete?

2. How am I framing the situation?

3. How is the present state defined?

4. What is/are the desired outcomes?

5. What outcomes do I have in mind given the diagnoses?

6. What is/are the gaps or complementary pairs (~) of outcomes and present states?

7. What are the clinical indicators of the desired outcomes?

8. On what scales or *tests* will the desired outcome be measured?

9. How will I know when the desired targeted outcomes are achieved?

Interventions

At the bottom of the OPT Model of Clinical Reasoning Worksheet, there is a box that indicates *Patient Care Interventions* (NIC), which are the evidence-based nursing care activities that will assist the patient to reach the outcome states. The nurse must make clinical decisions or choices about interventions that will help the patient transition from present state to the desired outcome state. As interventions are implemented, the nurse evaluates the degree to which outcomes are being achieved or not. Interventions are evidence-based and gathered from current resources such as the literature, recognized textbooks, and prototype examples. Rationales are listed and cited in a separate page column next to interventions. Listing the rationales for each intervention enhances understanding and justification for nursing activities. The interventions and the rationales for this case study are listed in Table 7.3 and include the measures of noninvasive pain relief methods and assessment, encouraging verbalization of feelings and reflection on life achievements, and facilitating resources to support spiritual care.

TABLE 7.3　INTERVENTIONS AND RATIONALES

Interventions	Rationales
1. a. **Collaborative:** When phototherapy is ordered, place seminude infant (diaper only) under prescribed amount of phototherapy (Ackley & Ladwig, 2017, p. 552). b. **Collaborative:** Collect and evaluate laboratory blood specimens (total serum bilirubin) while infant is undergoing phototherapy (Ackley & Ladwig, 2017, p. 552). 2. a. Provide time for clients to express expectations and concerns, and provide emotional support as needed (Ackley & Ladwig, 2017, p. 174). b. Explain myths and misconceptions (Carpenito, 2016). 3. Recommended techniques to promote bonding and infant nourishment: a. Increase skin-to-skin contact (kangaroo care). Provide practice times at breast for infant to "lick and learn." b. Express small amounts of milk into baby's mouth. c. Have mother pump breast after feeding to enhance milk production breastfeeding (Doenges, Moorhouse, & Murr, 2016, p. 106). 4. Monitor the infant for signs of deficient fluid volume, including sunken eyes, decreased tears, dry mucous membranes, poor skin turgor, and decreased urine output (Ackley & Ladwig, 2017, p. 390). 5. Teach parents about the use of in-patient phototherapy as prescribed, feedings, and assessment of hydration, body temperature, skin status, and urine and stool output (Ackley & Ladwig, 2017, p. 553).	1. a. Phototherapy is the primary therapy to treat mild to moderate neonatal indirect (unconjugated) hyperbilirubinemia; phototherapy enhances indirect bilirubin excretion (Blackburn, 2013; Stokowski, 2011, as cited in Ackley & Ladwig, 2017, p. 552). b. Transcutaneous bilirubin measurements do not provide an adequate estimate of serum bilirubin level and are not effective once phototherapy has been initiated (American Academy of Pediatrics, 2004, as cited in Ackley & Ladwig, 2017, p. 552). 2. Listening to the mother's and the partner's concerns can help prioritize them (Carpenito, 2016). 3. These measures promote optimal interaction between mother and infant and provide adequate nourishment for the infant, enhancing successful breastfeeding (Doenges, Moorhouse, & Murr, 2016, p. 106). 4. These assessment factors are more significant in identifying dehydration, a combination of physical examination findings is a better predictor than individual signs (Falszewska et al., 2014, as cited in Ackley & Ladwig, 2017, p. 390). 5. Information is provided to the parents of the infant undergoing phototherapy to prevent misinformation about the infant's condition and treatment and to decrease parental anxiety and stress (Hockenberry & Wilson, 2015).

STOP AND THINK

1. What clinical decisions or interventions help to achieve the outcomes?

2. What specific intervention activities will I implement?

3. Why am I considering these activities?

Judgments

The final step in constructing the OPT Model Worksheet is to reflect on the tests and interventions to determine whether the outcomes were achieved. The consequences of the tests are data one uses to make clinical judgments (Pesut, 2008). In the far-left column on the OPT Model of Clinical Reasoning Worksheet, judgments are listed for each outcome. *Judgments* are conclusions about outcome achievements. Each judgment requires four elements: 1) a contrast between present and desired state; 2) criteria associated with a desired outcome (i.e., a test); 3) consideration of the effects and influence of nurse interventions; and 4) a conclusion as to whether the intervention has been effective in the outcome achievement (Kuiper et al., 2009). Based on the analysis of tests, judgments are made as to whether the problem has been resolved. The nurse may have to reframe or attribute a different meaning to the facts in the patient-in-context story. Table 7.4 depicts the outcome states and judgments for this case study. A third column has been added within the table to provide the clinical reasoning used to guide each judgment statement. Exhibit 7.7 displays the judgments in this case.

EXHIBIT 7.7

Judgments

1. Bilirubin count decreased from 17.5 mg/dL to 9.2 mg/dL on day #5. Reticulocyte count 10%, hematocrit 37%.

2. Mother reports greater confidence in establishing satisfying, effective breastfeeding; verbalizes relaxed feelings during breastfeeding.

3. No further weight loss.

4. Increase in wet diapers (8 in past 24 hours), a weight gain of 2 oz. over past 3 days; no signs of dehydration.

5. Parents received information on the phototherapy, its impact on reducing the bilirubin levels. Parents instructed to have follow-up visit with the pediatrician.

STOP AND THINK

1. Given the tests that have been chosen, what is my clinical judgment of the evidence regarding reaching the outcome state?

2. Based on my judgment, have I achieved the outcome or do I need to reframe the situation?

3. How can I specifically take this experience and its lessons with me into the future as schema to reason about similar cases?

TABLE 7.4   TABLE OF OUTCOME STATES, JUDGMENTS, AND RATIONALES

Outcome State	Judgment	Notes
1. Newborn Adaptation: Infant will receive appropriate therapy to enhance indirect bilirubin excretion.	Bilirubin count has decreased from 17.5 mg/dL to 9.2 mg/dL on day 5 and after phototherapy sessions. Reticulocyte and hematocrit levels are also approaching normal levels, 10% and 37%, respectively, following phototherapy and the administration of intravenous fluids.	Day 5 has resulted in decreases in bilirubin level, but increases seen in reticulocyte and hematocrit levels. Breastfeeding has been established and intravenous fluids have been discontinued.
2. Anxiety Level: Mother will manifest positive self-esteem in relation to the infant feeding process.	Mother reports feeling greater confidence in establishing satisfying, effective breastfeeding. Verbalization of relaxed feelings during feedings.	Mother is able to have both breasts emptied at each breastfeeding session.
3. Breastfeeding Maintenance: Infant will not experience further weight loss while hospitalized.	No further weight loss has occurred.	Breastfeeding has been established, resulting in no additional weight loss and an increase in wet diapers.

4. **Fluid Balance:** Infant will maintain hydration (moist buccal membranes, four to six wet diapers in 24 hours, and weight loss no greater than 10% of birth weight) within 5 days of delivery.

Infant shows signs of adequate intake: increase in wet diapers to eight within the past 24 hours, weight gain of 2 oz. over the past 3 days, no signs of dehydration.

Blood glucose levels are stable. Infant is breastfeeding every 2–3 hours and mother is pleased with infant's progress. Intravenous fluids have been discontinued.

5. **Client Satisfaction:** Parents will receive information on neonatal jaundice prior to discharge.

Both mother and father have received information on the goal of phototherapy and its impact on reducing the levels of bilirubin. Parents have been provided information on having their infant seen by the pediatrician for a follow-up physical assessment and the importance of continuation of breastfeeding.

Parents were also provided information as to when to call the physician if infection and/or other complications arise.

Community lactation support information was also provided to ensure adequacy of intake of breast milk.

The Completed OPT Model of Clinical Reasoning

A completed OPT Model of Clinical Reasoning for a neonatal jaundice patient is displayed in Figure 7.3.

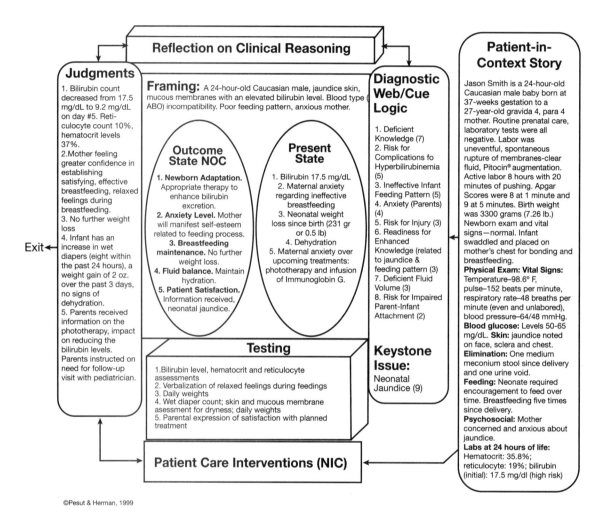

Reflection on Clinical Reasoning

Patient-in-Context Story

Jason Smith is a 24-hour-old Caucasian male baby born at 37-weeks gestation to a 27-year-old gravida 4, para 4 mother. Routine prenatal care, laboratory tests were all negative. Labor was uneventful, spontaneous rupture of membranes-clear fluid, Pitocin® augmentation. Active labor 8 hours with 20 minutes of pushing. Apgar Scores were 8 at 1 minute and 9 at 5 minutes. Birth weight was 3300 grams (7.26 lb.) Newborn exam and vital signs—normal. Infant swaddled and placed on mother's chest for bonding and breastfeeding.
Physical Exam: Vital Signs: Temperature–98.6° F, pulse–152 beats per minute, respiratory rate–48 breaths per minute (even and unlabored), blood pressure–64/48 mmHg.
Blood glucose: Levels 50-65 mg/dL.
Skin: jaundice noted on face, sclera and chest.
Elimination: One medium meconium stool since delivery and one urine void.
Feeding: Neonate required encouragement to feed over time. Breastfeeding five times since delivery.
Psychosocial: Mother concerned and anxious about jaundice.
Labs at 24 hours of life: Hematocrit: 35.8%; reticulocyte: 19%; bilirubin (initial): 17.5 mg/dl (high risk)

Judgments
1. Bilirubin count decreased from 17.5 mg/dL to 9.2 mg/dL on day #5. Reticulocyte count 10%, hematocrit levels 37%.
2. Mother feeling greater confidence in establishing satisfying, effective breastfeeding, relaxed feelings during breastfeeding.
3. No further weight loss
4. Infant has an increase in wet diapers (eight within the past 24 hours), a weight gain of 2 oz. over the past 3 days, no signs of dehydration.
5. Parents received information on the phototherapy, impact on reducing the bilirubin levels. Parents instructed on need for follow-up visit with pediatrician.

Exit ←

Framing: A 24-hour-old Caucasian male, jaundice skin, mucous membranes with an elevated bilirubin level. Blood type (ABO) incompatibility. Poor feeding pattern, anxious mother.

Outcome State NOC
1. **Newborn Adaptation.** Appropriate therapy to enhance bilirubin excretion.
2. **Anxiety Level.** Mother will manifest self-esteem related to feeding process.
3. **Breastfeeding maintenance.** No further weight loss.
4. **Fluid balance.** Maintain hydration.
5. **Patient Satisfaction.** Information received, neonatal jaundice.

Present State
1. Bilirubin 17.5 mg/dL
2. Maternal anxiety regarding ineffective breastfeeding
3. Neonatal weight loss since birth (231 gr or 0.5 lb)
4. Dehydration
5. Maternal anxiety over upcoming treatments: phototherapy and infusion of Immunoglobin G.

Diagnostic Web/Cue Logic
1. Deficient Knowledge (7)
2. Risk for Complications fo Hyperbilirubinemia (5)
3. Ineffective Infant Feeding Pattern (5)
4. Anxiety (Parents) (4)
5. Risk for Injury (3)
6. Readiness for Enhanced Knowledge (related to jaundice & feeding pattern (3)
7. Deficient Fluid Volume (3)
8. Risk for Impaired Parent-Infant Attachment (2)

Testing
1. Bilirubin level, hematocrit and reticulocyte assessments
2. Verbalization of relaxed feelings during feedings
3. Daily weights
4. Wet diaper count; skin and mucous membrane asessment for dryness; daily weights
5. Parental expression of satisfaction with planned treatment

Keystone Issue:
Neonatal Jaundice (9)

Patient Care Interventions (NIC)

©Pesut & Herman, 1999

Figure 7.3   OPT Model of Clinical Reasoning for Neonatal Health Issues (Neonatal Jaundice).

SUMMARY

Clinical reasoning for young patients experiencing physiological challenges of extrauterine life and for their concerned families begins with an understanding of who the patient is and what the family concerns are. Using the OPT Model as a conceptual framework and the Clinical Reasoning Web as a tool helps develop the clinical reasoning associated with a particular case. The OPT Model of Clinical Reasoning provides a visual illustration of where the patient is (present state) and where the nurse hopes the patient to be (outcome state), all of which is framed through identification of background issues of the patient's story (framing). Through "spinning and weaving" of the web, the nurse can determine the priority of care through the generation of hypotheses and thinking out loud (self-talk) to make explicit functional relationships between and among competing nursing care needs. Once the priority issue (the keystone) is identified, planning can begin. In this case study the identified keystone issue is Neonatal Jaundice.

The OPT Model of Clinical Reasoning provides a visual illustration of where the newborn patient is as well as the family (present state). Five present-state items were identified: an elevated bilirubin level, maternal anxiety regarding ineffective breastfeeding, newborn weight loss, dehydration, and maternal anxiety regarding prescribed treatment. From this point the nurse was able to establish where he or she hoped the patient to be (outcome state). In this case study the nurse was able to determine these outcomes (using NOC terminology) to be newborn adaptation, anxiety level (in the mother), breastfeeding maintenance, fluid balance in the newborn, and client satisfaction on the part of the parents.

The present-state and outcome-state items are framed through identification of background issues of the patient's story (framing). The nurse framed this patient and family situation as a 24-hour-old Caucasian male with jaundice, an elevated bilirubin level, blood type incompatibility, and an inadequate feeding pattern. Ultimately the nurse must determine what evidence supports evaluations (tests) that bridge the gap between the two states and make decisions (judgments) of patient progress in meeting the outcomes. The nurse identified these tests to consider: various blood tests (a bilirubin level, hematocrit, and reticulocyte counts), daily weights, wet diaper counts, skin assessments, and parental verbalizations of feelings and their degree of satisfaction of care and education provided. Experience with case studies of this nature enhances a nurse's experience and adds a clinical reasoning skill set that can be activated with future cases of a similar nature.

KEY POINTS

- Clinical reasoning for a neonatal patient who is experiencing elevated levels of bilirubin secondary to ABO incompatibility and difficulties with establishing effective breastfeeding can be promoted with the OPT Model.

- A step-by-step approach is used in this case study involving a patient who has hyperbilirubinemia and will undergo recommended medical treatment. This approach can be used for similar schema and prototypes of a neonatal patient in other health settings.

- Various thinking reflection strategies are used throughout the clinical reasoning process to complete the Clinical Reasoning Web and OPT Model of Clinical Reasoning.

STUDY QUESTIONS AND ACTIVITIES

1. Describe the benefits of using the OPT Model of Clinical Reasoning to plan and evaluate patient care.

2. How does this model differ from other nursing plans of care models?

3. What thinking strategies would you use in spinning and weaving the Reasoning Web?

4. Are there other nursing diagnoses you would assign to this case study involving a jaundiced neonate? If so and given the patient data presented in the case study, what would you suggest?

5. Are there other priorities you would give to this case study? In other words, is there a different keystone issue you would recommend in planning care?

6. What other tests would you consider appropriate to bridge the gap between present state and outcome state in this patient scenario?

References

Ackley, B., & Ladwig, G. (2017). *Nursing diagnosis handbook: An evidence-based guide to planning care* (11th ed.). St. Louis, MO: Mosby Elsevier.

American Academy of Pediatrics (AAP). (2004). Treatment of hyperbilirubinemia in the newborn infant 35 or more weeks of gestation. *Pediatrics, 114*(1), 297–316.

Bhutani, V. K., Johnson, L., and Sivieri, E. M. (1999). Predictive ability of a predischarge hour-specific serum bilirubin for subsequent significant hyperbilirubinemia in healthy term and near-term newborns. *Pediatrics, 103*, 6–14.

Blackburn, S. T. (2013). *Maternal, fetal, & neonatal physiology: A clinical perspective* (4th ed.). St. Louis, MO: Elsevier.

Butcher, H. K., Bulechek, G. M., Dochterman, J. M., & Wagner, C. M. (in press). *Nursing Interventions Classification (NIC)* (7th ed.). St. Louis, MO: Mosby Elsevier.

Butcher, H., & Johnson, M. (2012). Use of linkages for clinical reasoning and quality improvement. In M. Johnson, S. Moorhead, G. Bulechek, H. Butcher, M. Maas, & E. Swanson (Eds.), *NOC and NIC linkages to NANDA-I and clinical conditions* (3rd ed.), pp. 11–23. Maryland Heights, MO: Elsevier.

Carpenito, L. J. (2016). *Nursing diagnosis: Application to clinical practice* (15th ed.). Philadelphia, PA: Wolters Kluwer Health.

Clark, M. (2013). Clinical update: Understanding jaundice in the breastfed infant. *Community Practitioner, 86*(6), 42–45.

Doenges, M. E., Moorhouse, M. F., & Murr, A. C. (2017). *Nursing diagnosis manual: Planning, individualizing, and documenting client care* (11th ed.). St. Louis, MO: Elsevier.

Herdman, T. H., & Kamitsuru, S. (Eds.). (2014). *NANDA International nursing diagnoses: Definition and classifications, 2015-2017.* Oxford, England: Wiley Blackwell.

Hockenberry, M. J., & Wilson, D. (2015). *Wong's nursing care of infants and children* (10th ed.). St. Louis, MO: Elsevier.

Jaundice. (2016). *The American Heritage Dictionary of the English Language* (5th ed.). Retrieved from https://ahdictionary.com/word/search.html?q=jaundice

Johnson, M., Moorhead, S., Bulechek, G., Butcher, H., Maas, M., & Swanson, E. (Eds.). (2012). *NOC and NIC linkages to NANDA-I and clinical conditions* (3rd ed.). Maryland Heights, MO: Elsevier.

Kuiper, R. A., Pesut, D. J., & Arms, T. (2016). *Clinical reasoning and care coordination in advanced practice nursing.* New York, NY: Springer Publishing Company.

Kuiper, R., Pesut, D., & Kautz, D. (2009). Promoting the self-regulation of clinical reasoning skills in nursing students. *The Open Nursing Journal, 3,* 76–85. Retrieved from http://doi.org/10.2174/1874434600903010076

Lantzy, A. (2016). Neonatal hyperbilirubinemia (jaundice in neonates). *Merck Manuals.* Kenilworth, UK: Merck & Co., Inc. Retrieved from http://www.merckmanuals.com/professional/pediatrics/metabolic,-electrolyte,-and-toxic-disorders-in-neonates/neonatal-hyperbilirubinemia

Maisels, M. J., & McDonagh, A. F. (2008). Phototherapy for neonatal jaundice. *The New England Journal of Medicine, 358*(9), 921–928.

Maisels, J., & Watchko, J. F. (2012). Treatment of hyperbilirubinemia. In G. Buonocore, R. Bracci, & M. Windling (Eds.), *Neonatology: A practical approach to neonatal diseases* (pp. 629–640). Milan, Italy: Springer-Verlag Mailand. Digital edition. Retrieved from http://www.springer.com.liblink.uncw.edu/us/book/9788847014046?wt_mc=ThirdParty.SpringerLink.3.EPR653.About_eBook

Martin, S., Jerome, R. N., Epelbaum, M., Williams, A. M., & Walsh, W. (2008). Addressing hemolysis in an infant due to mother-infant ABO blood incompatibility. *Journal of the Medical Library Association, 96*(3), 183–188.

MedlinePlus. (2015). Hemolytic disease of the newborn. U.S. National Library of Medicine. Retrieved from https://medlineplus.gov/ency/article/001298.htm

MedlinePlus. (2016). Newborn jaundice. U.S. National Library of Medicine. Retrieved from https://medlineplus.gov/ency/article/001559.htm

Moorhead, S., Johnson, M., Maas, M. O., & Swanson, E. (Eds.). (2013). *Nursing Outcomes Classification (NOC): Measurement of health outcomes* (5th ed.). St. Louis, MO: Elsevier.

Pesut, D. (2008). Thoughts on thinking with complexity in mind. In C. Lindberg, S. Nash, & C. Lindberg (Eds.), *On the edge: Nursing in the age of complexity* (pp. 211–238). Bordentown, NJ: PlexusPress.

Porter, M., & Dennis, B. L. (2002). Hyperbilirubinemia in the term newborn. *American Family Physician, 15*(65), 599–607. Retrieved from http://www.aafp.org/afp/2002/0215/p599.html

Preer, G. L., & Philipp, B. L. (2011). Understanding and managing breast milk jaundice. *Archives of Disease in Childhood (Fetal and Neonatal Edition), 96*(6), F461–F466. doi:10.1136/adc.2010.184416

Shortland, D. B., & Hussey, M. (2008). Understanding neonatal jaundice: UK practice and international profile. *The Journal of the Royal Society for the Promotion of Health, 128*(4), 202–206. doi:10.1177/1466424008092229

Stokowski, L. A. (2011). Fundamentals of phototherapy for neonatal jaundice. *Advances in Neonatal Care, 11*(55), S10–S21.

CHAPTER **8**

CLINICAL REASONING AND ADOLESCENT HEALTH ISSUES

LEARNING OUTCOMES

- Explain the components of the OPT Model used to reason about the problems, interventions, and outcomes of an adolescent patient who has recently experienced a traumatic injury or accident.

- Identify relevant nursing diagnoses specific to the health issues of the patient with a traumatic injury.

- Identify outcomes appropriate for the health problems assessed in an adolescent with a traumatic injury.

- Describe relevant tests and clinical judgments used to reason about present-state to outcome-state changes for an adolescent who has suffered a traumatic injury.

- Describe the different thinking processes that support clinical reasoning skills and strategies to determine priorities and desired outcomes for an adolescent with traumatic injuries.

This chapter presents a case study involving a 16-year-old Caucasian male who was admitted to the emergency department after rolling over his all-terrain vehicle (ATV) and crushing his right lower extremity. He suffers from the complications of compartment syndrome. At this time, he is awaiting an additional surgery to close fasciotomy sites on the right lower leg.

ATVs have been implicated in the death of more than 10,000 individuals and caused injury to hundreds of thousands more since the mid-1980s, mainly due to turnovers of a vehicle (Myers, 2016). One of the resulting injuries of ATV rollovers is a crush injury. Crush injuries occur due to compression of the extremities or other parts of the body, which result in muscle swelling and/or neurological disturbances in the affected areas (Centers for Disease Control and Prevention, 2009). Lower extremities are the most common area of the body affected by crush injuries, with 74% of cases involving the lower extremities. Crush injuries can result in permanent disability or death as well as severe complications such as compartment syndrome, rhabdomyolysis, and renal failure (Sahjian & Frakes, 2007; Wallin, Nguyen, Russell, & Lee, 2016).

Compartment syndrome can occur due to an increase in the contents of a compartment, for example bleeding, and/or the decrease in size of a compartment, for instance a splint or cast that inhibits swelling from occurring (Taylor, Sullivan, & Mehta, 2016). These changes in the compartment disrupt interstitial compartment pressure (ICP). When the ICP exceeds perfusion pressure, the tissues can no longer be perfused, resulting in ischemia, cellular anoxia, and, ultimately, cellular death (Taylor et al., 2016). There is an increased risk of compartment syndrome in males and individuals 35 years of age and younger (Taylor et al., 2016). In addition, Wallin and colleagues (2016) suggest that there should be high index of suspicion of compartment syndrome in the pediatric population when there is a lower extremity injury.

Compartment syndrome, although overwhelmingly caused by trauma, can also occur due to overexertion, such as weightlifting. Regardless of how the compartment syndrome develops, the treatment involves alleviating the pressure to reduce the lack of perfusion, cell death, and loss of function.

Compounding the physiologic concerns are concurrent developmental factors often associated with the care of an adolescent, such as the individual described in the current case. Adolescence is a time when, statistically speaking, health-compromising, risky, and sometimes reckless behaviors reach their peak (Centers for Disease Control and Prevention, 2014). According to Steinberg (2008), adolescents and young adults are more likely than adults to binge drink, use drugs, have casual sex, and get into serious accidents. The behaviors exhibited by this adolescent, riding the ATV without a helmet, could have had more dire consequences.

THE PATIENT STORY

Meet Mr. Brian Crane, a 16-year-old Caucasian male who was admitted 8 days ago after a rollover ATV accident that occurred on his family's farm. He was transported by EMS (Emergency Medical Services) to the local community hospital. Once there he was transferred via critical care transport to the regional medical center for care in the pediatric intensive care unit for his severe lower right extremity crush injuries. Mr. Crane was not wearing his helmet and fortunately suffered only scalp lacerations. There were no head or neck injuries and no loss of consciousness. On the day after his admission, Mr. Crane developed compartment syndrome from a 500 mL hematoma behind the right knee and underwent two 25 cm fasciotomies on both the medial and lateral aspects of the right calf. Vacuum assisted closure devices (wound VACs) were placed to both sites. On day 4 of his admission, he was transferred to the pediatric floor. On day 8 of his admission, he is scheduled for closure of both fasciotomy sites in the operating room with possible skin grafting.

Medical History

Mr. Crane's history includes a hand fracture due to an earlier skateboarding accident and multiple emergency department visits for stitches, abrasions, and strains. He has never smoked, states he is a social drinker (fewer than four drinks per week), and denies illicit drug use. However, his toxicology screen on admission was positive for marijuana (THC).

Physical Assessment

Mr. Crane is awake, alert, and oriented to person, place, time, and situation. He is currently lying in bed with his legs elevated on pillows. He has many visitors in his room waiting for the surgical procedure today to close the fasciotomy sites. He is restless, agitated, has some abdominal discomfort, and complaining of pain: 8 on a scale of 0 to 10. Mr. Crane's height is 5'10" and he weighs 230 lbs. His body mass index (BMI) is 33 (obese). Vital signs are as follows: blood pressure is 134/84 mmHg (left arm); temperature is 99°F; heart rate is 80 beats per minute and regular; respirations are 14 breaths per minute; and oxygen saturation is 99% on room air.

Laboratory Test Results

Laboratory tests include toxicology screen, complete blood count, coagulation studies, serum electrolyte levels, and renal function studies. Abnormal laboratory values are hemoglobin 9.6 gm/dL, hematocrit 27%, white blood cell count 13,000 cells/L, platelet count 150,000/mcL, and the toxicology screen is positive for THC (marijuana).

Other Diagnostic Tests

The results of a computed tomography (CT) scan of Mr. Crane's head upon admission to the emergency department reveal no bleeding or fractures. X-ray images of his lower extremities reveal no fractures.

Medications

Medications include Vicodin 1–2 tablets every 4 hours for pain; morphine sulfate PCA 1mg/ml (PCA dose: 0.5 mg, Lockout: 10 minutes hourly maximum dose 3mg); heparin 5000 units subcutaneous every 8 hours; multivitamin with iron 1 tablet daily; cefazolin 1gram intravenous every 8 hours. Mr. Crane has no drug allergies.

Psychosocial Assessment

Mr. Crane states he is sexually active with his girlfriend but does not use condoms because "she is on birth control." He is the middle child of seven children. He denies having a formal religion, but does feel he is spiritual and feels "connected to the earth and all living things." He works for his father on their farm on weekends and school holidays.

Current Physical Condition

Mr. Crane has spent a significant amount of time in the hospital for treatment and recovery from his injuries in the emergency department, the pediatric intensive care unit, and currently on the pediatric unit. He admits to reckless behaviors and poor decision-making. Mr. Crane is limited with his weight-bearing ability and is currently using a rollator walker during physical therapy sessions. The current treatment plan is for closure of the fasciotomies in the operating room and discharge to home, with outpatient physical therapy and follow-up care. He has expressed anxiety over the upcoming surgery to close his fasciotomy sites and is worried about whether the surgeons will be able to close both sites. He is concerned about the possibility of physical limitations or disfigurements afterwards. The issue of the positive toxicology screen must be addressed with counseling regarding his risky behaviors, which is a concern of his parents. Finally, he has been asking questions about nutrition and expresses concern over his weight and appearance such as, "I still have all my baby fat."

PATIENT-CENTERED PLAN OF CARE USING THE OPT MODEL OF CLINICAL REASONING

The patient story in this case study has been obtained from all possible sources, including a physical examination, a current list of medications, and care conferences. The lists of patient problems and relevant nursing diagnoses support the creation of the Clinical Reasoning Web Worksheet and the OPT Model of Clinical Reasoning that help the nurse begin to filter the assessment data and information, frame the context of the story, and focus on the priority care needs and outcomes (Butcher & Johnson, 2012).

Patient Problems and Nursing Diagnoses Identification

The first step of care planning is to identify the various problems and cues presented by the patient and select the nursing diagnoses whose defining characteristics capture these cues and problems. The medical diagnosis for this patient is post-accident with injury to right lower leg and compartment syndrome.

Nursing Care Priority Identification

The nurse identifies the cues and problems collected from the physiologic assessment, psychosocial assessment, and the medical record. The similar problems and cues are clustered for interpretation and meaning. Then relevant nursing diagnoses that "fit" the cluster of cues and problems are identified based on definitions and defining characteristics of each nursing diagnosis. An assessment worksheet listing the major taxonomy domains, classes of each domain, patient cues and problems, relevant NANDA-I diagnoses with definitions (Herdman & Kamitsuru, 2014), Nursing Outcomes Classification (NOC) (Moorhead, Johnson, Maas, & Swanson, 2013), and Nursing Interventions Classification (NIC) (Butcher, Bulechek, Dochterman, & Walker [in press]) labels has been created. This worksheet is designed to assist the nurse in organizing patient care issues and to generate appropriate nursing diagnoses. An example of a completed table of the taxonomy domains, classes, patient cues and problems, relevant nursing diagnoses, and suggested NOC and NIC labels for this case study is presented in Table 8.1.

STOP AND THINK

1. What taxonomy domains are affected, and which diagnoses have I generated?

2. What cues/evidence/data from the patient and evidence from the patient assessment support the diagnoses?

CREATING A CLINICAL REASONING WEB

The *Clinical Reasoning Web* is a means by which the nurse analyzes and reasons through complex patient stories for the purpose of finding and prioritizing key healthcare issues. Using the web, the nurse defines problems based on patient cues in the data, identifies nursing diagnoses to address and define the various problems, and determines relationships among these diagnoses (Kuiper, Pesut, & Kautz, 2009). The web is a visual representation and iterative analysis of the functional relationships among diagnostic hypotheses and results in a keystone issue that requires nursing care. In other words, the Clinical Reasoning Web represents a graphic illustration of how the elements of the patient's story and issues relate to one another and is depicted by sketching lines of association among the nursing diagnoses (Kuiper, Pesut, & Arms, 2016). Whereas medical diagnoses are consistent labels for a cluster of symptoms, patient stories vary; each Clinical Reasoning Web is written to reflect the patient's unique story and the human response to actual or potential health problems that are best represented in nursing diagnoses. For example, given two patients with identical medical diagnoses, the nurse may determine that different nursing diagnoses and keystone issues are the priority for each based on thinking strategies and diagnostic hypotheses associated with each case.

Constructing the Clinical Reasoning Web

After the problems are identified from the assessment data, evidence, and cues and the nursing diagnoses are chosen, the Clinical Reasoning Web is constructed using the following steps:

1. Place a general description of the patient in the central oval with the primary medical diagnoses. In this case study it is a 16-year-old Caucasian male post ATV rollover accident who has suffered a compartment syndrome of the right lower leg with complications. He is currently hospitalized awaiting further surgery.

TABLE 8.1 DOMAINS, CLASSES (NANDA-I TAXONOMY II), PATIENT CUES/PROBLEMS, NURSING DIAGNOSES, NOC AND NIC LABELS

Domain	Classes	Identified Patient Problems
Health Promotion: The awareness of well-being or normality of function and the strategies used to maintain control of and enhance that well-being or normality of function	**Health Management:** Identifying, controlling, performing, and integrating activities to maintain health and well-being	• Does not use protective equipment while riding ATV • Admits to reckless driving • Early sexual activity • Positive drug screen
		• Asking questions about better diet choices • Stated he should probably wear his helmet in the future while riding ATV
Nutrition: The activities of taking in, assimilating, and using nutrients for the purposes of tissue maintenance, tissue repair, and the production of energy	**Ingestion:** Taking food or nutrients into the body	• BMI 33 • States poor food choices
Elimination/Exchange: Secretion and excretion of waste products from the body	**Gastrointestinal function:** The process of absorption and excretion of the end products of digestion	• Has not had a bowel movement for 4 days • Receiving oral and IV opiates for pain
Activity/Rest: The production, conservation, expenditure, or balance of energy resources	**Activity/Exercise:** Moving parts of the body (mobility), doing work, or performing actions often (but not always) against resistance	• Post right lower extremity crush injury • Two fasciotomies to treat compartment syndrome

NANDA-I Nursing Diagnoses	Nursing Outcomes Classifications (NOC)	Nursing Intervention Classifications (NIC)
Risk Prone Health Behavior: Impaired ability to modify lifestyle/ behaviors in a manner that improves health status	• Psychosocial Adjustment: Life Change • Risk Detection	• Self-efficacy enhancement
Readiness for Enhanced Health Management: A pattern of regulating and integrating into daily living a therapeutic regimen for the treatment of illness and its sequelae, which can be strengthened	• Adherence Behavior • Compliance Behavior • Knowledge: Treatment Regimen	• Mutual Goal Setting • Self-Modification Assistance • Health Education • Teaching: Individual • Nutritional Counseling
Obesity: A condition in which an individual accumulates abnormal or excessive fat for age and gender that exceeds overweight	• Nutrient Intake • Weight loss behavior	• Weight management • Nutrition management
Constipation: Decrease in normal frequency of defecation, accompanied by difficult or incomplete passage of stool and/or passage of excessively hard, dry stool	• Bowel Elimination	• Constipation/ • Impaction Management
Impaired Physical Mobility: A limitation in independent, purposeful physical movement of the body or of one or more extremities	• Ambulation	• Exercise therapy: Ambulation

continues

TABLE 8.1 DOMAINS, CLASSES (NANDA-I TAXONOMY II), PATIENT CUES/PROBLEMS, NURSING DIAGNOSES, NOC AND NIC LABELS (CONTINUED)

Domain	Classes	Identified Patient Problems
Perception/Cognition: The human information processing system including attention, orientation, sensation, perception, cognition, and communication	**Cognition:** Use of memory, learning, thinking, problem-solving, abstraction, judgment, insight, intellectual capacity, calculation, and language	• Needs education regarding recovery process, bowel regimen, weight loss diet • Does not understand risk of STIs if not using condoms; only concerned about pregnancy
Coping/Stress Tolerance: Contending with life events/life processes	**Coping Responses:** The process of managing environmental stress	• Expressed worry over the surgery to close fasciotomy sites and subsequent scarring • Concern he has not moved his bowels
Safety/Protection: Principles underlying conduct, thought, and behavior about acts, customs, or institutions viewed as being true or having intrinsic worth	**Infection:** Host responses following pathogenic invasion	• Fasciotomy sites • Laceration from ATV accident • Unprotected sexual activity
	Physical Injury: Bodily harm or hurt	• Two fasciotomy sites right lower leg • Scalp laceration
Comfort: Freedom from danger, physical injury, or immune system damage; preservation from loss; and protection of safety and security	**Physical Comfort:** Sense of well-being or ease and/or freedom from pain	• Pain level 8/10 • Pain is not responding well to current treatment

*Butcher, H., Bulechek, G., Dochterman, J., & Wagner, C. M. (in press).
Herdman, T. H., & Kamitsuru, S. (Eds.). (2014).
Moorhead, S., Johnson, M., Maas, M. O., & Swanson, E. (Eds.). (2013).

NANDA-I Nursing Diagnoses	Nursing Outcomes Classifications (NOC)	Nursing Intervention Classifications (NIC)
Knowledge, Deficient: Absence or deficiency of cognitive information related to a specific topic	• Knowledge: Disease process • Knowledge: Health Behavior • Healthy Diet, Medication, Personal Safety	• Teaching: Disease process, Individual, Learning facilitation
Anxiety: A vague uneasy feeling of discomfort or dread accompanied by perceptions of a real or imagined threat to one's existence	• Anxiety Self-Control	• Anxiety reduction
Risk for Infection: At increased risk for being invaded by pathogenic organisms	• Wound Healing: Primary Intention • Tissue Integrity: Skin • Risk control: Sexually Transmitted Diseases	• Incision Site Care • Infection Control • Risk Identification • Surveillance Teaching: Safe Sex • Wound Care
Impaired Skin Integrity: Altered epidermis and/or dermis	• Tissue Integrity: Skin and Mucous Membranes • Wound Healing: Primary Intention	• Incision site care, Pain management, Skin surveillance
Acute Pain: Unpleasant sensory and emotional experience arising from actual or potential tissue damage or described in terms of such damage; sudden or slow onset of any intensity from mild to severe with an anticipated or predictable end	• Pain Level	• Pain management • Analgesic administration • Patient-Controlled Analgesia Assistance

2. Place each NANDA-I nursing diagnosis generated from the patient cues in the ovals surrounding the middle circle.

3. Under each nursing diagnosis, list supporting data that was gathered from the patient's story and assessment.

4. Because each nursing diagnosis is directly related to the center oval containing a brief description of the patient's situation, the nurse draws a line from the central oval to each of the outlying nursing diagnosis ovals. Figure 8.1 displays the beginning steps of constructing the Clinical Reasoning Web for this case study.

Spinning and Weaving the Reasoning Web

In spinning and weaving the Clinical Reasoning Web, the nurse must analyze and explain the relationships among the nursing diagnoses. This process involves thinking out loud; using self-talk; schema search; hypothesizing; if-then, how-so thinking; and comparative analysis, as described in Chapter 3 of this book. In doing so, the nurse determines possible connections and relationships among the nursing diagnoses contained in the outlying ovals.

The nurse must consider how each of the nursing diagnoses and related healthcare issues it defines relates to the other diagnoses. If there is a functional relationship between two diagnoses, then a line with a one-directional arrow is drawn to indicate a one-way connection; a line with two-directional arrows is drawn to indicate a two-way connection. For example, what is the relationship between Impaired Physical Mobility and Acute Pain? How are these two diagnoses related? How do they influence one another? In the case of Mr. Crane, the nurse would consider whether Impaired Physical Mobility would cause Acute Pain, or in a reciprocal fashion whether the feeling of Acute Pain would contribute to Impaired Physical Mobility. For this relationship, there is a one-way connection between Acute Pain and Impaired Physical Mobility. Another example would be to consider how the nursing diagnosis Risk for Infection relates to the issue of Anxiety. In this situation, there is no relationship. Therefore, no connection is made between these two diagnoses.

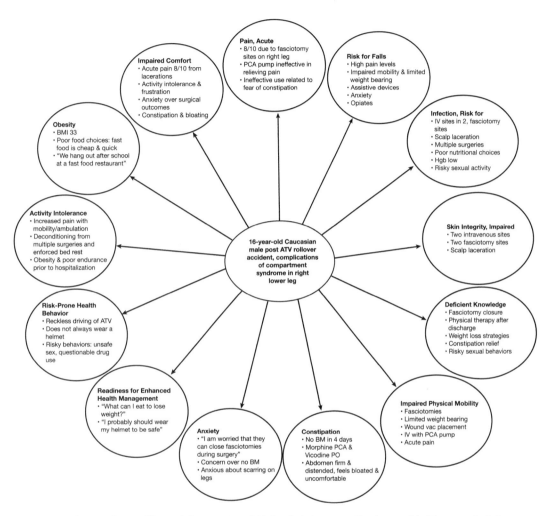

Figure 8.1 Clinical Reasoning Web: Adolescent Patient with Traumatic Injury: Connections from Medical Diagnosis to Nursing Diagnoses.

The nurse continues to spin and weave using the following steps:

1. The first step is iterative, recursive, and repeated with each of the other ovals to determine relationships for connections. If there are functional relationships, connections are drawn until the process is exhausted. Visually, the web emerges.

2. When all connections are made, the lines leading to and from each oval with nursing diagnoses are counted and recorded. The numbers can be recorded on the Clinical Reasoning Web Worksheet. A table showing the hierarchy of priorities of Mr. Crane's problems based on the number of connections is displayed in Table 8.2.

3. The nursing diagnosis with the most connecting lines radiating to and from that oval becomes the *keystone* issue. Figure 8.2 displays a completed Clinical Reasoning Web for this case.

TABLE 8.2 NURSING DOMAINS, NURSING DIAGNOSES, AND CONNECTIONS

Domain	Class	Nursing Diagnoses	Web Connections
Comfort	Physical Comfort	Acute Pain	8
Elimination Exchange	Gastrointestinal Function	Constipation	7
Nutrition	Ingestion	Obesity	7
Safety/Protection	Physical Injury	Impaired Skin Integrity	7
Comfort	Physical Comfort	Impaired Comfort	6
Coping/Stress Tolerance	Coping Response	Anxiety	6
Activity/Rest	Activity/Exercise	Impaired Physical Mobility	6
Perception/Cognition	Cognition	Knowledge Deficit	5
Safety/Protection	Physical Injury	Risk for Falls	5
Health Promotion	Health Management	Readiness for Enhanced Health Management	3
	Health Management	Risk-Prone Health Behavior	3
Activity/Rest	Activity/Exercise	Activity Intolerance	6
Safety/Protection	Infection	Risk for Infection	3

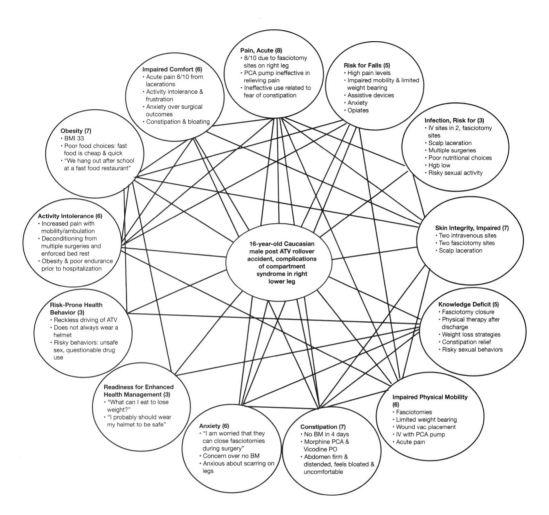

Figure 8.2 Clinical Reasoning Web: Adolescent Patient with Traumatic Injury: Connections Between Nursing Diagnoses.

The *keystone* issue, defined as the nursing diagnosis with the most connections, emerges as a priority problem. It is the basis for defining the patient's present state, which is contrasted with a desired outcome state (Kuiper et al., 2009). Identifying the keystone issue guides clinical reasoning by identifying the central NANDA-I diagnosis that needs to be addressed first and enables the nurse to focus on subsequent care planning (Butcher & Johnson, 2012). After a keystone issue is identified, there is continued knowledge work to identify the complementary nature of the problems ~ outcomes using the juxtaposing thinking strategy. The keystone issue in this case is Acute Pain.

Interventions are chosen to assist Mr. Crane with coping and resolving his acute pain issues. In doing so, these interventions are likely to influence other issues that are identified on the web.

STOP AND THINK

1. What are the relationships between and among the identified problems (diagnoses)?

2. What keystone issue(s) emerge?

COMPLETING THE OPT MODEL OF CLINICAL REASONING

After the Reasoning Web has been completed with identification of the keystone and cue logic, the OPT Model of Clinical Reasoning can be completed. All sections of the OPT Model are completed with the case study described in this chapter.

Patient-in-Context Story

Exhibit 8.1 displays the patient-in-context story for the adolescent Brian Crane. On the far-right side of the OPT Model in Figure 8.3, the patient-in-context story is recorded. This story underscores the patient demographics, medical diagnoses, and current situation. The information placed in this box is presented in a brief format with some relevant facts that support the rest of the model.

EXHIBIT 8.1

Patient-in-Context Story

16-year-old white male, ATV accident with crush injury to right lower leg. Compartment syndrome from a hematoma behind the right R knee, 2 - 25cm fasciotomies performed. Closure of both sites with possible skin grafting on day 8.

Past Medical History: Previous fractures, stitches, abrasions, and strains after accidents

Physical Exam: Neuromuscular: right foot - decreased sensation on the dorsum, decreased range of motion of toes; right lower leg - weak muscle strength. Cardiovascular: 3+ edema of right lower leg distal to knee. 1+- DP & PT pulses right side

Height/Weight: 5'10" /230 lbs. BMI: 33 (obese).

Skin: scalp laceration with sutures. GI: firm abdomen, hypoactive bowel sounds in 4 quadrants, + flatus

Psychosocial: Social drinker, sexually active, does not use condoms, admits to reckless behaviors and poor decision-making.

Vital Signs: Temperature 99°F; Pulse 80 bpm, regular; Respirations 14 bpm; O2 saturation 99% on room air; Blood pressure 134/84 mmHg; Pain 8/10 in right leg and abdominal discomfort.

Laboratory Tests: Hgb 9.6 gm/dL, Hct 27%, WBC: 13,000 cells/L, Platelet count 150, 000/mcL, positive drug screen for marijuana (THC)

Medications: Vicodin and morphine sulfate for pain, heparin, multivitamin, cefazolin.

Diagnostic Cluster/Cue Logic

The next step in the care planning process is completing the *diagnostic cluster/cue logic*. The keystone issue is placed at the bottom of the column with all the other identified nursing diagnoses and listed above it, in priority order. At this point, the nurse reflects on this list to ask whether there is evidence to support these nursing diagnoses and whether the keystone issue is correctly identified. *Cue logic* is the deliberate structuring of patient-in-context data to discern the meaning for nursing care (Butcher & Johnson, 2012). In this case study, the nursing diagnoses depicted in the outlying ovals on the Reasoning Web are recorded under diagnostic cluster/cue logic on the OPT Model Clinical Reasoning Worksheet along with the number of arrows radiating to/from each diagnosis. Exhibit 8.2 displays the identified keystone issue—in this case, Acute Pain—and it is listed directly below the other nursing diagnoses.

EXHIBIT 8.2

Diagnostic Cluster/Cue Logic

1. Constipation (7)
2. Skin Integrity Impaired (7)
3. Obesity (7)
4. Impaired Comfort (6)
5. Impaired Physical Mobility (6)
6. Knowledge Deficit (5)
7. Risk for Falls (5)
8. Readiness for Enhanced Health (3)
9. Risk Prone Health Behavior (3)
10. Risk for Infection (3)

Keystone Issue/Theme
Acute Pain (8)

EXHIBIT 8.3

Frame

16-year-old male, with traumatic right leg injury, compartment syndrome, awaiting surgery. Pain level 8/10 and restless. Discharge to home with outpatient physical therapy.

Framing

In the center and top of the worksheet is a box to indicate the *frame* or theme that best represents the background issue(s) regarding the patient-in-context story. The frame of this case is a 16-year-old male, who suffered a traumatic leg injury with complications, who is awaiting additional surgery. Currently, he is resting in bed with a pain level 8 out of 10, verbalized discomfort and restlessness. Several visitors are present. The discharge plan is to be discharged home with outpatient physical therapy. This frame helps to organize the present state and outcome state and illustrate the gaps between them to provide insights about essential care needs. The frame is the lens or background view to help the nurse differentiate this patient schema and prototype from others dealt with in the past. The interventions and tests that will be used in this care plan are specific to the frame that is identified. Exhibit 8.3 displays the frame in the case of Mr. Crane.

Present State

The *present state* is a description of the patient-in-context or the initial condition of the patient (Butcher & Johnson, 2012). The items listed in this section change over time as a result of nursing actions and the patient's situation. The cues and problems identified for the patient listed under the keystone issue capture the present state of the patient. These are the problems in which the care of the patient will be planned, implemented, and evaluated. The present-state items are listed in the oval of the identified keystone issue and, in this case, there are five primary issues related to the keystone issue: 1) reporting throbbing pain 8 out of 10, 2) minimal use of the PCA because the patient is concerned about the side effects of the medication, 3) no bowel movement for 4 days, 4) expressed anxiety over the lack of a bowel movement with the need for continued pain medications, and 5) limited mobility, up to bathroom only. Exhibit 8.4 displays the list of present-state issues that relate to the keystone issue and will be subjected to tests to determine whether the identified outcomes are achieved.

Outcome State

Given a defined present state, consideration must be given to desired outcomes that will be achieved to resolve the keystone issue. In other words, one outcome state or goal is listed for each present-state item, and each can be tested and achieved through nursing and collaborative interventions. In this case study, the outcome states with NOC labels (in bold) aim to assist Mr. Crane to 1) have pain control, 2) become more satisfied with the effectiveness of his pain management regimen, 3) improve his comfort level related to his bowel movements, 4) decrease his anxiety and concern about the side effects of his pain management regimen, and 5) manage the disruptive effects of his acute pain on his ability to return to normal functioning and independence in activities of daily living.

EXHIBIT 8.4

Present State

1. Reporting pain 8/10, throbbing.

2. Minimal response to PCA, afraid of side effects with higher dose.

3. No bowel movement in 4 days.

4. Expressed anxiety over bowel movements and need for continued pain medications.

5. Limited mobility: up to bathroom only.

EXHIBIT 8.5

Outcome State

1. **Pain Level:** Reports pain level 4/10 within 2 hours.

2. **Patient Satisfaction:** Pain Management: Reports pain management regimen achieves pain goal, no higher than 4, without increased side effects in 24 hours.

3. **Discomfort Level:** Elimination pattern normal for patient in 24 hours.

4. **Pain Management:** Decreased anxiety in 24 hours.

5. **Pain Disruptive Effects:** Walking with aid of a walker around hall in 24 hours.

Since each present state and its corresponding outcome state directly relate to each other, they are placed next to each other for juxtaposition. This placement assists the nurse with comparative analysis and reflection while exercising clinical reasoning in this care situation. Exhibit 8.5 displays the outcome states for this case study.

Tests

The differences or gaps between the present state and outcome state become the foci of concern in the next step of care planning. The nurse must consider what tests and related interventions are most appropriate to fill the gap between the present state and the desired outcomes. Based on these clinical decisions, the nurse considers evidence that might indicate whether the gaps have been filled. In collaboration with other healthcare providers and the patient, tests are conducted to measure changes and gather data. The nurse asks what and if clinical indicators are available for each desired outcome state; that is, what to consider as to whether the desired outcome is achieved. The tests chosen in this case include 1) the pain scale, 2) number of PCA attempts, 3) intake and output, 4) Hospital Anxiety and Depression scale, and 5) distance ambulated. The tests for Mr. Crane are displayed in Exhibit 8.6.

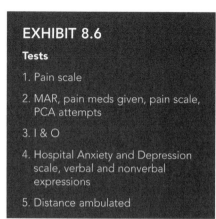

EXHIBIT 8.6

Tests

1. Pain scale

2. MAR, pain meds given, pain scale, PCA attempts

3. I & O

4. Hospital Anxiety and Depression scale, verbal and nonverbal expressions

5. Distance ambulated

STOP AND THINK

1. Is the patient-in-context story complete?

2. How am I framing the situation?

3. How is the *present state* defined?

4. What is/are the desired outcomes?

5. What outcomes do I have in mind given the diagnoses?

6. What is/are the gaps or complementary pairs (~) of outcomes and present states?

7. What are the clinical indicators of the desired outcomes?

8. On what scales or tests will the desired outcome be measured?

9. How will I know when the desired targeted outcomes are achieved?

Interventions

At the bottom of the OPT Model of Clinical Reasoning Worksheet, there is a box that indicates *Patient Care Interventions* (NIC), which are the evidence-based nursing care activities that will assist the patient to reach the outcome states. The nurse must make clinical decisions or choices about interventions that will help the patient transition from present state to the desired outcome state. As interventions are implemented, the nurse evaluates the degree to which outcomes are being achieved. Interventions are evidence-based and gathered from current resources such as the literature, recognized textbooks, and prototype examples. Rationales are listed and cited in a separate page column next to interventions. Listing the rationales for each intervention enhances understanding and justification for nursing activities. The interventions and the rationales for this case study are listed in Table 8.3 and include the measures of noninvasive pain relief methods and assessment, encouraging verbalization of feelings and reflection on life achievements, and facilitating resources to support spiritual care.

STOP AND THINK

1. What clinical decisions or interventions help to achieve the outcomes?

2. What specific intervention activities will I implement?

3. Why am I considering these activities?

TABLE 8.3 INTERVENTIONS AND RATIONALES

Interventions	Rationales

1. Pain Management:
  a. Teach the use of non-pharmacological techniques along with other pain relief measures. Use guided imagery and breathing exercises to cope with increased pain levels.
  b. Control environmental factors that may influence the patient's response to discomfort. Obtain fan from facilities management to decrease room temperature; minimize number of visitors in the room.
 	
2. Analgesic Administration:
  a. Instruct patient to request PRN medications before the pain is severe. Advised to call for medications if needed when notices increase in pain and do this in addition to use of the PCA.
  b. Reinforce education on correct use of PCA pump and correct any myths/misconceptions on its use.
  c. Administer adjuvant analgesics when needed to potentiate analgesia. Give ordered Flexeril to supplement PCA and Vicodin.
 	
3. Medication Management:
  a. Determine what drugs are needed, and administer according to prescriptive authority and/or protocol. Report of no BM for 4 days, determine the use of laxative needed and administer appropriate medications (i.e., suppository and implement stool softener regimen).
  b. Monitor patient for therapeutic effect of medication. To report BM occurrence and amount.
	1. Relaxation techniques provide individuals with self-control when discomfort or pain occurs, reversing the physical and emotional stress of pain (Potter, Perry, Stockert, & Hall, 2017). Non-pharmacological interventions are used to complement, not replace, pharmacological interventions (American Pain Society [APS], 2008). The nurse can control room temperature, ventilation, noise, and odors to create a more comfortable environment (Potter et al., 2017).
	
	2. Nursing principles for administering analgesics include administering them as soon as pain occurs and before it increases in intensity (Pasero, Quinn, Portenoy, McCaffery, & Rizos, 2011; Potter et al., 2017). Reinforce the importance of taking pain medications to maintain the comfort-function goal (McCaffery, Herr, & Pasero, 2011 as cited in Ackley & Ladwig, 2017). Manage acute pain using a multimodal approach (APS, 2008 as cited in Ackley & Ladwig, 2017). Muscle relaxants may be ordered with opioids to enhance pain control or relieve other symptoms related to pain (Potter et al., 2017).
	
	3. Laxatives should be used with caution, and a step-wise progression of laxatives is recommended (Hinrichs, Huseboe, Tang, & Titler, 2001). Recognize that opioids cause constipation. If the client is receiving temporary opioids (e.g., for acute postoperative pain), request an order for laxative if the patient develops constipation (Ackley & Ladwig, 2017). Outcome is reached when the client is able to report the passage of soft, formed brown stools (Potter et al., 2017).

Interventions	Rationales

4. Anxiety Reduction:
 	
  a. Provide factual information concerning diagnosis, treatment and prognosis. Review use of medications and non-pharmacological interventions (i.e., abdominal massage, moving to chair, leg lifts) to promote bowel movement.
 	
  b. Rule out withdrawal from alcohol and other substances as a cause of the anxiety.
 	
  c. Provide complementary and alternative non-pharmacological measures to reduce anxiety. Explore options that he is willing to implement to reduce anxiety, such as distraction with music, guided imagery, yoga or meditation, or backrubs/massage, therapeutic touch.
 	
5. Exercise Therapy: Ambulation
 	
  a. Encourage patient to sit in bed, on side of bed, or in chair as tolerated. Advise that more movement will increase movement of bowels. Encourage minimum of sitting OOB in chair three times a day and progressively work toward ambulating.
 	
  b. Instruct in availability of assistive devices, if appropriate. Ordered to ambulate TID with walker. Make sure one is available in the room and encourage usage.
	4. Explain all activities, procedures, and issues that involve the client using non-medical terms and slow calm speech (Finke et al., 2008 as cited in Ackley & Ladwig, 2017).
	
	5. According to McCabe and colleagues (2011) participants exhibited elevated levels of anxiety and nervousness when withdrawing from sedatives and/or alcohol. Massage, therapeutic touch guided imagery, yoga, backrubs alleviate anxiety (Labrique-Walusis, Keister, & Russell, 2010; Parlak, Polant, & Nuran, 2010; Thomas & Sethares, 2010). Music also had a positive effect on reducing anxiety in many studies studying music listening and post-operative anxiety (Nilsson, 2008).
	
	6. For individuals who are unable to walk, chair or bed exercises such as pelvic tilt, low trunk rotation, and single leg lifts are recommended (Hinrichs et al., 2001). Physical activity promotes peristalsis, whereas immobilization depresses peristalsis (Potter et al., 2017).

Judgments

The final step in constructing the OPT Model Worksheet is to reflect on the tests and interventions to determine if the outcomes were achieved. The consequences of the tests are data one uses to make clinical judgments (Pesut, 2008). In the far-left column on the OPT Model of Clinical Reasoning Worksheet, judgments are listed for each outcome. *Judgments* are conclusions about outcome achievements.

EXHIBIT 8.7

Judgments

1. Pain level not at 4/10 within 2 hours but level improving, currently 8/10.

2. Now using PCA pump to stay ahead of pain level decreasing, should get to goal of 4/10 within the next 24 hours.

3. No bowel movement, interventions being implemented, started on medication regimen with dietary changes.

4. Expressed decreased anxiety about bowels but still anxious about surgery and recovery, using music and distraction to help alleviate anxiety.

5. Not walking, 0 distance ambulated, working on pain management, sitting in chair doing exercises, waiting for surgery.

Each judgment requires four elements: 1) a contrast between present and desired state, 2) criteria associated with a desired outcome (i.e., test), 3) consideration of the effects and influence of nurse interventions, and 4) a conclusion as to whether the intervention has been effective in the outcome achievement (Kuiper et al., 2009). Based on the analysis of tests, judgments are made about progress on the outcome states. The nurse may have to reframe or attribute a different meaning to the facts in the patient-in-context story. Table 8.4 depicts the outcome states and judgments for this case study. A third column has been added within the table to provide the clinical reasoning used to guide each judgment statement. Exhibit 8.7 displays the judgments in this case.

TABLE 8.4　TABLE OF OUTCOME STATES, JUDGMENTS, AND RATIONALES

Outcome State	Judgment	Clinical Reasoning
Pain Level: Reports pain level 4/10 within 2 hours.	Pain level not at 4/10 within 2 hours but level improving, currently 8/10 on the pain scale.	Pain scale score is decreasing with current management strategies and patient's increased understanding of how to manage the pain; however, he is returning to the OR for closure of the fasciotomies and will need reminders about the importance of staying ahead of the pain.
Patient Satisfaction: Pain Management: Reports that pain management regimen achieves pain goal, no higher than 4, without side effects within 24 hours.	Has begun using the PCA pump to stay ahead of pain and the pain level is decreasing; should reach goal of 4/10 within the next 8 hours.	Review of PCA shows the patient has an increase in the number of attempts, MAR indicates he is taking the Flexeril and Vicodin PRN; pain scale score is improving, though not currently at goal.

Outcome State	Judgment	Clinical Reasoning
Discomfort Level: Elimination pattern within patient is normal within the next 48 hrs.	Currently has not had a normal BM for him. Interventions being implemented and started on medication regimen with dietary changes.	Review of his intake and output show no bowel movement recorded. Bowel regimen implemented and once he returns from surgery and can start oral intake again, will increase fiber and offer natural stimulants such as apple juice or prunes/prune juice.
Pain Management: Decreased anxiety within 24 hours.	Expressed decreased anxiety about bowels but still anxious about surgery and recovery. Using music and distraction to help alleviate anxiety.	Still verbally expressing his anxiety over surgery and outcomes. Nonverbally, remains restless and distracted although not as severe with music and distraction interventions. Hospital Anxiety and Depression anxiety subscale score high at 15 indicating moderate anxiety is present.
Pain Disruptive Effects: Walking with walker around hall within 24 hours.	Has not been able to walk, still working on pain management, agreed to sit in chair, doing exercises, waiting for return to operating room.	Distance ambulated is 0 feet, still in too much pain and too anxious about surgery. After he has this last surgery to close the fasciotomies, physical therapy can work with him intensely to increase ambulation using a device for support.

STOP AND THINK

1. Given the tests that have been chosen, what is my clinical judgment of the evidence regarding reaching the outcome state?

2. Based on my judgment, have I achieved the outcome or do I need to reframe the situation?

3. How can I specifically remember this experience and take the schema into the future when I reason about similar cases?

The Completed OPT Model of Clinical Reasoning

The completed OPT Model of Clinical Reasoning for an adolescent patient post-traumatic injury is displayed in Figure 8.3.

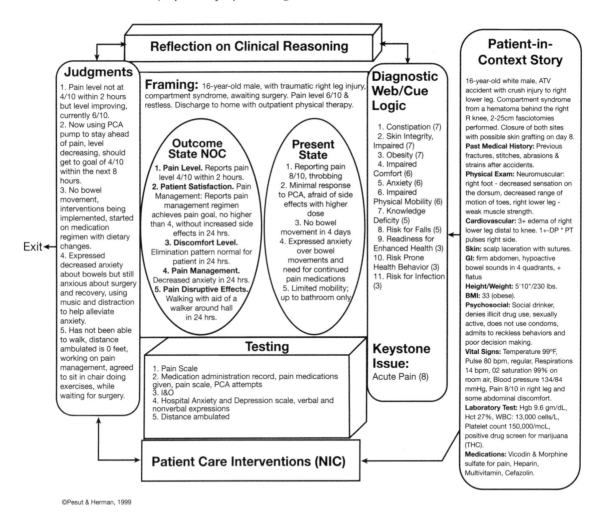

©Pesut & Herman, 1999

Figure 8.3   OPT Model of Clinical Reasoning for an Adolescent with Traumatic Injury.

SUMMARY

Clinical reasoning for adolescent patients who are hospitalized for illness and present with risk-taking behaviors begins with an understanding of who is the patient and what is his or her story given the context of the family dynamics. Using the OPT Model as a conceptual framework and the Clinical Reasoning Web as a tool helps develop the clinical reasoning associated with a particular case. The OPT Clinical Reasoning Model provides a visual illustration of where the patient is (present state) and where the nurse hopes the patient to be (outcome state), all of which is framed through identification of background issues of the patient's story (framing).

Through "spinning and weaving" of the web, the nurse can determine the priority of care through the generation of hypotheses and thinking out loud (self-talk) to make explicit functional relationships between and among competing nursing care needs. Once the priority issue (the keystone) is identified, planning can begin. Ultimately the nurse must determine what evidence supports evaluations (tests) that bridge the gap between the two states and make decisions (judgments) of patient progress in meeting the outcomes. Experience with case studies of this nature augments the nurse's experience and adds to her clinical reasoning skill set that can be activated with future cases of a similar nature.

KEY POINTS

- Clinical reasoning for an adolescent trauma patient who is experiencing physical, developmental, and psychosocial challenges can be promoted with the OPT Model.

- A step-by-step approach is used in this case study involving an adolescent patient who has recently experienced a traumatic injury and is receiving medical treatment. This approach can be used for similar schema and proto-types of adolescent patients in other health settings.

- Various thinking and reflection strategies are used throughout the clinical reasoning process to complete the Clinical Reasoning Web and OPT Model of Clinical Reasoning.

STUDY QUESTIONS AND ACTIVITIES

1. Describe the benefits of using the OPT Clinical Reasoning Model to plan and evaluate patient care given the case described in this chapter.

2. How does this model differ from other nursing plans of care models?

3. What thinking strategies would you use in spinning and weaving the Clinical Reasoning Web?

4. Are there other nursing diagnoses you would assign to this case study involving an adolescent trauma patient? If so and given the patient data presented in the case study, what would you suggest?

5. Are there other priorities you would give to this case study? In other words, is there a different keystone issue you would recommend in planning care?

6. What other tests would you consider appropriate to bridge the gap between the present state and the outcome state in this patient scenario?

References

Ackley, B., & Ladwig, G. (2017). *Nursing diagnosis handbook: An evidence-based guide to planning care* (11th ed.). St. Louis, MO: Mosby Elsevier.

American Pain Society (APS). (2008). *Principles of analgesic use in acute and chronic pain* (6th ed.). Glenview, Il: American Pain Society.

Butcher, H. K., Bulechek, G. M., Dochterman, J. M., & Wagner, C. M. (in press). *Nursing Interventions Classification (NIC)* (7th ed.). St. Louis, MO: Mosby Elsevier.

Butcher, H., & Johnson, M. (2012). Use of linkages for clinical reasoning and quality improvement. In M. Johnson, S. Moorhead, G. Bulechek, H. Butcher, M. Maas, & E. Swanson (Eds.), *NOC and NIC linkages to NANDA-I and clinical conditions* (3rd ed.), pp. 11–23. Maryland Heights, MO: Elsevier.

Centers for Disease Control and Prevention (CDC). (2009). Blast injuries: Crush injury and crush syndrome. Retrieved from https://www.acep.org/uploadedFiles/ACEP/Practice_Resources/disater_and_EMS/disaster_preparedness/BlastInjury_Crush_Eng.pdf

Centers for Disease Control and Prevention (CDC). (2014). Morbidity and mortality weekly report: Youth risk behavior surveillance: United States, 2013. *Surveillance Summaries, 63*(4), 1–168.

Herdman, T. H., & Kamitsuru, S. (Eds.). (2014). *NANDA International nursing diagnoses: Definitions and classification, 2015–2017.* Oxford, England: Wiley Blackwell.

Hinrichs, M., Huseboe, J., Tang, J. H., & Titler, M. G. (2001). Research based protocol: Management of constipation. *Journal of Gerontological Nursing, 27*(2), 17–28.

Ignatavicius, D., & Workman, L. (2016). *Medical-surgical nursing: Patient-centered collaborative care* (8th ed.). St. Louis, MO: Elsevier.

Johnson, M., Moorhead, S., Bulechek, G., Butcher, H., Maas, M. & Swanson, E. (Eds.). (2012). *NOC and NIC linkages to NANDA-I and clinical conditions* (3rd ed.). Maryland Heights, MD: Elsevier.

Kuiper, R. A., Pesut, D. J., & Arms, T. (2016). *Clinical reasoning and care coordination in advanced practice nursing.* New York, NY: Springer Publishing.

Kuiper, R., Pesut, D., & Kautz, D. (2009). Promoting the self-regulation of clinical reasoning skills in nursing students. *The Open Nursing Journal, 3*, 76–85. Retrieved from http://doi.org/10.2174/1874434600903010076

Labrique-Walusis, F., Keister, K., & Russell, A. (2010). Massage therapy for stress management: Implications for nursing practice. *Orthopaedic Nursing, 29*(4), 254–257.

McCabe, S., West, B., Cranford, J., Ross-Durow, P., Young, A., Teter, C., & Boyd, C. (2011). Medical misuse of controlled medications among adolescents. *Archives of Pediatric and Adolescent Medicine, 165*(8), 729–735.

Moorhead, S., Johnson, M., Maas, M. O., & Swanson, E. (Eds.). (2013). *Nursing Outcomes Classification (NOC): Measurement of health outcomes* (5th ed.). St. Louis, MO: Elsevier.

Myers, M. (2016). ATV overturns: Engineering controls to prevent crush injuries. *Professional Safety, 61*(8), 36–43.

Nilsson, U. (2008). The anxiety and pain reducing effects of music interventions: A systematic review. *AORN Journal, 87*(4), 780–807.

Parlak, G., Polat, S., & Nuran, A. (2010). Itching, pain, and anxiety levels are reduced with massage therapy, yoga stretching in burned adolescents. *Journal of Burn Care Research, 31*(3), 429–432.

Pasero, C., Quinn, T. E., Portenoy, R., McCaffery, M., & Rizos, A. (2011). Opioid analgesics. In C. Pasero & M. McCaffery (Eds.), *Pain assessment and pharmacologic management* (pp. 277–622). St. Louis, MO: Mosby/Elsevier.

Pesut, D. (2008). Thoughts on thinking with complexity in mind. In C. Lindberg, S. Nash, & C. Lindberg (Eds.), *On the edge: Nursing in the age of complexity* (pp. 211–238). Bordentown, NJ: Plexus Press.

Potter, P.A., Perry, A. G., Stockert, P., & Hall, A. (2017). *Fundamentals of nursing* (9th ed.). St Louis, MO: Elsevier.

Sahjian, M., & Frakes, M. (2007). Crush injuries: Pathophysiology and current treatment. *Advanced Emergency Nursing Journal, 29*(2), 145–150.

Steinberg, L. (2008). A social neuroscience perspective on adolescent risk-taking. *Developmental Review, 28*(1), 78–106.

Taylor, R., Sullivan, M., & Mehta, S. (2016). Acute compartment syndrome: Obtaining diagnosis, providing treatment and minimizing medicolegal risk. *Current Reviews in Musculoskeletal Medicine, 5*(3), 206–213.

Thomas, K., & Sethares, K. (2010). Is guided imagery effective in reducing pain and anxiety in postoperative total joint arthroplasty patients? *Orthopaedic Nursing, 29*(6), 393–399.

Wallin, K., Nguyen, H., Russell, L., & Lee, D. (2016). Acute traumatic compartment syndrome in pediatric foot: A systematic review and case report. *The Journal of Foot and Surgery, 55*(4), 817–820.

C H A P T E R

9

CLINICAL REASONING AND YOUNG ADULT HEALTH ISSUES

LEARNING OUTCOMES

- Explain the components of the OPT Model that are essential to the reflective clinical reasoning to manage the problems, interventions, and outcomes of a patient undergoing caregiver strain.

- Identify relevant nursing diagnoses specific to the health issues of the caregiver role.

- Identify outcomes appropriate for the health problems assessed in a caregiving scenario.

- Describe relevant tests and clinical judgments used to reason about present-state to outcome-state changes for an individual in the caregiving role.

- Describe the different thinking processes that support clinical reasoning skills and strategies to determine priorities and desired outcomes for a caregiver.

This chapter presents a case study involving a young 26-year-old adult who has served as the primary caregiver for her terminally ill mother and has recently assumed the guardianship role for her two siblings, ages 15 and 13 years.

On an annual basis, there are approximately 43.5 million adults in this country who provide unpaid care for someone with a serious health condition (National Institutes of Health [NIH], 2015). Informal caregiving implies various activities and experiences involved in assisting individuals who are unable to provide help and assistance for themselves. Two factors are involved in caregiving: the affective component, which is "caring," and the behavioral component known as "caregiving" (Pearlin, Mullan, Semple, & Skaff, 1990).

Providing assistance to others often includes complex care activities, and it takes a toll on the health and well-being of the caregiver. Many suffer physical and emotional strain and feelings of being overwhelmed. For those engaged in full-time employment, the demands become even more complex. Caregivers working at least 30 hours a week are more likely to report having workday interruptions as a result of caregiving responsibilities (National Alliance of Caregiving and AARP, 2015).

Caregivers are diverse in age, gender, socioeconomic status, race, and ethnicity, but they share many commonalities in the stress and strain of providing care. The degree of strain and burden felt by caregivers due to their caregiving role is linked to symptoms of depression and anxiety. Caregivers with a reduced amount of social support report greater depressive symptoms, anxiety, and impaired sleep quality (Phillips, Gallagher, Hunt, Der, & Carroll, 2009).

Caregivers' needs differ depending upon the various aspects of the care recipients' conditions and needs as well as the caregivers' own problems, strengths, and resources. In one study, 84% of caregivers state they could use more information or help on caregiving topics (National Alliance of Caregiving and AARP, 2015). Most commonly they want information about keeping the care recipients safe at home and about managing their own stress (National Alliance of Caregiving and AARP, 2015).

A new diagnosis, *Caregiver Role Strain,* was accepted by NANDA-I in 1992. Earlier diagnoses that addressed caregiver strain were Ineffective Family Coping and Fatigue. The more recent diagnosis of Caregiver Role Strain presented a well-described family phenomenon that can be measured and predicted (Burns, Archbold, Stewart, & Shelton, 1993). The diagnosis of Caregiver Role Strain was updated in 1998 and 2000. The current definition is "difficulty in performing family or significant-other caregiver role" (Herdman & Kamitsuru, 2014, p. 279). Defining characteristics identify several dimensions of the diagnosis that include caregiving activities; physiological, emotional, socioeconomic relationship; and family process issues related to the diagnosis. Nurses play an important part in preventing its occurrence or reducing the role strain that caregivers feel. This diagnosis also lends itself to a significant societal issue that needs to be addressed by nurses working in a variety of settings.

THE PATIENT STORY

Meet Miss Darlene Davis, a 26-year-old female who has served for the past 6 months as the primary caregiver for her 53-year-old mother who is diagnosed with stage IV ovarian cancer. Miss Davis is the oldest daughter of three. She has been close to her mother throughout her life and supported her mother through two divorces and deteriorating health. Her mother has been receiving palliative care since her cancer diagnosis in 2015 and has been receiving at-home hospice care for the past month. Currently her mother is semi-responsive, and her pain, according to her nonverbal responses, is being controlled.

Miss Davis was granted guardianship a month ago for her two younger sisters, ages 15 and 13 years. The biological father of the two younger siblings refused to assume these responsibilities due to health concerns of his own and living out of state. A full family assessment had been conducted earlier and revealed no issues with the custodial arrangements. Arrangement for financial support has been established to assist Miss Davis with the financial responsibilities of the family. Due to the rapid deterioration of her condition, Miss Davis's mother is not expected to live beyond 2 weeks.

Miss Davis has confided in two nurses that over the past couple of months she has experienced depression, anxiety, fear of the unknown, grief, and loss of personal freedom related to the impending death of her mother. She has also experienced physical, emotional, and social burdens of caring for both her mother and younger siblings. She suffers from sleep disturbances and is irritable most of the day.

Miss Davis has been engaged for the past 6 months to her long-term boyfriend and indicates that she does not spend as much time with her fiancé or friends as she had 3 months prior. This is due to fatigue and lack of sleep. She spends most of her free time assisting her mother and assuming custodial responsibilities for her sisters. Miss Davis states that she is willing to continue to care for her younger siblings and asks for advice and assistance on caregiving responsibilities, such as meal planning, household maintenance, providing transportation, and paying bills. She also wants to become more involved in her siblings' school activities when she has the available time. She has told the nurses that she hopes to one day regain feelings of optimism.

Physical Assessment

The physical examination reveals that Miss Davis's height is 5'9", her weight is 120 lb. with a reported weight loss of 8 lb. over the past 7 weeks. Her BMI is 18.2 (underweight). Her vital signs are (a) temperature of 98.4°F, (b) heart rate of 80 beats per minute and irregular, (c) respirations of 18 breaths per minute, and (d) blood pressure of 132/90 mmHg, which is slightly elevated from normal blood pressure readings for her age (American Heart Association, 2017). Currently she is not experiencing any pain but reports occasional tension headaches. Miss Davis is current on all vaccinations and has had no prior trauma. Her father had a history of alcoholism and has been deceased since 2010. Her mother was diagnosed with stage IV ovarian cancer in 2015 and is currently receiving hospice care at home.

Psychosocial Assessment

Miss Davis verbalizes feelings of depression, grief, anxiety, fatigue, despair, and social isolation. She reports not having "much of an appetite" and has lost 8 lbs. over the past 7 weeks.

Medications

Miss Davis's medications include birth control pills and ibuprofen as needed for tension headaches. There are no known drug allergies.

PATIENT-CENTERED PLAN OF CARE USING THE OPT MODEL OF CLINICAL REASONING

The patient story in this case study has been obtained from all possible sources, including a physical examination, a current list of medications, and care conferences. The lists of patient problems and relevant nursing diagnoses support the creation of the Clinical Reasoning Web Worksheet and the OPT Model of Clinical Reasoning that help the nurse begin to filter the assessment data and information, frame the context of the story, and focus on the priority care needs and outcomes (Butcher & Johnson, 2012).

PATIENT PROBLEMS AND NURSING DIAGNOSES IDENTIFICATION

The first step of care planning is to identify the various problems and cues presented by the patient and select the nursing diagnoses whose defining characteristics capture these cues and problems. The medical diagnosis for this patient is depression related to being a primary caregiver for her terminally ill mother.

Nursing Care Priority Identification

Although there is no formal medical diagnosis in this case study, the patient has reported feelings of depression, anxiety, grief, fatigue, and social isolation. The nurse identifies the cues and problems collected from the physiologic assessment, psychosocial assessment, and medical record. The similar problems and cues are clustered for interpretation and meaning. Then relevant nursing diagnoses that "fit" the cluster of cues and problems are identified based on definitions and defining characteristics of each nursing diagnosis.

An assessment worksheet listing the major taxonomy domains, classes of each domain, patient cues and problems, relevant NANDA-I diagnoses with definitions (Herdman & Kamitsuru, 2014), Nursing Outcomes Classification (NOC) (Moorhead, Johnson, Maas, & Swanson, 2013), and Nursing Interventions Classification (NIC) (Butcher, Bulechek, Dochterman, & Walker [in press]) labels has been created. This worksheet is designed to assist the nurse in organizing patient care issues and to generate appropriate nursing diagnoses. An example of a completed table of the taxonomy domains, subcategories, patient cues and problems, relevant nursing diagnoses, and suggested NOC and NIC labels for this case study is presented in Table 9.1.

STOP AND THINK

1. What taxonomy domains are affected, and which diagnoses have I generated?

2. What cues/evidence/data from the patient and evidence from the patient assessment support the diagnoses?

CREATING A CLINICAL REASONING WEB

The *Clinical Reasoning Web* is a means by which the nurse analyzes and reasons through complex patient stories for the purpose of finding and prioritizing key healthcare issues. Using the web, the nurse defines problems based on patient cues in the data, identifies nursing diagnoses to address and define the various problems, and determines relationships among these diagnoses (Kuiper, Pesut, & Kautz, 2009). The web is a visual representation of the functional relationships among the NANDA-I diagnoses describing the present state and results in a keystone issue that requires nursing care (Butcher & Johnson, 2012). In other words, the Clinical Reasoning Web represents a graphic illustration of how the elements of the patient's story and issues relate to one another and is depicted by sketching lines of association among the nursing diagnoses (Kuiper, Pesut, & Arms, 2016). Whereas medical diagnoses are consistent labels for a cluster of symptoms, patient stories vary, and each Clinical Reasoning Web is written to reflect the patient's unique story and the human response to actual or potential health problems represented in nursing diagnoses. For example, given two patients with identical medical diagnoses, the nurse may determine that different nursing diagnoses and keystone issues are the priority for each based on thinking strategies and diagnostic hypotheses associated with each case.

TABLE 9.1 DOMAINS, CLASSES (NANDA-I TAXONOMY II), PATIENT CUES/PROBLEMS, NURSING DIAGNOSES, NOC, AND NIC LABELS

Domain	Classes	Identified Patient Problems
Activity/Rest: The production, conservation, expenditure, or balance of energy resources	**Sleep/Rest:** Slumber, repose, ease, relaxation, or inactivity	• Sleep disturbance: difficulty falling and remaining asleep • Mood alterations
Role Relationship: The positive and negative connections or associations between people or groups of people and the means by which those connections are demonstrated	**Caregiving Roles:** Socially expected behavior patterns by people providing care who are not healthcare professionals	• Expressed desire to enhance parenting skills; family wishes to enhance home environment after death of mother • Fatigue and sad affect • Insufficient recreation and social activities • Lack of parenting skills • Feelings of depression • Compromised work performance
	Family Relationships: Associations of people who are biologically related or related by choice	• Family members grieving over mother's impending death • Family role change, prolonged illness of mother • Lack of extended family support for grief-stricken children
Coping/Stress Tolerance: Contending with life events/life processes	**Coping Responses:** The process of managing environmental stress	• Feelings of stress related to the unknown • Imminent death of mother • Compromised performance at work due to strain of caregiving

NANDA-I Nursing Diagnoses	Nursing Outcomes Classifications (NOC)	Nursing Intervention Classifications (NIC)
Disturbed Sleep Pattern: Time-limited interruptions of sleep amount and quality due to external factors	• Rest	• Sleep Enhancement • Relaxation Therapy
Readiness for Enhanced Family Processes: A pattern of family functioning that is sufficient to support the well-being of family members and can be strengthened	• Family Coping • Family Functioning	• Family Integrity Promotion
Caregiver Role Strain: Difficulty in performing family/significant other caregiver role	• Caregiver Emotional Health • Caregiver Well-Being • Parenting Performance • Coping • Caregiver Physical Health • Caregiver Social Involvement	• Caregiver Support • Parenting Promotion • Coping Enhancement • Respite Care • Support System Enhancement
Interrupted Family Processes: Change in family relationships and and/or functioning	• Family Normalization	• Coping • Family Integrity Promotion
Anxiety: Vague, uneasy feeling of discomfort or dread accompanied by an autonomic response; a feeling of apprehension caused by anticipation of danger. It is an alerting signal that warns of impending danger and enables the individual to take measures to deal with threat	• Anxiety Level • Coping	• Anxiety Reduction

continues

TABLE 9.1 DOMAINS, CLASSES (NANDA-I TAXONOMY II), PATIENT CUES/PROBLEMS, NURSING DIAGNOSES, NOC, AND NIC LABELS (CONTINUED)

Domain	Classes	Identified Patient Problems
		• Chronic worry and anxiety, poor concentration, fatigue and sleep disturbance
		• Sadness over mother's impending death, despair and helplessness, desire to find meaning in mother's illness
		• Expressed desire to enhance coping skills, lessen stressors related to caregiving, and find additional social support
Comfort: Freedom from danger, physical injury, or immune system damage; preservation from loss; and protection of safety and security	**Social Comfort:** Sense of well-being or ease with one's social situation	• Expressed feelings of social isolation due to demands of parenting and caregiving for mother • Little time to spend with fiancé

Butcher, H., Bulechek, G., Dochterman, J., & Wagner, C. M. (in press).
Herdman, T. H., & Kamitsuru, S. (Eds.). (2014).
Moorhead, S., Johnson, M., Maas, M. O., & Swanson, E. (Eds.). (2013).

NANDA-I Nursing Diagnoses	Nursing Outcomes Classifications (NOC)	Nursing Intervention Classifications (NIC)
Ineffective Coping: Inability to form a valid appraisal of the stressors, inadequate choices of practiced responses and/or inability to use available resources	• Coping	• Coping Enhancement • Emotional Support
Grieving: A normal complex process that includes emotional, physical, spiritual, social, and intellectual responses and behaviors by which individuals, families, and communities incorporate an actual, anticipated, or perceived loss into their daily lives	• Coping • Grief Resolution • Family Resiliency	• Family Support • Coping Enhancement • Emotional Support
Readiness for Enhanced Coping: A pattern of cognitive and behavioral efforts to manage demands that is sufficient for well-being and can be strengthened	• Self-Awareness • Coping	• Coping Enhancement
Risk for Loneliness: At risk for experiencing discomfort associated with a desire or need for more contact with others	• Loneliness • Social Involvement	• Socialization Enhancement

Constructing the Clinical Reasoning Web

After the problems are identified from the assessment data, evidence, and cues and the nursing diagnoses are chosen, the Clinical Reasoning Web is constructed using the following steps:

1. Place a general description of the patient in the central oval with the primary medical diagnoses. In this case study it is a 26-year-old white female who is caring for her terminally ill mother diagnosed with end-stage ovarian cancer and who has recently been appointed guardianship of her two younger siblings. There is no formal medical diagnosis other than patient reports of feelings of depression, anxiety, and fatigue.

2. Place each NANDA-I nursing diagnosis generated from the patient cues in the ovals surrounding the middle circle.

3. Under each nursing diagnosis, list supporting data that was gathered from the patient's story and assessment.

4. Because each nursing diagnosis is directly related to the center oval containing a brief description of the patient's situation, the nurse draws a line from the central oval to each of the outlying nursing diagnosis ovals. Figure 9.1 displays the beginning steps of constructing the Clinical Reasoning Web for this case study.

Spinning and Weaving the Reasoning Web

In spinning and weaving the Clinical Reasoning Web, the nurse must analyze and explain the relationships among the nursing diagnoses. This process involves thinking out loud; using self-talk; schema search; hypothesizing; if-then, how-so thinking; and comparative analysis, as described in Chapter 3 of this book. In doing so, the nurse determines possible connections and relationships among the nursing diagnoses contained in the outlying ovals.

The nurse continues to spin and weave using the following steps:

1. Consider how each of the nursing diagnoses and related healthcare issues it defines relates to all the other diagnoses. If there is a functional relationship between two diagnoses, then a line with a one-directional arrow is drawn to indicate a one-way connection; lines with two-directional arrows are drawn to indicate two-way connections. For example, what is the relationship between decreased Caregiver Role Strain and Anxiety? How are these two diagnoses related? How do they influence one another? In the case of Miss Davis, the nurse would consider whether Caregiver Role Strain would cause Anxiety or in a reciprocal fashion whether the feeling of Anxiety would contribute to Caregiver Role Strain. In this case, there are two-way connections between Caregiver Role Strain and Anxiety. Another example would be to consider how the nursing diagnosis Risk for Loneliness relates to the issue of Readiness for Enhanced Parenting. In this case, there is no relationship; therefore, no connection is made between these two diagnoses.

2. The first step is repeated with each of the other ovals to determine relationships for connections. If there are functional relationships, connections are drawn until the process is exhausted; visually, the web emerges.

3. When all connections are made, the lines leading to and from each oval with nursing diagnoses are counted and recorded. The numbers can be recorded on the Clinical Reasoning Web Worksheet. The hierarchy of priorities of Miss Davis's problems based on the number of connections is displayed in Table 9.2.

4. The nursing diagnosis with the most connecting lines radiating to and from that oval becomes the *keystone issue*. Figure 9.2 displays a completed Clinical Reasoning Web for this case.

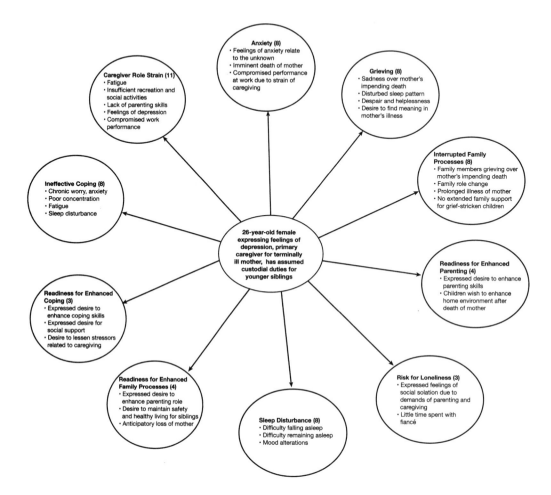

Figure 9.1   Clinical Reasoning Web: Young Adult and Mental Health Issues: Connections from Medical Diagnosis to Nursing Diagnoses.

TABLE 9.2 NURSING DOMAINS, NURSING DIAGNOSES, AND CONNECTIONS

Nursing Domain	Class	Nursing Diagnoses	Web Connections
Psychosocial Domain	Roles/Relationships	Caregiver Role Strain	11
		Interrupted Family Processes	8
	Coping	Ineffective Coping	10
	Emotion	Grieving	8
	Knowledge	Readiness for Enhanced Coping	10
		Readiness for Enhanced Parenting	5
		Readiness for Enhanced Family Processes	4
Functional Domain	Comfort	Anxiety	7
	Sleep/Rest	Disturbed Sleep Pattern	8
Environmental Domain	Risk Management	Risk for Loneliness	3
Physiological Domain			

The keystone issue, the nursing diagnosis with the most connections, emerges as a priority problem. It is the basis for defining the patient's present state, and this in turn is contrasted with a desired outcome state (Kuiper et al., 2009). Identifying the keystone issue guides clinical reasoning by identifying the central NANDA-I diagnosis that needs to be addressed first and enables the nurse to focus on subsequent care planning (Butcher & Johnson, 2012; Herdman & Kamitsuru, 2014). After a keystone issue is identified, there is continued knowledge work to identify the complementary nature of the problems ~ outcomes using the juxtaposing thinking strategy. The keystone issue and nursing diagnosis, in this case, is Caregiver Role Strain. Interventions are chosen to assist Miss Davis with coping and resolving mental conflicts. These interventions are likely to influence other issues that are identified on the web.

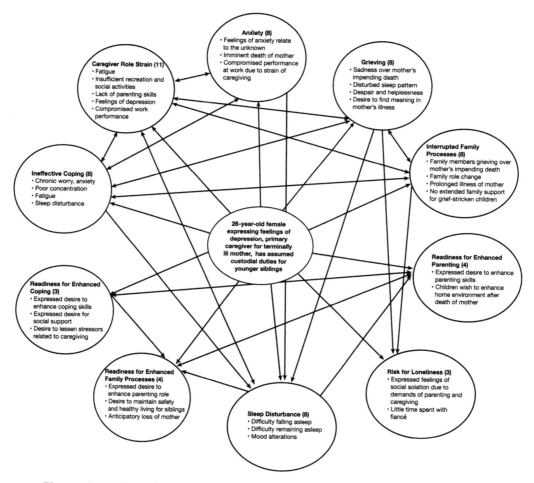

Figure 9.2   Clinical Reasoning Web: Young Adult and Mental Illness: Connections Among Nursing Diagnoses.

STOP AND THINK

1. What are the relationships between and among the identified problems (diagnoses)?

2. What keystone issue(s) emerge?

COMPLETING THE OPT CLINICAL REASONING MODEL

After the Reasoning Web has been completed with identification of the keystone and cue logic, the OPT Model of Clinical Reasoning can be completed. All sections of the OPT Model are completed with the case study described in this chapter.

Patient-in-Context Story

Exhibit 9.1 displays the patient-in-context story for the young adult Darlene Davis. On the far-right side of the OPT Model in Figure 9.3, the patient-in-context story is recorded. This story underscores the patient demographics, medical diagnoses, and current situation. The information placed in this box is presented in a brief format with some relevant facts that support the rest of the model.

EXHIBIT 9.1

Patient-in-Context Story

Miss Davis, a 26-year-old female, has served for the past 6 months as the primary caregiver for her terminally ill 53-year-old mother who has stage IV ovarian cancer. Miss Davis, the oldest of three children, was recently granted guardianship of her two younger siblings (ages 15 and 13 years). Her mother has been receiving hospice care at home due to her rapidly deteriorating condition. Miss Davis has been the primary caregiver for her mother since her diagnosis.

Miss Davis has reported that over the past 2 months she has experienced feelings of depression, anxiety, fear of the unknown, a loss of personal freedom, and grief related to the impending death of her mother.

Social: Miss Davis has been engaged for the past 6 months to her long-term boyfriend but has not spent much time with him for the past 3 months and has not seen close friends. She has confided to the nurses that she hopes she can regain feelings of optimism.

Diagnostic Cluster/Cue Logic

The next step in the care planning process is completing the *diagnostic cluster/cue logic*. The keystone issue is placed at the bottom of the column with all the other identified nursing diagnoses listed above it, in priority order. At this point, the nurse reflects on this list to ask if there is evidence to support these nursing

EXHIBIT 9.2

Diagnostic Cluster/Cue Logic

1. Ineffective Coping (10)

2. Social Isolation (8)

3. Grieving (8)

4. Interrupted Family Processes (8)

5. Disturbed Sleep Pattern (8)

6. Anxiety (7)

7. Readiness for Enhanced Parenting (5)

8. Readiness for Enhanced Family Processes (4)

9. Risk for Loneliness (3)

Keystone Issue/Theme
Caregiver Role Strain (11)

EXHIBIT 9.3

Frame

26-year-old Caucasian female who has served as the caregiver for her terminally ill mother and has recently taken on custodial responsibilities for her two siblings who are younger than 18 years. Expressed feelings of sadness, fatigue, social isolation, sleep disturbance, and weight loss.

diagnoses and whether the keystone issue is correctly identified. *Cue logic* is the deliberate structuring of patient-in-context data to discern the meaning for nursing care (Butcher & Johnson, 2012). In this case study, the nursing diagnoses depicted in the outlying ovals on the reasoning web are recorded under diagnostic cluster/cue logic on the OPT Model Clinical Reasoning Worksheet along with the number of arrows radiating to/from each diagnosis. Exhibit 9.2 displays the identified keystone issue—in this case, Caregiver Role Strain—and it is listed directly below the other nursing diagnoses.

Framing

In the center and top of the worksheet is a box to indicate the *frame* or theme that best represents the background issue(s) regarding the patient-in-context story. The frame of this case is a 26-year-old Caucasian female who has served as the caregiver for her terminally ill mother and has recently taken on custodial responsibilities for her two younger siblings. She has expressed feelings of sadness, fatigue, social isolation, sleep disturbances, and weight loss. This frame helps to organize the present state and outcome state, and it illustrates the gaps between them to provide insights about essential care needs. The frame is the lens or background view to help the nurse differentiate this patient schema and prototype from others the nurse might have dealt with in the past. The interventions and tests that will be used in this care plan are specific to the frame that is identified. Exhibit 9.3 displays the frame in the case of Miss Davis.

Present State

The *present state* is a description of the patient-in-context story or the initial condition of the patient (Butcher & Johnson, 2012). The items listed in this section change over time as a result of nursing actions and the patient's situation. The cues and problems identified for the patient listed under the keystone issue capture the present state of the patient. These are the problems in which the care of the patient will be planned, implemented, and evaluated. The present-state items are listed in the oval of the identified keystone issue and, in this case, there are six primary issues related to the keystone issue: 1) fatigue and sad affect, 2) insufficient recreational and social activities, 3) expressed lack of parenting skills, 4) feelings of depression, 5) compromised performance at work, and 6) lack of leisure time to spend with fiancé and siblings. Exhibit 9.4 displays the list of present-state issues that relate to the keystone issue and will be subjected to tests to determine whether the identified outcomes are achieved.

Outcome State

Given a defined present state, consideration must be given to desired outcomes that will be achieved to resolve the keystone issue (see Exhibit 9.5). In other words, one outcome state or goal is listed for each present-state item, and each can be tested and achieved through nursing and collaborative interventions. In

EXHIBIT 9.4

Present State

1. Fatigue and sad affect

2. Insufficient recreational and social activities

3. Lack of parenting skills

4. Feelings of depression

5. Compromised performance at work

6. Lack of leisure time to spend with fiancé and siblings

EXHIBIT 9.5

Outcome State

1. **Caregiver Emotional Health:** Identifies means to achieve respite care.

2. **Caregiver Well-Being:** Participation in social and self-care activities.

3. **Parenting Performance:** Identification of resources and support to develop parenting skills.

4. **Coping:** Identification of effective coping strategies.

5. **Anxiety:** Identifies strategies and seeks means in which to alleviate distress at work including financial resources that allow for reduction in work hours.

6. **Caregiver Social Involvement:** Participation in leisure activities with fiancé and sisters.

this case study, the outcome states with NOC labels (in bold) aim to assist Miss Davis to 1) identify means to achieve respite care, 2) participate in social and self-care activities, 3) identify resources and support to develop parenting skills, 4) identify effective coping strategies, 5) identify strategies and seek means in which to alleviate distress at work including financial resources that allow for reduction in work hours, and 6) participate in leisure activities with fiancé and sisters.

Because each present state and its corresponding outcome state directly relate to each other, they are placed next to each other for juxtaposition. This placement assists the nurse with comparative analysis and reflection while exercising clinical reasoning in this care situation.

Tests

The differences or gaps between the present state and outcome state become the foci of concern in the next step of care planning. The nurse must consider what tests and related interventions are most appropriate to fill the gap between the present state and the desired outcomes. Based on these clinical decisions, the nurse considers evidence that might indicate whether the gaps have been filled. In collaboration with other healthcare providers and the patient, tests are conducted to measure changes and gather data. The nurse asks what and if clinical indicators are available for each desired outcome state—that is, what to consider as to whether the desired outcome is achieved. The tests chosen in this case include 1) the Fatigue Severity Scale and respite care, 2) self-reports of access to community resources, 3) Modified Caregiver Strain Risk Index, 4) utilization of financial resources and community support, 5) evidence of a reduced work schedule, and 6) leisure activity participation. The tests for Miss Davis are displayed in Exhibit 9.6.

EXHIBIT 9.6

Tests

1. Fatigue Severity Scale; respite care

2. Self-reports of community resource access

3. Modified Caregiver Strain Risk Index

4. Utilization of financial resources & community support

5. Evidence of a reduced work schedule

6. Leisure activity participation

STOP AND THINK

1. Is the patient-in-context story complete?

2. How am I framing the situation?

3. How is the *present state* defined?

4. What is/are the desired outcomes?

5. What outcomes do I have in mind given the diagnoses?

6. What is/are the gaps or complementary pairs (~) of outcomes and present states?

7. What are the clinical indicators of the desired outcomes?

8. On what scales or tests will the desired outcome be measured?

9. How will I know when the desired targeted outcomes are achieved?

Interventions

At the bottom of the OPT Model of Clinical Reasoning Worksheet, there is a box that indicates *Patient Care Interventions* (NIC), which are the evidence-based nursing care activities that will assist the patient to reach the outcome state. The nurse must make clinical decisions or choices about interventions that will help the patient transition from present state to the desired outcome state. As interventions are implemented, the nurse evaluates the degree to which outcomes are being achieved. Interventions are evidence-based and gathered from current resources such as the literature, recognized textbooks, and prototype examples. Rationales are listed and cited in a separate page column next to interventions.

Listing the rationales for each intervention enhances understanding and justification for nursing activities. The interventions and the rationales for this case study are listed in Table 9.3 and include the measures of noninvasive pain relief methods and assessment, encouraging verbalization of feelings and reflection on life achievements, and facilitating resources to support spiritual care.

STOP AND THINK

1. What clinical decisions or interventions help to achieve the outcomes?

2. What specific intervention activities will I implement?

3. Why am I considering these activities?

TABLE 9.3   INTERVENTIONS AND RATIONALES

Interventions	Rationales

1. a. Screen for caregiver role strain at the onset of the care situation, at regular intervals throughout the care situation, and with changes in care recipient status and care transitions (Ackley & Ladwig, 2017).
 	
   b. Regularly monitor signs of depression, anxiety, burden and deteriorating physical health in the caregiver throughout the care situation (Ackley & Ladwig, 2017).
 	
2. a. Assist caregiver to find personal time to meet her needs, learn stress management techniques and to schedule regular respite time (Ackley & Ladwig, 2017).
 	
   b. Teach the caregiver stress-reducing techniques (Gulanick & Myers, 2014).
	1. Caregiver assessment should be done at regular intervals throughout the care trajectory (Adelman et al., 2014, as cited in Ackley & Ladwig, 2017, p. 202).
	
	2. a. Interventions to provide support for family caregivers have shown improvements in caregiver health (Basu et al., 2013, as cited in Ackley & Ladwig, 2017, p. 202).
	
	   b. It is important that the caregiver has the opportunity to relax and reenergize emotionally throughout the day to be able to emotionally and physically assume care responsibilities (Gulanick & Myers, 2014, p. 42).

Interventions	Rationales
3. a. Support groups can be used to gain mutual and educational support (Ackley & Ladwig, 2017). b. Regularly monitor social support for the caregiver and help the caregiver identify and use appropriate support systems for varying times in the care situation (Ackley & Ladwig, 2017). 4. a. Assist the client to expect positive outcomes and recognize the pathways to achieve the positive outcomes. b. Identify agencies that may be helpful, such as support groups, psychotherapists, and grief specialists (Carpenito, 2016). 5. a. Help the caregiver identify competing occupational demands and potential benefits to maintaining work as a way of providing normalcy. Guide caregivers to seek ways to maintain employment through mechanisms such as job sharing or decreasing hours at work (Ackley & Ladwig, 2017). b. Suggest ways for caregiver to use time more efficiently (Ralph & Taylor, 2014). 6. Stress the importance of taking care of self (rest-exercise balance, stress management, supportive social networks, maintaining a sense of humor, and advising caregiver to initiate phone contacts or visits for friends) (Carpenito, 2016, p. 132).	3. a. Support groups can improve depressed symptoms and burden, particularly for female caregivers (Chien et al., 2011, as cited in Ackley & Ladwig, 2017, p. 203). b. Lower levels of perceived support can cause caregiver to feel abandoned and increase their distress (Hwang et al., 2011, as cited in Ackley & Ladwig, 2017, p. 202). 4. a. Research shows that these actions facilitate the development of hope as a strength (Proctor et al., 2011, as cited in Ackley & Ladwig, 2017, p. 464). b. People with few supportive relationships have more difficulty grieving (Leming & Dickinson, 2010; Varcarelis, 2011, as cited in Carpenito, 2016, p. 351). 5. Employed caregivers report that work can provide a sense of fulfillment, refuge, and satisfaction (Eldh & Carlsson, 2011, as cited in Ackley & Ladwig, 2017, p. 203). 6. Numerous researchers have identified consistent social supports as the single most significant factor that reduces or prevents caregiver role strain (Clipp & George, 1990; Pearlin et al., 1990; Sheifld, 1992, as cited in Carpenito, 2016, p. 132).

Judgments

The final step in constructing the OPT Model Worksheet is to reflect on the tests and interventions to determine whether the outcomes were achieved. The consequences of the tests are data one uses to make clinical judgments (Pesut, 2008). In the far-left column on the OPT Model of Clinical Reasoning Worksheet,

EXHIBIT 9.7

Judgments

1. Patient has verbalized means in which to take time for herself away from caregiving and parental responsibilities.

2. Patient has joined a physical fitness facility. Patient reports that she is getting more sleep than before.

3. Patient identified community and school resources for parenting support.

4. Patient has listed activities to facilitate relaxation, means in which to become engaged in recreational activities and leisure events involving the whole family.

5. Patient has met with her supervisor at work and has negotiated a weekly reduction in work hours.

6. Patient has engaged in leisure activities with her fiancé and siblings twice in the past week.

judgments are listed for each outcome. *Judgments* are conclusions about outcome achievements. Each judgment requires four elements: 1) a contrast between present and desired state, 2) criteria associated with a desired outcome (i.e., test), 3) consideration of the effects and influence of nurse interventions, and 4) a conclusion as to whether the intervention has been effective in the outcome achievement (Kuiper et al., 2009). Based on the analysis of tests, judgments are made as to whether the problem has been resolved or not. The nurse may have to reframe or attribute a different meaning to the facts in the patient-in-context story. Table 9.4 depicts the outcome states and judgments for this case study. Exhibit 9.7 displays the judgments in this case.

TABLE 9.4 TABLE OF OUTCOME STATES AND JUDGMENTS

Outcome State	Judgment
Caregiver Emotional Health: Patient will identify means to achieve respite care.	Fatigue Severity Scale Score: 34 (most likely not suffering from fatigue).
	Patient has verbalized three means in which to take time for herself away from caregiving and parental responsibilities.
Caregiver Well-Being: Patient will take part in social and self-care activities.	Patient has joined a physical fitness facility. Patient reports that she is getting more sleep than before.
Social Support: Patient will identify resources and support to develop parenting skills.	Modified Strain Risk Scale score: 14/26.
	Patient has listed community resources and church members for parenting support.
Coping: Patient will identify effective coping strategies.	Patient has listed activities to facilitate relaxation, means in which to become engaged in recreational activities, and leisure events involving the whole family.
Anxiety: Patient will seek strategies to alleviate distress at work including financial resources to allow for reduction in work hours.	Patient has met with her supervisor at work and has negotiated a weekly reduction in work hours.
Caregiver Emotional Health & Social Involvement: Patient will participate in leisure activities with fiancé and sisters.	Patient has engaged in leisure activities with both her fiancé and siblings twice within the past week.

STOP AND THINK

1. Given the tests that I choose, what is my clinical judgment of the evidence regarding reaching the outcome state?

2. Based on my judgment, have I achieved the outcome or do I need to reframe the situation?

3. How can I specifically take this experience and learning with me into the future as schema to reason about similar cases?

The Completed OPT Model of Clinical Reasoning

The completed OPT Model of Clinical Reasoning for a young adult caregiver with health issues is displayed in Figure 9.3.

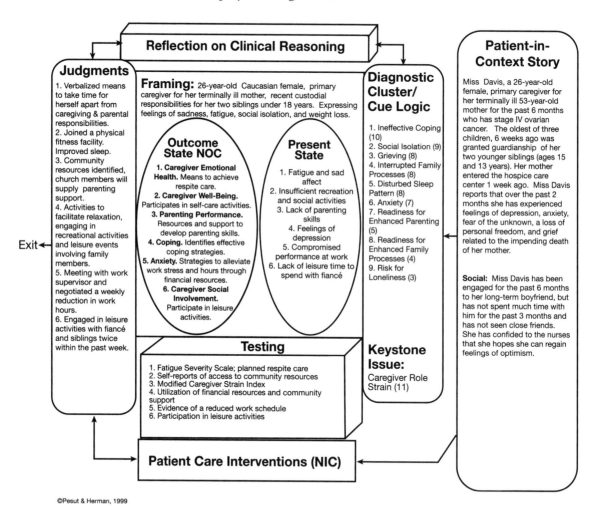

©Pesut & Herman, 1999

Figure 9.3 OPT Model of Clinical Reasoning for Young Adult and Mental Health Issues.

SUMMARY

Clinical reasoning for patients and family members who are experiencing Caregiver Role Strain associated with working with terminally ill patients receiving palliative care begins with an understanding of the patient's condition and the impact of care and emotional stress placed on the caregiver given the context of the family dynamics. Using the OPT Model as a conceptual framework and the Clinical Reasoning Web as a tool helps develop the clinical reasoning associated with a particular case. The OPT Clinical Reasoning Model provides a visual illustration of where the patient is (present state) and where the nurse hopes the patient to be (outcome state), all of which is framed through identification of background issues of the patient's story (framing). Through "spinning and weaving" of the web, the nurse can determine the priority of care through the generation of hypotheses and thinking out loud (self-talk) to make explicit functional relationships between and among competing nursing care needs. After the priority issue (the keystone) is identified, planning can begin. In this case study, the identified keystone is Caregiver Role Strain.

The OPT Clinical Reasoning Model provides a visual illustration of where the caregiver in this situation is (present state). Six present state items were identified: 1) fatigue and sad affect, 2) insufficient recreation and social activities, 3) lack of parenting skills, 4) depression, 5) compromised performance at work, and 6) lack of leisure time with significant other.

In this case study the nurse was able to determine these outcomes (using NOC terminology) to be: 1) caregiver emotional health, 2) caregiver well-being, 3) parenting performance, 4) coping, 5) anxiety, and 6) caregiver social involvement. The present-state and outcome-state items are framed through identification of background issues of the caregiver's story (framing). The nurse framed the caregiver situation as a 26-year-old Caucasian female who is the caregiver for her terminally ill mother and who has recently assumed custodial responsibilities of her two minor siblings. The caregiver has expressed feelings of sadness, fatigue, social isolation, and weight loss.

Ultimately the nurse must determine what evidence supports evaluations (tests) that bridge the gap between the two states and make decisions (judgments) of progress the caregiver has made in meeting the outcomes. The nurse identified tests to consider: 1) Fatigue Severity Scale, 2) self-reports of access to community resources, 3) Modified Caregiver Strain Index, 4) verbalized utilization of financial resources and community support, 5) evidence of reduced work hours, and 6) the caregiver's participation in leisure activities. Experience with case studies of this nature augments the nurse's experience and adds to her clinical reasoning skill set that can be activated with future cases of a similar nature.

KEY POINTS

- Clinical reasoning for a family member caring for patients receiving hospice and palliative care can be promoted with the OPT Model.

- A step-by-step approach is used in this case study involving a caregiver for a terminally ill patient receiving palliative and hospice care. This approach can be used for similar schema and prototypes of end-of-life care in other health settings.

- Various thinking and reflection strategies are used throughout the clinical reasoning process to complete the Clinical Reasoning Web and OPT Model of Clinical Reasoning.

STUDY QUESTIONS AND ACTIVITIES

1. Describe in your words the benefits of using the OPT Clinical Reasoning Model to plan and evaluate patient care given the scenario and case presented in this chapter.

2. How does this model differ from other nursing plans of care models?

3. What thinking strategies would you use in spinning and weaving the Reasoning Web?

4. Are there other nursing diagnoses you would assign to this case study involving a caregiver? If so and given the caregiver data presented in the case study, what would you suggest?

5. Are there other priorities you would give to this case study? In other words, is there a different keystone issue you would recommend in planning care?

6. What other tests would you consider appropriate to bridge the gap between present state and outcome state in this scenario?

References

AARP and the National Alliance for Caregiving. (2015). Caregiving in the U.S.: Special report. Retrieved from http://www.aarp.org/content/dam/aarp/ppi/2015/caregiving-in-the-united-states-2015-report-revised.pdf

Ackley, B., & Ladwig, G. (2017). *Nursing diagnosis handbook: An evidence-based guide to planning care* (11th ed.). St. Louis, MO: Mosby Elsevier.

American Heart Association. (Jan. 2017). Understanding blood pressure readings. Retrieved from http://www.heart.org/HEARTORG/Conditions/HighBloodPressure/KnowYourNumbers/Understanding-Blood-Pressure-Readings_UCM_301764_Article.jsp#.WJJjg6Yo4eE

Butcher, H. K., Bulechek, G. M., Dochterman, J. M., & Wagner, C. M. (in press). *Nursing Interventions Classification (NIC)* (7th ed.). St. Louis, MO: Mosby Elsevier.

Burns, C., Archbold, P., Stewart, B., & Shelton, K. (1993). New diagnosis: Caregiver role strain. *International Journal of Nursing Knowledge, 4*(2), 70–76.

Butcher, H., & Johnson, M. (2012). Use of linkages for clinical reasoning and quality improvement. In M. Johnson, S. Moorhead, G. Bulechek, H. Butcher, M. Maas, & E. Swanson (Eds.), *NOC and NIC linkages to NANDA-I and clinical conditions* (3rd ed.), p. 11–23. Maryland Heights, MO: Elsevier.

Carpenito, L. J. (2016). *Nursing diagnosis: Application to clinical practice* (15th ed.). Philadelphia, PA: Wolters Kluwer Health.

Clipp, E. C., & George, L. K. (1990). Caregiver needs and patterns of social support. *Journal of Gerontology, 45*(3), S102–S111.

Gulanick, M., & Myers, J. (2014). *Nursing care plans: Diagnoses, interventions and outcomes.* Maryland Heights, MO: Elsevier.

Herdman, T. H., & Kamitsuru, S. (Eds.). (2014). *NANDA International nursing diagnoses: Definition and classifications, 2015-2017.* Oxford, England: Wiley Blackwell.

Johnson, M., Moorhead, S., Bulechek, G., Butcher, H., Maas, M., & Swanson, E. (Eds.). (2012). *NOC and NIC linkages to NANDA-I and clinical conditions* (3rd ed.). Maryland Heights, MO: Elsevier.

Kuiper, R. A., Pesut, D. J., & Arms, T. (2016). *Clinical reasoning and care coordination in advanced practice nursing.* New York, NY: Springer Publishing Company.

Kuiper, R., Pesut, D., & Kautz, D. (2009). Promoting the self-regulation of clinical reasoning skills in nursing students. *The Open Nursing Journal, 3*, 76–85. Retrieved from http://doi.org/10.2174/1874434600903010076

Leming, M., & Dickinson, G. (2010). *Understanding dying, death, and bereavement* (7th ed.). Belmont, CA: Wadsworth Cengage Learning.

Moorhead, S., Johnson, M., Maas, M. O., & Swanson, E. (Eds.). (2013). *Nursing Outcomes Classification (NOC): Measurement of health outcomes* (5th ed.). St. Louis, MO: Elsevier.

National Institutes of Health. (2015). *Coping with caregiving: Take care of yourself while caring for others.* NIH News in Health newsletter. Retrieved from https://newsinhealth.nih.gov/issue/dec2015/feature1

Pearlin, L., Mullan, J., Semple, S., & Skaff, M. (1990). Caregiving and the stress process: An overview of concepts and their measures. *The Gerontologist, 30*(5), 583–594.

Pesut, D. (2008). Thoughts on thinking with complexity in mind. In C. Lindberg, S. Nash, & C. Lindberg (Eds.), *On the edge: Nursing in the age of complexity* (pp. 211–238). Bordentown, NJ: Plexus Press.

Phillips, A. C., Gallagher, S., Hunt, K., Der, G., & Carroll, D. (2009). Symptoms of depression in non-routine caregivers: The role of caregiver strain and burden. *British Journal of Clinical Psychology, 48*(4), 335–346.

Potter, P. A., Perry, A. G., Stockert, P., & Hall, A. (2017). *Fundamentals of nursing* (9th ed.). St Louis, MO: Elsevier.

Ralph, S. S., & Taylor, C. M. (2014). *Sparks and Taylor's nursing diagnosis pocket guide* (9th ed.). Philadelphia, PA: Wolters Kluwer Health, Lippincott Williams & Wilkins.

10

CLINICAL REASONING AND WOMEN'S HEALTH ISSUES

LEARNING OUTCOMES

- Explain the components of the OPT Model that are essential for clinical reasoning to manage the problems, interventions, and outcomes of a patient who has a women's health problem of endometriosis.

- Identify relevant nursing diagnoses specific to the health issues of a patient with endometriosis.

- Identify outcomes appropriate for a woman with the health problem of advanced endometriosis.

- Describe relevant tests and clinical judgments used to reason about present-state to outcome-state changes for a woman with advanced endometriosis and resultant surgical intervention.

- Describe the different thinking processes that support clinical reasoning skills and strategies to determine priorities and desired outcomes for a woman with advanced endometriosis and ensuing surgical intervention.

This chapter presents a case study involving a 40-year-old female who was admitted after having a robot-assisted total vaginal hysterectomy with bilateral salping-oophorectomy and colostomy creation due to severe, stage IV endometriosis. For years, she has suffered with the painful effects of endometriosis, many times avoiding particular treatments due to beliefs about medications. At this time, she is on the medical-surgical unit recovering from surgery with her husband at the bedside.

Endometriosis is a common benign condition in childbearing women, particularly during their 30s and 40s. It is estimated that 1 in 10 women are affected by endometriosis (American Society for Reproductive Medicine [ASRM], 2012). Endometriosis occurs when the lining of the uterus, the endometrium, implants outside of the uterus. One theory about its development is that some of the endometrial cells that are shed during monthly menses flow backward onto the ovaries and pelvis via the fallopian tubes (ASRM, 2012). These implants can end up on the bladder, bowel, ovaries, or even the diaphragm. This endometrial tissue responds to normal monthly hormonal changes in progesterone and estrogen by thickening, breaking down, and bleeding (Mayo Clinic, 2016). However, the tissue cannot be shed normally, which causes blood blisters to form, and those can further develop into cysts, scar tissue, or adhesions (Johns Hopkins, 2016). Adenomyosis occurs when endometrial tissue is within, or grows into, the muscle layer or myometrium of the uterus (Mayo Clinic, 2016). This process can cause an enlargement of the uterus.

Women experience varying symptoms of endometriosis and adenomyosis. It is important to note that symptoms do not necessarily correlate with the severity of the condition. For instance, some women experience no symptoms and have severe disease, whereas others have severe symptoms and minimal disease. Symptoms include pain that may be in the abdomen, lower back, or pelvic areas; heavy periods or irregular bleeding; painful menstrual cramps; painful intercourse; pain with bowel movements or urination worsened during menses; fatigue; nausea; constipation; diarrhea; and infertility. Many women describe a progression or worsening of symptoms over time.

Several factors put women at risk for developing endometriosis and include never having children, early onset of menses, menopause at an older age, shortened menstrual cycles (less than every 27 days), higher levels of estrogen, greater lifetime exposure to estrogen, alcohol use, and one or more first-degree relatives with endometriosis (mother, sister, or aunt) (Mayo Clinic, 2016). Complications from endometriosis and adenomyosis include infertility, ovarian cancer, and endometriosis-associated adenocarcinoma.

Diagnosing endometriosis begins with a thorough history and physical assessment, a pelvic examination, and direct visualization via laparoscopy. Additional tests might include ultrasound, hysterosalpingography, transvaginal ultrasound, a complete blood count, and cancer antigen-125. "Endometriosis is classified into one of four stages (I-minimal, II-mild, III-moderate, and IV-severe) depending on location, extent, and depth of endometriosis implants; presence and severity of adhesions; and presence and size of ovarian endometriomas" (ASRM, 2012, paragraph 6). Women are treated either medically with pain medications, hormone therapy, or surgery. Surgery may entail conservative efforts aimed at preserving childbearing ability or radical interventions such as a total hysterectomy with or without removal of the ovaries and fallopian tubes. Depending on the life stage and health history, a woman with the history of an estrogen receptor positive breast cancer who undergoes total hysterectomy might not be a candidate to receive hormone therapy to treat the sudden onset of surgical menopause.

THE PATIENT STORY

Meet Mrs. Virginia Graham, a 40-year-old African-American female who was admitted to the surgical unit after scheduled robotic-assisted laparoscopic total vaginal hysterectomy with bilateral salpingoophorectomy (TVH/BSO). She complained of heavy menstrual periods for years with severe cramping, passing clots, painful intercourse, and fatigue, which have worsened over time. She was initially referred for surgical evaluation after a hysteroscopy, which revealed small fibroids. An exploratory laparoscopy 6 months ago revealed severe endometriosis, a large endometrioma on her left ovary, which was incised and drained, and findings consistent with adenomyosis. The endometriosis was so severe (stage IV) that her uterus had adhered to her pelvic wall, and her vagina had adhered to her rectum and lower sigmoid colon. Following the hysterectomy, the gynecologist referred her for evaluation by a colorectal surgeon for a possible resection and colostomy.

Medical History

Mrs. Graham refused other more conservative medicinal therapies prior to her exploratory laparoscopy. Obstetric history reveals gravida 3, para 2, and one abortion. She has never had any sexually transmitted diseases and is monogamous in sexual activity with her husband, but it has decreased over time due to pain with intercourse. Mrs. Graham stated during the pre-operative evaluation that "she is pretty certain she does not want any more children."

Physical Assessment

For this case, the assessment took place in the post-anesthesia care unit (PACU). She is sleepy, pale, rouses to verbal stimuli, and is oriented to person, place, and time once awake. She has periods of bradycardia and trace edema in bilateral lower extremities. Sequential compression devices are on her legs. There are five laparoscopic puncture sites on her abdomen, which are open to air and closed with Dermabond®. There is one small ecchymosis at the right upper quadrant puncture site; otherwise her abdomen is soft, slightly distended with hypoactive bowel sounds in all four quadrants. The colostomy is in the left lower quadrant with a small amount of bloody drainage. The stoma is beefy red and peristomal skin is intact. The peri-pad shows a small amount of blood. She is 5'4" tall and weighs 127 pounds. Her body mass index is 21.8 (normal). Vital signs include a temperature of 97.6° Fahrenheit, regular heart rate of 58 beats per minute, respirations at 12 breaths per minute, oxygen saturation of 99% on room air, and a blood pressure of 94/64 mmHg. Mrs. Graham rates her pain as 2 on a scale of 0 to 10 within the abdomen, which she describes as "pressure." She received 2 mg Dilaudid prior to leaving the PACU.

Laboratory Test Results

Laboratory tests include a hemoglobin of 10 gm/dL (low), hematocrit of 31% (low), and CA 125 (Cancer Antigen 125) of 274 u/mL (high).

Medications

Medications include oxycodone 5mg by mouth every 4 hours as needed for pain, hydromorphone (Dilaudid) 1mg intravenously every 2 hours if needed for pain, Estradiol transdermal patch 0.5 mg topically now, and then to be applied twice per week, and pitavastatin (Livalo) 2 mg orally every night at bedtime. Mrs. Graham has no drug allergies.

Psychosocial Assessment

Mrs. Graham is a nonsmoker and social drinker (<1 drink every week). She is Baptist and is very active in her church. Both parents and her younger brother are alive. She currently works at a community college and attends classes part time at the local university in the MBA program. She says she runs, bikes, walks for exercise, and likes to read books for relaxation.

Current Physical Condition

Mrs. Graham is currently recovering from an 8-hour surgery. Her husband is concerned about her reaction to surgery and the temporary colostomy. He is hopeful she will become pain-free, begin to enjoy her life, and that their intimacy will return when she is physically and emotionally ready. She will be discharged in a few days and follow up with both surgeons.

PATIENT-CENTERED PLAN OF CARE USING THE OPT MODEL OF CLINICAL REASONING

The patient story in this case study has been obtained from all possible sources, including a physical examination, a current list of medications, and care conferences. The lists of patient problems and relevant nursing diagnoses support the creation of the Clinical Reasoning Web Worksheet and the OPT Model of Clinical Reasoning that help the nurse begin to filter the assessment data and information, frame the context of the story, and focus on the priority care needs and outcomes (Butcher & Johnson, 2012).

PATIENT PROBLEMS AND NURSING DIAGNOSES IDENTIFICATION

The first step of care planning is to identify the various problems and cues presented by the patient and select the nursing diagnoses whose defining characteristics capture these cues and problems.

Nursing Care Priority Identification

The medical diagnosis for this patient is stage IV endometriosis, status post robotic-assisted total vaginal hysterectomy, bilateral salpingoophorectomy with colon resection, and the creation of a colostomy. The nurse identifies the cues and problems collected from the physiologic assessment, psychosocial assessment, and the medical record. Similar problems and cues are clustered for interpretation and meaning. Then relevant nursing diagnoses that "fit" the cluster of cues and problems are identified based on definitions and defining characteristics of each nursing diagnosis. An assessment worksheet listing the major taxonomy domains,

classes of each domain, patient cues and problems, relevant NANDA-I diagnoses with definitions (Herdman & Kamitsuru, 2014), Nursing Outcomes Classification (NOC) (Moorhead, Johnson, Maas, & Swanson, 2013), and Nursing Interventions Classification (NIC) (Butcher, Bulechek, Dochterman, & Wagner [in press]) labels has been created. This worksheet is designed to assist the nurse in organizing patient care issues and to generate appropriate nursing diagnoses. An example of a completed table of the taxonomy domains, classes, patient cues and problems, relevant nursing diagnoses, and suggested NOC and NIC labels for this case study is presented in
Table 10.1.

STOP AND THINK

1. What taxonomy domains are affected, and which diagnoses have I generated?

2. What cues/evidence/data from the patient and evidence from the patient assessment support the diagnoses?

TABLE 10.1 DOMAINS, CLASSES (NANDA-I TAXONOMY II), PATIENT CUES/PROBLEMS, NURSING DIAGNOSES, NOC AND NIC LABELS

Domain	Classes	Identified Patient Problems
Activity/Rest: The production, conservation, expenditure, or balance of energy resources	**Sleep/Rest:** Slumber, repose, ease, relaxation, or inactivity	• Difficulty staying asleep • Up with hot flashes and night sweats • Tired all day • Daily activities being affected • Expresses desire to improve sleep so she can go back to her normal functioning
	Energy Balance: A dynamic state of harmony between intake and expenditure of resources	• Chronic anemia • Hemoglobin 9.6 gm/dL • Difficulty getting through the workday and -week due to being exhausted and tired
Role Relationship: The positive and negative connections or associations between people or groups of people and the means by which those connections are demonstrated	**Family Relationships:** Associations of people who are biologically related or related by choice	• Hospital is 3 hours away from home • Not able to care for young children at home • Not able to drive for 4 weeks post-op • Husband took time off work to be with her during surgery but can't for recovery
	Role Performance: Quality of functioning in socially expected behavior patterns	• Supportive husband • Wants his wife to feel better because she has not been well in a long time • Anxious to see how their relationship is affected by the surgery

NANDA-I Nursing Diagnoses	Nursing Outcomes Classifications (NOC)	Nursing Intervention Classifications (NIC)
Disturbed Sleep Pattern: Time-limited interruptions of sleep amount and quality due to external factors	• Sleep	• Environmental Management: Comfort • Sleep Enhancement • Medication Management • Relaxation Therapy
Readiness for Enhanced Sleep: A pattern of natural, periodic suspension of relative consciousness to provide rest and sustain a desired lifestyle, which can be strengthened	• Sleep	• Environmental Management: Comfort • Sleep Enhancement • Medication Management • Relaxation Therapy
Fatigue: An overwhelming sustained sense of exhaustion and decreased capacity for physical and mental work at the usual level	• Endurance • Nutritional Status: Energy	• Energy Management • Nutrition Management
Interrupted Family Processes: Change in family relationships and/or functioning	• Family Coping • Family Functioning	• Coping Enhancement • Family Process Maintenance • Family Integrity Promotion
Readiness for Enhanced Relationship: A pattern of mutual partnership to provide for each other's needs, which can be strengthened	• Development: Middle Adulthood • Role Performance	• Role Enhancement

continues

TABLE 10.1 DOMAINS, CLASSES (NANDA-I TAXONOMY II), PATIENT CUES/PROBLEMS, NURSING DIAGNOSES, NOC AND NIC LABELS (CONTINUED)

Domain	Classes	Identified Patient Problems
Sexuality: Sexual identity, sexual function, and reproduction	**Sexual Identity:** The state of being a specific person in regard to sexuality and/or gender	• Pain with intercourse • Not as sexually active as she would like • Concerns about going through surgical menopause and its effects on sexuality • Wants sex life to improve
Coping/Stress Tolerance: Contending with life events/life processes	**Coping Responses:** The process of managing environmental stress	• Loss of childbearing ability • Sudden onset of menopause which she equates with "old lady" • Concerned she is not going to be an attractive "woman" anymore • Husband worried about wife's reaction to colostomy and how this will affect her

NANDA-I Nursing Diagnoses	Nursing Outcomes Classifications (NOC)	Nursing Intervention Classifications (NIC)
Sexual Dysfunction: The state in which an individual experiences a change in sexual function during the sexual response phases of desire, excitation, and/or orgasm, which is viewed as unsatisfying, unrewarding, or inadequate	• Physical Aging • Sexual Functioning	• Hormone Replacement Therapy • Emotional Support • Body Image Enhancement
Grieving: A normal complex process that includes emotional, physical, spiritual, social, and intellectual responses and behaviors by which individuals, families, and communities incorporate an actual, anticipated, or perceived loss into their daily lives	• Coping • Psychosocial Adjustment: Life Change	• Anticipatory Guidance • Coping Enhancement • Resiliency Promotion • Spiritual Support
Anxiety: Vague, uneasy feeling of discomfort or dread accompanied by an autonomic response (the source is often nonspecific or unknown to the individual); a feeling of apprehension caused by anticipation of danger It is an alerting sign that warns of impending danger and enables the individual to take measures to deal with that threat	• Anxiety Level • Anxiety Self-Control • Coping	• Anxiety Reduction • Coping Enhancement

continues

TABLE 10.1 DOMAINS, CLASSES (NANDA-I TAXONOMY II), PATIENT CUES/PROBLEMS, NURSING DIAGNOSES, NOC AND NIC LABELS   (CONTINUED)

Domain	Classes	Identified Patient Problems
Comfort: Freedom from danger, physical injury, or immune system damage; preservation from loss; and protection of safety and security	**Physical Comfort:** Sense of well-being or ease and/or freedom from pain	• Pelvic fullness and pressure • Rates pain between 2-6/10 • Requesting Dilaudid every 3 hours • "Gas pains" • Painful menses and pressure for years • Painful, non-pleasurable intercourse
Safety/Protection: Principles underlying conduct, thought, and behavior about acts, customs, or institutions viewed as being true or having intrinsic worth	**Physical Injury:** Bodily harm or hurt	• Laparoscopic puncture sites x 5 • New colostomy

Butcher, H., Bulechek, G., Dochterman, J., & Wagner, C. M. (in press).
Herdman, T. H., & Kamitsuru, S. (Eds.). (2014).
Moorhead, S., Johnson, M., Maas, M. O., & Swanson, E. (Eds.). (2013).

NANDA-I Nursing Diagnoses	Nursing Outcomes Classifications (NOC)	Nursing Intervention Classifications (NIC)
Acute Pain: Unpleasant sensory and emotional experience arising from actual or potential tissue damage or described in terms of such damage; sudden or slow onset of any intensity from mild to severe with an anticipated or predictable end	• Pain Level	• Pain management • Analgesic administration
Chronic Pain: Unpleasant sensory and emotional experience arising from actual or potential tissue damage or described in terms of such damage; sudden or slow onset of any intensity from mild to severe with an anticipated or predictable end and a duration of > 6 months		
Impaired Skin Integrity: Altered epidermis and/or dermis	• Tissue Integrity: Skin and Mucous Membranes • Wound Healing: Primary Intention	• Incision site care, Pain management, Skin surveillance

CREATING A CLINICAL REASONING WEB

The *Clinical Reasoning Web* is a means by which the nurse analyzes and reasons through complex patient stories for the purpose of finding and prioritizing key healthcare issues. Using the web, the nurse defines problems based on patient cues in the data, identifies nursing diagnoses to address and define the various problems, and determines relationships among these diagnoses (Kuiper, Pesut, & Kautz, 2009). The web is a visual representation and iterative analysis of the functional relationships among diagnostic hypotheses and results in a keystone issue that requires nursing care. In other words, the Clinical Reasoning Web represents a graphic illustration of how the elements of the patient's story and issues relate to one another and is depicted by sketching lines of association among the nursing diagnoses (Kuiper, Pesut, & Arms, 2016). Whereas medical diagnoses are consistent labels for a cluster of symptoms, patient stories vary; each Clinical Reasoning Web is written to reflect the patient's unique story and the human response to actual or potential health problems that are best represented in nursing diagnoses. For example, given two patients with identical medical diagnoses, the nurse might determine that different nursing diagnoses and keystone issues are the priority for each based on thinking strategies and diagnostic hypotheses associated with each case.

Constructing the Clinical Reasoning Web

After the problems are identified from the assessment data, evidence, and cues and the nursing diagnoses are chosen, the Clinical Reasoning Web is constructed using the following steps:

1. Place a general description of the patient in the central oval with the primary medical diagnoses. In this case study, the patient is a 40-year-old African-American female with stage IV endometriosis, status post robotic-assisted laparoscopic total vaginal hysterectomy with bilateral salpingoophorectomy (TVH/SBO) with colon resection and ostomy creation. She is currently hospitalized recovering from surgery.

2. Place each NANDA-I nursing diagnosis generated from the patient cues in the ovals surrounding the middle circle.

3. Under each nursing diagnosis, list supporting data that was gathered from the patient's story and assessment.

4. Because each nursing diagnosis is directly related to the center oval containing a brief description of the patient's situation, the nurse draws a line from the central oval to each of the outlying nursing diagnosis ovals. Figure 10.1 displays the beginning steps of constructing the Clinical Reasoning Web for this case study.

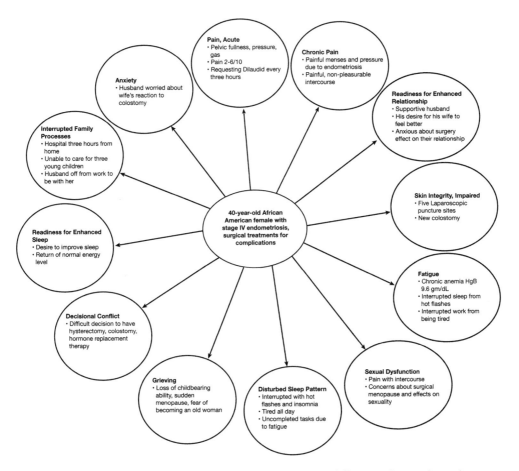

Figure 10.1   Clinical Reasoning Web: Middle-Aged Female with Endometriosis and Surgical Intervention: Connections from Medical Diagnosis to Nursing Diagnoses.

Spinning and Weaving the Reasoning Web

In spinning and weaving the Clinical Reasoning Web, the nurse must analyze and explain the relationships among the nursing diagnoses. This process involves thinking out loud; using self-talk; schema search; hypothesizing; if-then, how-so thinking; and comparative analysis, as described in Chapter 3 of this book. In doing so, the nurse determines possible connections and relationships among the nursing diagnoses contained in the outlying ovals.

The nurse continues to spin and weave using the following steps:

1. Consider how each of the nursing diagnoses and related healthcare issues it defines relates to all the other diagnoses. If there is a functional relationship between two diagnoses, then a line with a one-directional arrow is drawn to indicate a one-way connection; lines with two-directional arrows are drawn to indicate two-way connections. For example, what is the relationship between Anxiety and Disturbed Sleep Pattern? How are these two diagnoses related? How do they influence one another? In the case of Mrs. Graham, the nurse would consider whether Anxiety would cause Disturbed Sleep Patterns, or in a reciprocal fashion whether having Disturbed Sleep Patterns would contribute to the feelings of Anxiety. In this case, there is a two-way connection between Anxiety and Disturbed Sleep Pattern. Another example would be to consider how the nursing diagnosis Fatigue relates to the issue of Sexual Dysfunction. In this case, there is a one-way connection between them with Fatigue contributing to Sexual Dysfunction, but no relationship between Sexual Dysfunction and Fatigue. Therefore, a one-way connection is made from Fatigue to Sexual Dysfunction.

2. The first step is repeated with each of the other ovals to determine relationships for connections. If there are functional relationships, connections are drawn until the process is exhausted; visually, the web emerges.

3. When all connections are made, the lines leading to and from each oval with nursing diagnoses are counted and recorded. The numbers can be recorded on the Clinical Reasoning Web Worksheet. A table showing the hierarchy of priorities of Mrs. Graham's problems based on the number of connections is displayed in Table 10.2.

4. The nursing diagnosis with the most connecting lines radiating to and from that oval becomes the *keystone* issue. Figure 10.2 displays a completed Clinical Reasoning Web for this case.

TABLE 10.2 NURSING DOMAINS, NURSING DIAGNOSES, AND CONNECTIONS

Domain	Class	Nursing Diagnoses	Web Connections
Activity/Rest	Sleep/Rest	Disturbed Sleep Pattern	12
Activity/Rest	Energy Balance	Fatigue	11
Coping/Stress Tolerance	Coping Response	Grieving	11
Comfort	Physical Comfort	Chronic Pain	9
Sexuality	Sexual Function	Sexual Dysfunction	7
Roles/Relationships	Family Relationships	Interrupted Family Processes	7
Comfort	Physical Comfort	Acute Pain	7
Life Principles	Value/Belief/Action Congruence	Decisional Conflict	6
Activity/Rest	Sleep/Rest	Readiness for Enhanced Sleep	6
Roles/Relationships	Role Performance	Readiness for Enhanced Relationship	5
Coping/Stress Tolerance	Coping Response	Anxiety	5
Safety/Protection	Physical Injury	Impaired Skin Integrity	5

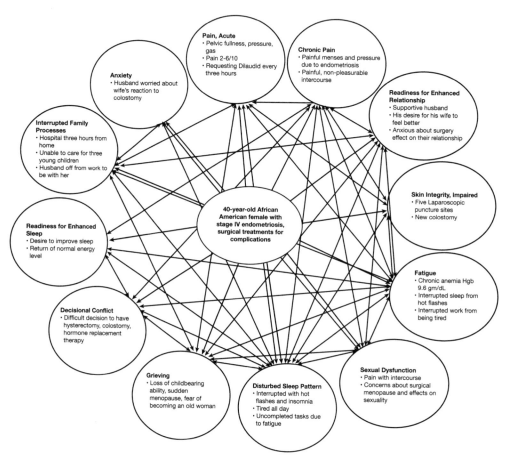

Figure 10.2 Clinical Reasoning Web: Middle-Aged Female with Endometriosis and Surgical Intervention: Connections Among Nursing Diagnoses.

The keystone issue, the nursing diagnosis with the most connections, emerges as a priority problem. It is the basis for defining the patient's present state, and this in turn is contrasted with a desired outcome state (Kuiper et al., 2009). Identifying the keystone issue guides clinical reasoning by identifying the central NANDA-I diagnosis that needs to be addressed first and enables the nurse to focus on subsequent care planning (Butcher & Johnson, 2012). After a keystone issue is identified, there is continued knowledge work to identify the complementary nature of the problems ~ outcomes using the juxtaposing thinking strategy. The keystone issue in this case is Disturbed Sleep Pattern. Interventions are chosen to assist

Mrs. Graham with coping and resolving her disturbed sleep patterns. In doing so, these interventions are likely to influence other issues that are identified on the web.

STOP AND THINK

1. What are the relationships between and among the identified problems (diagnoses)?

2. What *keystone* issue(s) emerge?

COMPLETING THE OPT MODEL OF CLINICAL REASONING

After the Clinical Reasoning Web has been completed with identification of the keystone and cue logic, the OPT Model of Clinical Reasoning can be completed. All sections of the OPT Model are completed with the case study described in this chapter.

Patient-in-Context Story

Exhibit 10.1 displays the patient-in-context story for the adult patient Virginia Graham. On the far-right side of the OPT Model in Figure 10.3, the patient-in-context story is recorded. This story underscores the patient demographics, medical diagnoses, and current situation. The information placed in this box is presented in a brief format with some relevant facts that support the rest of the model.

EXHIBIT 10.1

Patient-in-Context Story

Mrs. Graham, 40-year-old married African-American female, stage IV endometriosis and surgery.

Medical History: Obstetric history: gravida 3, para 2, abortions 1. Fractures of right great toe, left fibula. Hypercholesterolemia, Anemia

Surgical History: Exploratory laparotomy 6 months ago, endometriomas and endometriosis

Review of Systems: Cardiovascular: Trace edema bilateral lower extremities, 5 laparotomy puncture sites on abdomen, Dermabond®, small ecchymosis at RUQ site. GI: abdomen soft, distended, hypoactive bowel sounds 4 quadrants, colostomy bag to LLQ, small amount bloody drainage, stoma pink GU: Small amount blood on peri-pad. Height/Weight: 5'4"/127 lbs. BMI: 21.8 (normal).

Psychosocial: Active at Baptist church and works full time, Currently in MBA program. Children ages 9 and 11.

Vital Signs: Temperature 97.6F; Pulse 58 bpm, regular; Respirations 12 bpm; O2 sauration: 99% on room air; blood pressure: 134/84 mmHg; pain: 2/10 in abdomen, "pressure."

Laboratory Tests: Hgb 10 gm/dL, HCT 31%, CA 125- 274 u/mL

Medications: Oxycodone & Dilaudid PRN pain, Estradiol transdermal patch, Livalo 2mg

Diagnostic Cluster/Cue Logic

The next step in the care planning process is completing the *diagnostic cluster/cue logic*. The keystone issue is placed at the bottom of the column with all the other identified nursing diagnoses listed above it, in priority order. At this point, the nurse reflects on this list to ask whether there is evidence to support these nursing diagnoses and the keystone issue is correctly identified. *Cue logic* is the deliberate structuring of patient-in-context data to discern the meaning for nursing care (Butcher & Johnson, 2012). In this case study, the nursing diagnoses depicted in the outlying ovals on the Reasoning Web are recorded under diagnostic cluster/ cue logic on the OPT Model Clinical Reasoning Worksheet along with the number of arrows radiating to/from each diagnosis. Exhibit 10.2 displays the identified keystone issue, in this case as Disturbed Sleep Pattern, and it is listed directly below the other nursing diagnoses.

Framing

In the center and top of the worksheet is a box to indicate the *frame* or theme that best represents the background issue(s) regarding the patient-in-context story. The frame of this case is a 40-year-old woman post-operative total vaginal hysterectomy with bilateral salpingoophorectomy and colostomy who suffered pain and fatigue secondary to many years of endometriosis. She is drowsy. Mr. Graham is concerned how his wife will react to the surgeries. This frame helps organize the present state and outcome state, and it illustrates the gaps between them to provide insights about essential care needs. The frame is the lens or background view to help the nurse differentiate this patient schema and prototype from others the nurse might have dealt with in the past. The interventions and tests that will be used in this care plan are specific to the frame that is identified. Exhibit 10.3 displays the frame in the case of Mrs. Graham.

Present State

The *present state* is a description of the patient-in-context story or the initial condition of the patient (Butcher & Johnson, 2012). The items listed in this section change over time as a result of

EXHIBIT 10.2

Diagnostic Cluster/Cue Logic

1. Fatigue (11)
2. Grieving (11)
3. Pain, Chronic (9)
4. Sexual Dysfunction (7)
5. Interrupted Family Processes (7)
6. Pain, Acute (7)
7. Decisional Conflict (6)
8. Readiness for Enhanced Sleep (6)
9. Readiness for Enhanced Relationship (5)
10. Anxiety (5)
11. Impaired Skin Integrity (5)

Keystone Issue/Theme
Disturbed Sleep Pattern (12)

EXHIBIT 10.3

Frame

A 40-year-old woman post surgeries for endometriosis for many years. Her husband is present and concerned about wife's reaction to and aftermath of surgery.

nursing actions and the patient's situation. The cues and problems identified for the patient listed under the keystone issue capture the present state of the patient. These are the problems in which the care of the patient will be planned, implemented, and evaluated. The present-state items are listed in the oval of the identified keystone issue and, in this case, there are five primary issues related to the keystone issue, including 1) reports difficulty staying asleep, 2) hot flashes and night sweats during sleep, 3) sleeping 5 to 6 hours a night, and feeling tired all day, 4) feels like she can't get everything done due to being tired, and 5) chronic anemia (Hgb 9.6 gm/dL). Exhibit 10.4 displays the list of present-state issues that relate to the keystone issue and will be subjected to selected tests to determine whether the identified outcomes are achieved.

EXHIBIT 10.4

Present State

1. Reports difficulty staying asleep

2. Hot flashes and night sweats during sleep

3. Only sleeping 5-6 hours a night and tired all day

4. Feels like she can't get everything done due to being tired

5. Chronic anemia Hgb 9.6 gm/dL

EXHIBIT 10.5

Outcome State

1. **Sleep:** Will remain asleep throughout the night by 2-week follow-up visit.

2. **Sleep:** Decreased episodes of hot flashes and night sweats that interrupt sleep by 2-week follow-up visit.

3. **Sleep:** Will increase hours of sleep to at least 7 hours by 2-week follow-up visit.

4. **Endurance:** Be less sleepy during the day allowing for achievement of activities once sleep patterns are improved.

5. **Nutritional Status:** Energy. Achieve a hemoglobin within normal limits within 3 months.

Outcome State

Given a defined present state, consideration must be given to desired outcomes that will be achieved to resolve the keystone issue. In other words, one outcome state or goal is listed for each present-state item, and each can be tested and achieved through nursing and collaborative interventions. Exhibit 10.5 displays the outcome states for this case study. The outcome states with NOC labels (in bold) aim to assist Mrs. Graham to 1) remain asleep throughout the night by the 2-week follow-up visit, 2) have decreased episodes of hot flashes and night sweats that interrupt sleep by the 2-week follow-up visit, 3) increase hours of sleep to at least 7 hours by the 2-week follow-up visit, 4) be less sleepy during the day allowing for achievement of activities once sleep patterns are improved, and 5) achieve a hemoglobin within normal limits in 3 months.

Because each present state and its corresponding outcome state directly relate to each other, they are placed next to each other for juxtaposition. This placement assists the nurse with comparative analysis and reflection while exercising clinical reasoning in this care situation.

Tests

The differences or gaps between the present state and outcome state become the foci of concern in the next step of care planning. The nurse must consider what tests and related interventions are most appropriate to fill the gap between the present state and the desired outcomes. Based on these clinical decisions, the nurse considers evidence that might indicate whether the gaps have been filled. In collaboration with other healthcare providers and the patient, tests are conducted to measure changes and gather data. The nurse asks what and if clinical indicators are available for each desired outcome state—that is, what to consider as to whether the desired outcome is achieved. The tests chosen in this case include: 1) sleep diary, partner reports of sleep pattern, pain scale, 2) frequency chart of hot flashes and night sweats, hormone levels, sleep quality, 3) hours slept nightly, sleep diary, time to bed/awakening, 4) activity and energy levels, feeling rejuvenated on awakening, verbal and nonverbal expressions, and 5) complete blood count (CBC), which includes hematocrit and hemoglobin results. The tests for Mrs. Graham are displayed in Exhibit 10.6.

EXHIBIT 10.6

Tests

1. Sleep diary, partner reports of sleep pattern, pain scale

2. Frequency chart of hot flashes and night sweats, hormone levels, sleep quality

3 & 4. Activity and energy levels, feeling rejuvenated on awakening, verbal and nonverbal expressions

5. CBC

STOP AND THINK

1. Is the patient-in-context story complete?

2. How am I framing the situation?

3. How is the *present state* defined?

4. What is/are the desired outcomes?

5. What outcomes do I have in mind given the diagnoses?

6. What is/are the gaps or complementary pairs (~) of outcomes and present states?

7. What are the clinical indicators of the desired outcomes?

8. On what scales or *tests* will the desired outcome be measured?

9. How will I know when the desired targeted outcomes are achieved?

Interventions

At the bottom of the OPT Model of Clinical Reasoning Worksheet, there is a box that indicates *Patient Care Interventions* (NIC), which are the evidence-based nursing care activities that will assist the patient to reach the outcome states. The nurse must make clinical decisions or choices about interventions that will help the patient transition from present state to the desired outcome state. As interventions are implemented, the nurse evaluates the degree to which outcomes are being achieved or not. Interventions are evidence-based and gathered from current resources such as literature, recognized textbooks, and prototype examples. Rationales are listed and cited in a separate page column next to interventions. Listing the rationales for each intervention enhances understanding and justification for nursing activities. The interventions and the rationales for this case study are listed in Table 10.3 and include the measures of noninvasive pain relief methods and assessment, encouraging verbalization of feelings and reflection on life achievements, and facilitating resources to support spiritual care.

STOP AND THINK

1. What clinical decisions or interventions help to achieve the outcomes?

2. What specific intervention activities will I implement?

3. Why am I considering these activities?

TABLE 10.3 INTERVENTIONS AND RATIONALES

Interventions	Rationales

1. Sleep Enhancement
  a. Obtain a sleep history including bedtime routines, number of times awakened during the night, noise and light level
  b. Assess environmental factors that interrupt sleep
  c. Keep environment quiet, room lighting dim, and bedding supportive. Consider white noise to help with relaxation
  d. Offer earplugs and eye mask as a method to help
  e. Establish a sleeping and waking routine with regular times and incorporate a relaxation technique at bedtime
2. Medication Management, Hormone Replacement Therapy
  a. Review alternatives to hormone replacement therapy and discuss with patient her preferences
  b. Review information regarding beneficial and adverse effects of the different hormonal components
  c. Review information regarding the different methods of administration
  d. Collaborate with PCP and pharmacist on chosen method of HRT and conduct a medication reconciliation to identify any interactions
  e. Facilitate the decision to start or abstain from hormone replacement therapy
	1. Assessment of sleep behaviors and patterns is an important part of any health status examination (Humphries, 2008; Salas & Gamaldo, 2008). Most adults who are satisfied with nighttime sleep average 7.5 to 9 hours of sleep per night (Floyd, 2002). Regular schedules help promote sleep initiation and sleep maintenance by maintaining a circadian rhythm of alertness/drowsiness. The nurse can control room temperature, ventilation, noise, and odors to create a more comfortable environment (Potter & Perry, 2016).
	
	2. Encourage women who are in menopause to discuss the benefits and risks of hormonal therapy (Ignatavicius & Workman, 2016). Delivery methods vary for different symptoms and can include an estrogen patch, pills, topical creams, and rings (National Institute on Aging, 2016). The efficacy of estrogens in treating vasomotor symptoms is well established. Findings show that other agents can ameliorate vasomotor symptoms, but none have estrogen's effectiveness (Grant et al., 2015).

continues

TABLE 10.3 INTERVENTIONS AND RATIONALES (CONTINUED)

Interventions	Rationales

3. Environmental Management: Comfort
 	
  a. Based on assessment, teach the listed sleep promotion techniques:
 	
    - Arise at the same time each day even if sleep the night before was poor
 	
    - Limit caffeine and alcohol use
 	
    - Engage in relaxing activities at bedtime such as a hot bath, reading a book
 	
    - Avoid screens, blue light such as iPads, telephones, televisions, and laptops; should also avoid keeping these electronic devices in the room if they go off during the night
	3. Although many factors can interfere with falling and staying asleep, forcing a regular arise time helps establish a circadian rhythm and ensue better sleep the following night (Woodward, 2012). Caffeine is one of the most widely consumed psychoactive substances and it has profound effects on sleep-wake function including soft drinks and chocolate (Roehrs & Roth, 2008). Limited alcohol use suppresses REM sleep, which can lead to REM rebound, a lighter, more fragmented sleep later in the night (Dean et al., 2010).

4. Energy Management
 	
  a. Encourage verbalization of feelings about limitations
 	
  b. Use valid instruments to measure fatigue such as the Fatigue Impact Scale
 	
  c. Monitor nutritional intake to ensure adequate energy resources particularly in the post-operative period
 	
  d. Encourage regular exercise during the day to aid in stress control/release of energy
 	
  e. Assist the patient in assigning priority to activities to accommodate energy levels
 	
  f. Encourage the patient to choose activities that gradually build endurance
 	
  g. Assist the patient to identify tasks that the family and friends can perform in the home to prevent/relieve fatigue
	4. The Fatigue Impact Scale has good internal reliability, is brief, and has good psychometric properties and has been shown to detect changes in fatigue over time (Whitehead, 2009). Patients who feel as if they have control over their fatigue and its impact on their lives have lower levels of fatigue (Primdahl, Wagner, & Horslev-Petersen, 2011 as cited in Ackley & Ladwig, 2017).

5. Nutrition Therapy
 	
  a. Assess adequacy of nutrition
 	
  b. Evaluate vitamin B12 and iron intake
 	
  c. Offer foods rich in iron and vitamin B12, vitamin C, and folic acid
 	
  d. Monitor food intake, encourage small frequent meals, and consider supplementation. Collaborate with primary care provider and nutritionist
 	
  e. Consider social factors that may interfere with nutrition
	5. Inadequate nutrition can also contribute to fatigue, particularly if anemia is present (Minton, Richardson, Sharpe, Hotopf, & Stone, 2008 as cited in Ackley & Ladwig, 2017). Iron in meat, fish, and poultry is absorbed more readily than iron in plants. Vitamin C increases the solubility of iron. Vitamin B12 and folic acid are necessary for erythropoiesis (Nix, 2016).

Judgments

The final step in constructing the OPT Model Worksheet is to reflect on the tests and interventions to determine whether the outcomes were achieved. The consequences of the tests are data one uses to make clinical judgments (Pesut, 2008). In the far-left column on the OPT Model of Clinical Reasoning Worksheet, judgments are listed for each outcome. *Judgments* are conclusions about outcome achievements. Each judgment requires four elements: 1) a contrast between present and desired state, 2) criteria associated with a desired outcome (i.e., test), 3) consideration of the effects and influence of nurse interventions, and 4) a conclusion as to whether the intervention has been effective in the outcome achievement (Kuiper et al., 2009). Based on the analysis of tests, judgments are made as to whether the problem has been resolved. The nurse might have to reframe or attribute a different meaning to the facts in the patient-in-context story. Table 10.4 depicts the outcome states and judgments for this case study. A third column has been added within the table to provide the clinical reasoning used to guide each judgment statement. Exhibit 10.7 displays the judgments in this case.

EXHIBIT 10.7

Judgments

1. Partially met, long-term goal, evaluate at followup treatment of menopause and symptoms interfering with sleep. Pain currently well controlled, 2/10 with Dilaudid.

2. Met, monitor at followup, no hot flashes or night sweats wearing estradiol patch.

3. Partially met, long-term goal, evaluate at followup. Slept 10 hours on day of surgery.

4. Long-term goal, evaluate at follow up, slept 10 hours on day of surgery.

5. Long-term goal, evaluate trends of Hgb to assess for bleeding.

TABLE 10.4 TABLE OF OUTCOME STATES, JUDGMENTS, AND RATIONALES

Outcome State	Judgment	Clinical Reasoning
Sleep: Will remain asleep throughout the night by 2-week follow-up visit.	Long-term goal, will evaluate at follow up, should be met pending decision on treatment of menopause and symptoms currently interfering with sleep. Pain currently well controlled, 2/10 with Dilaudid.	Pain scale score reflects that acute pain is well controlled with Dilaudid; transition to oral analgesia for discharge. Slept through the night on day of surgery due to anesthetics and analgesia. Evaluate sleep at follow-up appointments.
Sleep: Decreased episodes of hot flashes and night sweats that interrupt sleep by 2-week follow-up visit.	Long-term goal, will evaluate at follow up, slept through the night day of surgery, no hot flashes or night sweats wearing estradiol patch.	Assess sleep patterns post-surgery. No reports of hot flashes or night sweats the night of surgery. Estradiol topical therapy has been initiated and will continue until 2-week follow-up visit, at which time long-term plans and considerations will be discussed.
Sleep: Will increase hours of sleep to at least 7 hours by 2-week follow-up visit.	Long-term goal, will evaluate at follow up. Slept 10 hours from 9pm-7am on day of surgery.	This outcome has been met, but assessment of sleep patterns after discharge is necessary. Hot flashes and night sweats are monitored while on hormonal therapy.
Endurance: Be less sleepy during the day allowing for achievement of activities once sleep patterns are improved.	Long-term goal, will evaluate at follow up, should be met if able to correct sleep pattern disturbances with control of menopausal symptoms and improved sleep hygiene.	This is a long-term goal and will need to be monitored at 2- and 6-week visits to gynecologist and primary care physician. Fatigue Impact Scale should be administered at 2-week visit for baseline data.
Nutritional Status: Achieve a hemoglobin within normal limits within 3 months.	Long-term goal, will evaluate at follow up but should be met now that her uterus has been removed and her menses will cease. Hgb 9.0 gm/dL on post-op day 1.	Baseline hemoglobin was low and had surgical blood loss, which should recover with the ceasing of menses and improved nutritional intake.

STOP AND THINK

1. Given the tests that have been chosen, what is my clinical judgment of the evidence regarding reaching the outcome state?

2. Based on my judgment, have I achieved the outcome or do I need to reframe the situation?

3. How can I specifically remember this experience and take the schema into the future when I reason about similar cases?

The Completed OPT Model of Clinical Reasoning

The completed OPT Model of Clinical Reasoning for a middle-aged female experiencing women's health problems is displayed in Figure 10.3.

SUMMARY

Clinical reasoning for women experiencing female health problems may encounter long-lasting effects of prescribed treatment. It begins with an understanding of who the patient is and her story given the context of the family dynamics. Using the OPT Model of Clinical Reasoning as a conceptual framework and the Clinical Reasoning Web as a tool helps develop the clinical reasoning associated with a particular case. The OPT Model of Clinical Reasoning provides a visual illustration of where the patient is (present state). Five present-state items were identified: difficulty staying asleep, hot flashes and night sweats during sleep, sleeping 5 to 6 hours a night and tired all day, feeling like she can't get everything done due to being tired, and chronic anemia (a hemoglobin value of 9.6 gm/dL). From these present states, the nurse was able to establish where he or she hoped the patient to be (outcome state). In this case study, the nurse was able to determine the following outcomes (using NOC terminology): sleep ~ endurance and nutritional status ~ energy.

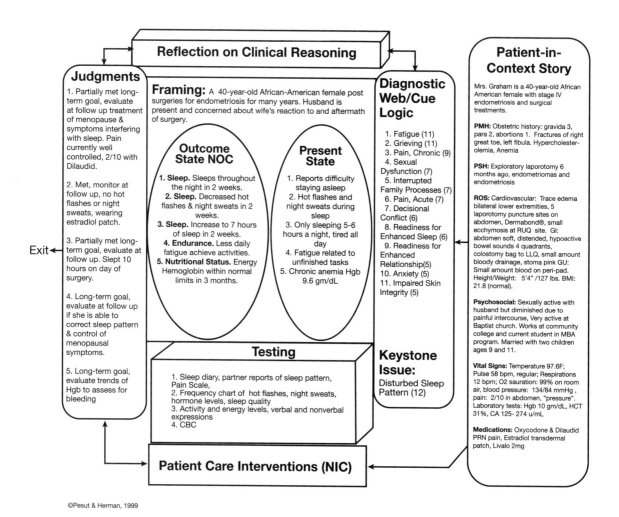

Reflection on Clinical Reasoning

Judgments
1. Partially met long-term goal, evaluate at follow up treatment of menopause & symptoms interfering with sleep. Pain currently well controlled, 2/10 with Dilaudid.

2. Met, monitor at follow up, no hot flashes or night sweats, wearing estradiol patch.

3. Partially met long-term goal, evaluate at follow up. Slept 10 hours on day of surgery.

4. Long-term goal, evaluate at follow up if she is able to correct sleep pattern & control of menopausal symptoms.

5. Long-term goal, evaluate trends of Hgb to assess for bleeding

Exit ◄───

Framing: A 40-year-old African-American female post surgeries for endometriosis for many years. Husband is present and concerned about wife's reaction to and aftermath of surgery.

Outcome State NOC
1. **Sleep.** Sleeps throughout the night in 2 weeks.
2. **Sleep.** Decreased hot flashes & night sweats in 2 weeks.
3. **Sleep.** Increase to 7 hours of sleep in 2 weeks.
4. **Endurance.** Less daily fatigue achieve activities.
5. **Nutritional Status.** Energy Hemoglobin within normal limits in 3 months.

Present State
1. Reports difficulty staying asleep
2. Hot flashes and night sweats during sleep
3. Only sleeping 5-6 hours a night, tired all day
4. Fatigue related to unfinished tasks
5. Chronic anemia Hgb 9.6 gm/dL

Testing
1. Sleep diary, partner reports of sleep pattern, Pain Scale,
2. Frequency chart of hot flashes, night sweats, hormone levels, sleep quality
3. Activity and energy levels, verbal and nonverbal expressions
4. CBC

Diagnostic Web/Cue Logic
1. Fatigue (11)
2. Grieving (11)
3. Pain, Chronic (9)
4. Sexual Dysfunction (7)
5. Interrupted Family Processes (7)
6. Pain, Acute (7)
7. Decisional Conflict (6)
8. Readiness for Enhanced Sleep (6)
9. Readiness for Enhanced Relationship(5)
10. Anxiety (5)
11. Impaired Skin Integrity (5)

Keystone Issue:
Disturbed Sleep Pattern (12)

Patient-in-Context Story

Mrs. Graham is a 40-year-old African American female with stage IV endometriosis and surgical treatments.

PMH: Obstetric history: gravida 3, para 2, abortions 1. Fractures of right great toe, left fibula. Hypercholesterolemia, Anemia

PSH: Exploratory laporotomy 6 months ago, endometriomas and endometriosis

ROS: Cardiovascular: Trace edema bilateral lower extremities, 5 laporotomy puncture sites on abdomen, Dermabond®, small ecchymosis at RUQ site. GI: abdomen soft, distended, hypoactive bowel sounds 4 quadrants, colostomy bag to LLQ, small amount bloody drainage, stoma pink GU: Small amount blood on peri-pad. Height/Weight: 5'4" /127 lbs. BMI: 21.8 (normal).

Psychosocial: Sexually active with husband but diminished due to painful intercourse, Very active at Baptist church. Works at community college and current student in MBA program. Married with two children ages 9 and 11.

Vital Signs: Temperature 97.6F; Pulse 58 bpm, regular; Respirations 12 bpm; O2 sauration: 99% on room air, blood pressure: 134/84 mmHg , pain: 2/10 in abdomen, "pressure". Laboratory tests: Hgb 10 gm/dL, HCT 31%, CA 125- 274 u/mL

Medications: Oxycodone & Dilaudid PRN pain, Estradiol transdermal patch, Livalo 2mg

Patient Care Interventions (NIC)

©Pesut & Herman, 1999

Figure 10.3 OPT Model of Clinical Reasoning for Middle-Aged Female with Endometriosis and Surgical Intervention.

All considerations for present state and outcome state are framed through identification of background issues of the patient's story (framing). The nurse framed this patient situation as a 40-year-old African-American woman post-op TVH / BSO and colostomy who suffered pain and fatigue due to endometriosis for many years. She is stable in the post-operative unit with her husband, who is concerned how the patient will react to surgical outcomes. The nurse must determine what evidence supports evaluations (tests) that bridge the gap between the two states and make decisions (judgments) of patient progress in meeting the outcomes. The nurse identified these tests to consider: 1) sleep diary, partner reports of sleep pattern, pain scale; 2) frequency chart of hot flashes and night sweats, hormone levels, sleep quality; 3) hours slept nightly, time to bed/awakening; 4) activity and energy levels, feeling rejuvenated on awakening, verbal and nonverbal expressions; and 5) complete blood counts. Experience with case studies of this nature augments the nurse's experience and adds to her clinical reasoning skill set that can be activated with future cases of a similar nature.

KEY POINTS

- Clinical reasoning for a middle-aged female who is experiencing physical, developmental, and psychosocial challenges can be promoted with the OPT Model.

- A step-by-step approach is used in this case study involving a middle-aged woman who has recently experienced a major surgical intervention with life-changing ramifications and who will need continued medical treatment and follow up. This approach can be used for similar schema and prototypes of women in other health settings.

- Various thinking and reflection strategies are used throughout the clinical reasoning process to complete the Clinical Reasoning Web and OPT Model of Clinical Reasoning.

STUDY QUESTIONS AND ACTIVITIES

1. Describe the benefits of using the OPT Clinical Reasoning Model to plan and evaluate patient care given the case study presented in this chapter.

2. How does this model differ from other nursing plans of care models?

3. What thinking strategies would you use in spinning and weaving the Reasoning Web?

4. Are there other nursing diagnoses you would assign to this case study involving a middle-aged female with endometriosis and subsequent surgical interventions? If so and given the patient data presented in the case study, what would you suggest?

5. Are there other priorities you would give to this case study? In other words, is there a different keystone issue you would recommend in planning care?

6. What other tests would you consider appropriate to bridge the gap between present state and outcome state in this patient scenario?

References

Ackley, B., & Ladwig, G. (2017). *Nursing diagnosis handbook: An evidence-based guide to planning care* (11th ed.). St. Louis, MO: Mosby Elsevier.

American Society of Reproductive Medicine (ASRM). (2012). *Endometriosis. A guide for patients.* Patient Information Series, American Society for Reproductive Medicine.

Butcher, H. K., Bulechek, G. M., Dochterman, J. M., & Wagner, C. M. (in press). *Nursing Interventions Classification (NIC)* (7th ed.). St. Louis, MO: Mosby Elsevier.

Butcher, H., & Johnson, M. (2012). Use of linkages for clinical reasoning and quality improvement. In M. Johnson, S. Moorhead, G. Bulechek, H. Butcher, M. Maas, & E. Swanson (Eds.), *NOC and NIC linkages to NANDA-I and clinical conditions* (3rd ed.), pp. 11–23. Maryland Heights, MO: Elsevier.

Carpenito, L. J. (2016). *Nursing diagnosis: Application to clinical practice* (15th ed.). Philadelphia, PA: Wolters Kluwer Health.

Dean, G., Finnell, D., Scribner, M., Wand, Y. J., Steinbrenner, L., & Gooneratne, N. (2010). Sleep in lung cancer: The role of anxiety, alcohol and tobacco. *Journal of Addictions Nursing, 21*(2–3), 130–138.

Doenges, M. E., Moorhouse, M. F., & Murr, A. C. (2016). *Nursing diagnosis manual: Planning, individualizing and documenting client care* (5th ed.). Philadelphia, PA: F. A. Davis Company.

Floyd, J. A. (2002). Sleep and aging. *Nursing Clinics of North America, 37*(7), 719–731.

Grant, M., Marbella, A., Wang, A., Pines, E., Hoag, J., Bonnell, C., & Aronson, N. (2015). *Menopausal symptoms: Comparative effectiveness of therapies.* Agency for Healthcare Research and Quality, Report No. 15-EHC005-EF. Rockville, MD.

Gulanick, M., & Myers, J. L. (2014). *Nursing care plans: Diagnoses, interventions, and outcomes.* Philadelphia, PA: Mosby Elsevier.

Herdman, T. H., & Kamitsuru, S. (Eds.). (2014). *NANDA International nursing diagnoses: Definition and classifications, 2015-2017.* Oxford, England: Wiley Blackwell.

Humphries, J. D. (2008). Sleep disruption in hospitalized adults. *Medsurg Nursing, 17*(6), 391–395. Retrieved from http://search.proquest.com.liblink.uncw.edu/docview/230527288?accountid=14606

Ignatavicius, D. D., & Workman, M. L. (2016). *Medical surgical nursing: Patient-centered collaborative care* (8th ed.). St. Louis, MO: Elsevier.

Johns Hopkins. (2016). *Health library: Endometriosis.* Retrieved from http://www.hopkinsmedicine.org/healthlibrary/conditions/gynecological_health/endometriosis_85,p00573/

Kuiper, R. A., Pesut, D. J., & Arms, T. (2016). *Clinical reasoning and care coordination in advanced practice nursing.* New York, NY: Springer Publishing Company.

Kuiper, R., Pesut, D., & Kautz, D. (2009). Promoting the self-regulation of clinical reasoning skills in nursing students. *The Open Nursing Journal, 3*, 76–85. Retrieved from http://doi.org/10.2174/1874434600903010076

Labrique-Walusis, F., Keister, K., & Russell, A. (2016). Massage therapy for stress management: Implications for nursing practice. *Orthopaedic Nursing, 29*(4), 254–257.

Mayo Clinic. (2016). Endometriosis. Retrieved from http://www.mayoclinic.org/diseases-conditions/endometriosis/home/ovc-20236421

Minton, O., Richardson, A., Sharpe, M., Hotopf, M., & Stone, P. (2008). A systemic review and meta-analysis of the pharmacological treatment of cancer-related fatigue. *Journal of the National Cancer Institute, 100*(16), 1155–1166. doi:10.1093/jnci/djn250

Moorhead, S., Johnson, M., Maas, M. O., & Swanson, E. (Eds.). (2013). *Nursing Outcomes Classification (NOC): Measurement of health outcomes* (5th ed.). St. Louis, MO: Elsevier.

National Institute on Aging. (2016). Menopause. Retrieved from https://www.nia.nih.gov/health/publication/hormones-and-menopause

Nilsson, U. (2008). The anxiety- and pain-reducing effects of music interventions: A systematic review. *AORN Journal, 87*(4), 780–807.

Nix, S. (2016). *Williams' basic nutrition and diet therapy* (15th ed.). St. Louis, MO: Elsevier.

Pesut, D. (2008). Thoughts on thinking with complexity in mind. In C. Lindberg, S. Nash, & C. Lindberg (Eds.), *On the edge: Nursing in the age of complexity* (pp. 211–238). Bordentown, NJ: PlexusPress.

Potter, P. A., & Perry, A. G. (2016). *Fundamentals of nursing* (8th ed.). St. Louis, MO: Elsevier.

Primdahl, J., Wagner, L., & Horslev-Petersen, K. (2011). Being an outpatient with rheumatoid arthritis — A focus group study on patients' self-efficacy and experiences from participation in a short course and one of three different outpatient settings. *Scandinavian Journal of Caring Sciences, 25*(2), 394–403. doi:10.1111/j.1471-6712.2010.00854.x

Ralph, S. S., & Taylor, C. M. (2014). *Nursing diagnosis reference manual* (9th ed.). Philadelphia, PA: Wolters Kluwer/Lippincott Williams & Wilkins.

Roehrs, T., & Roth, R. (2008). Caffeine: Sleep and daytime sleepiness. *Sleep Medicine Reviews, 12*(1), 153–162. Retrieved from http://dx.doi.org.liblink.uncw.edu/10.1016/j.smrv.2007.07.004

Salas, R., & Gamaldo, S. (2008). Adverse effects of sleep deprivation in the ICU. *Critical Care Clinics, 24*(3), 461–476.

Whitehead, L. (2009). The measurement of fatigue in chronic illness: A systematic review of unidimensional and multidimensional fatigue measures. *Journal of Pain and Symptom Management, 37*(1), 107–128. Retrieved from http://dx.doi.org.liblink.uncw.edu/10.1016/j.jpainsymman.2007.08.019

Woodward, M. (2012). Sleep in older people. *Reviews in Clinical Gerontology, 22*(2), 130–149. Retrieved from http://dx.doi.org.liblink.uncw.edu/10.1017/S0959259811000232

CHAPTER 11

CLINICAL REASONING AND MEN'S HEALTH ISSUES

LEARNING OUTCOMES

- Explain the components of the OPT Model that are essential to reflective clinical reasoning to manage the problems, interventions, and outcomes of a patient who has a men's health problem of benign prostatic hyperplasia (BPH) with the possible complication of pyelonephritis.

- Identify relevant nursing diagnoses specific to the health issues of a patient with BPH.

- Identify outcomes appropriate for a man with the health problem of BPH.

- Describe relevant tests and clinical judgments used to reason about present-state to outcome-state changes for a man with BPH with the possible complication of pyelonephritis.

- Describe the different thinking processes that support clinical reasoning skills and strategies to determine priorities and desired outcomes for a man with BPH with the possible complication of pyelonephritis.

This chapter presents a case study involving a 61-year-old male who presents to the clinic with complaints of difficulty urinating, urinary hesitancy, and nocturia. He has had these symptoms for approximately a year, but because of finances he could not get to the clinic. He finally sought care because he is feeling run down, has some lower back pain, pain with urination, and feels nauseated. Now, he is being evaluated for benign prostatic hyperplasia (BPH) versus prostate cancer as well as the complication of pyelonephritis due to obstructed urine flow. His urine dipstick analysis shows leukocyte casts, which is consistent with pyelonephritis, making the diagnosis more likely.

BPH is the most common benign neoplasm in men, with 50% of 50-year-olds and 80 to 90% of 80-year-olds having BPH diagnosed histologically (Teichman, 2001). The cause of BPH is a change in androgen levels and aging (Roberts & Hartlaub, 1999). BPH is an enlarged prostate gland. The prostate gland surrounds the urethra. As the prostate gets larger, it may squeeze or partly block the urethra. This often causes problems with urination. Common urinary symptoms include difficulty initiating a urine stream; an obstructed urine stream (dribbling); feeling the need to urinate, which may wake men at night; or a weak urine stream or sensation that the bladder is not completely empty after urinating. In aging men, BPH is the most common cause of urinary complaints and can cause obstruction, eventually leading to urinary infection. BPH does not cause prostate cancer or erectile dysfunction; however, if the prostate causes urinary obstruction, complications such as bladder infection, kidney infections, and urinary stones can occur. This patient has ignored his symptoms for more than a year and probably could have prevented this progression to pyelonephritis if he had sought treatment earlier. Symptoms of pyelonephritis include flank pain, costovertebral angle tenderness, nausea/vomiting, fever, and symptoms of cystitis (Miller & Hemphill, 2001). The patient has all of these symptoms.

THE PATIENT STORY

Meet Mr. Adam Freeman, a 61-year-old Native American male presented to the clinic today with complaints of difficulty urinating, urinary hesitancy, and nocturia. He has had these symptoms for approximately a year because he could not get to the clinic due to financial hardship. He is feeling run down with some lower back pain and pain with urination and feels nauseated. Adam does not have any insurance and does not have a primary care provider.

Medical History

Mr. Freeman has a history of hypertension, chronic obstructive pulmonary disease, and has recently gained a lot of weight. A family friend suggested he might have diabetes. He does not get routine physical examinations and has not had a flu or pneumonia vaccine.

Physical Assessment

Mr. Freeman appears tired, is guarding his back, and makes frequent trips to the bathroom. He is awake, alert, and oriented to person, place, time, and situation. He has no abnormal heart sounds or murmurs but has an irregular rhythm. The 12-lead electrocardiogram (EKG) reveals he has a sinus rhythm with occasional premature ventricular contractions. His skin is warm and dry with pink, dry mucous membranes. He complains of altered sensations in his feet and lower extremities. His abdomen is large, obese, but soft with normoactive bowel sounds in all four quadrants. His bladder is distended, and he has costovertebral angle tenderness on palpation. His urine is cloudy, amber, and foul smelling, but no obvious blood is noted. A digital rectal exam performed by the nurse practitioner reveals a uniformly enlarged, non-tender prostate. No nodules are palpated. Mr. Freeman is 6'2" tall and weighs 232 lb. His body mass index is 30 (obese).

Vital signs include a temperature of 100.6° Fahrenheit, irregular heart rate of 98 beats per minute, respirations at 18 breaths per minute, oxygen saturation of 96% on room air, and a blood pressure of 146/94 mmHg. Mr. Freeman rates his pain as 3 on a scale of 0 to 10 in the lower abdomen and lower back.

Laboratory Test Results

A urinalysis and urine culture were sent to the laboratory. Other laboratory tests include a urine dipstick that was positive for leukocyte esterase, nitrites, white blood cells, and protein with a specific gravity of 1.020. Prostate-specific antigen (PSA) is 3.1 ng/mL, blood urea nitrogen (BUN) is 27 mg/dL, and creatinine (Cr) is 2.4 mg/dL. A complete blood count (CBC) showed a white blood cell (WBC) count of 13,000, hemoglobin 11.6 gm/dL, and hematocrit of 33%.

Medications

Mr. Freeman's medications at home include hydrochlorothiazide 25 mg daily and Lisinopril 5 mg daily; however, he states he "rarely" takes his medicines.

Psychosocial Assessment

Mr. Freeman is widowed; his wife died of a heart attack 3 years ago. He currently lives with his three sons and one daughter-in-law in a "double-wide trailer" in one of the outlying rural counties. They all share a vehicle. He does not work and has been disabled due to a logging accident at work.

Current Physical Condition

Mr. Freeman is currently being evaluated for possible pyelonephritis and BPH. The healthcare team is discussing the need to admit him to the hospital for further diagnostic work-up and treatment with parenteral antibiotics.

PATIENT-CENTERED PLAN OF CARE USING THE OPT MODEL OF CLINICAL REASONING

The patient story in this case study has been obtained from all possible sources, including a physical examination, a current list of medications, and care conferences. The lists of patient problems and relevant nursing diagnoses support the creation of the Clinical Reasoning Web Worksheet and the OPT Model of Clinical Reasoning that help the nurse begin to filter the assessment data and information, frame the context of the story, and focus on the priority care needs and outcomes (Butcher & Johnson, 2012).

PATIENT PROBLEMS AND NURSING DIAGNOSES IDENTIFICATION

The first step of care planning is to identify the various problems and cues presented by the patient and select the nursing diagnoses whose defining characteristics capture these cues and problems. The medical diagnosis for this patient is benign prostatic hypertrophy.

Nursing Care Priority Identification

The nurse identifies the cues and problems collected from the physiologic assessment, psychosocial assessment, and the medical record. Similar problems and cues are clustered for interpretation and meaning. Then relevant nursing diagnoses that "fit" the cluster of cues and problems are identified based on definitions and defining characteristics of each nursing diagnosis. An assessment worksheet listing the major taxonomy domains, classes of each domain, patient cues and problems, relevant NANDA-I diagnoses with definitions (Herdman & Kamitsuru, 2014), Nursing Outcomes Classification (NOC) (Moorhead, Johnson, Maas, & Swanson, 2013), and Nursing Interventions Classification (NIC) (Butcher, Bulechek, Dochterman, & Wagner [in press]) labels has been created. This worksheet is designed to assist the nurse in organizing patient care issues and to generate appropriate nursing diagnoses. An example of a completed table of the taxonomy domains, classes, patient cues and problems, relevant nursing diagnoses, and suggested NOC and NIC labels for this case study is presented in Table 11.1.

STOP AND THINK

1. What taxonomy domains are affected, and which diagnoses have I generated?

2. What cues/evidence/data from the patient and evidence from the patient assessment support the diagnoses?

TABLE 11.1   DOMAINS, CLASSES (NANDA-I TAXONOMY II), PATIENT CUES/PROBLEMS, NURSING DIAGNOSES, AND NOC AND NIC LABELS

Domain	Classes	Identified Patient Problems
Activity/Rest: The production, conservation, expenditure, or balance of energy resources	**Sleep/Rest:** Slumber, repose, ease, relaxation, or inactivity	• Up every 2 hours to urinate • Because of frequent trips to the bathroom, sleeps later than normal and naps every day • Feeling run down • Cannot drink his routine "warm tea with brandy" at bed because limiting fluids at bedtime • Acute pain • Nocturia • States he gets up about every 2 hours during the night to urinate
	Activity/Exercise: Moving parts of the body (mobility), doing work, or performing actions often (but not always) against resistance	• Has complaints of low back and abdominal pain • Feeling "run down"; tires easily with walking short distances • Nausea
Health Promotion: The awareness of well-being or normality of function and the strategies used to maintain control of and enhance that well-being or normality of function	**Health Management:** Identifying, controlling, performing, and integrating activities to maintain health and well-being	• Limited finances • Lives in a rural area with limited access to care • Not insured, no primary care provider • Does not engage in preventive care (no flu or pneumonia vaccine) • Obesity BMI 30 • Drinks 3–4 beers per day • Noncompliant with medication regimen • Does not comply with physical activity recommendations

NANDA-I Nursing Diagnoses	Nursing Out-comes Classifica-tions (NOC)	Nursing Intervention Classifications (NIC)
Disturbed Sleep Pattern: Time-limited interruptions of sleep amount and quality due to external factors.	• Sleep	• Urinary Elimination Management • Pain Management
Insomnia: A disruption in amount and quality of sleep that impairs functioning.	• Fatigue Level • Personal Well-Being	• Sleep Enhancement • Energy Management • Urinary Elimination Management
Activity Intolerance: Insufficient physiological or psychological energy to endure or complete required or desired daily activities.	• Activity Tolerance • Energy Conservation • Self-Care: Activities of Daily Living	• Energy Management • Exercise Promotion • Sleep Enhancement
Ineffective Health Management: Pattern of regulating and integrating into daily living a therapeutic regimen for the treatment of illness and its sequelae that is satisfactory for meeting specific health goals.	• Alcohol Abuse Cessation • Cardiac Disease Self-Management • Health Beliefs Perceived Control • Participation in Healthcare Decisions	• Behavior Modification • Coping Enhancement • Teaching: Disease Process, Activity/Exercise, Prescribed Diet, Prescribed Medication • Immunization/Vaccination Management • Weight Management • Financial Resource Assistance

continues

TABLE 11.1 DOMAINS, CLASSES (NANDA-I TAXONOMY II), PATIENT CUES/PROBLEMS, NURSING DIAGNOSES, AND NOC AND NIC LABELS   (CONTINUED)

Domain	Classes	Identified Patient Problems
		• Says he "rarely" takes his medicines • Drinks alcohol despite hypertension diagnosis • Does not participate in physical activity even though he knows it is good for his blood pressure
Nutrition: The activities of taking in, assimilating, and using nutrients for the purposes of tissue maintenance, tissue repair, and the production of energy	**Ingestion:** Taking food or nutrients into the body	• Recent large amount of weight gain • Weighs 232 lb. • BMI of 30 • Sedentary lifestyle
Elimination and Exchange	**Urinary Function**	• Bladder distention • Post void residual (PVR) 325 mL • Cloudy, foul smelling urine • Bladder distention • PVR 325 mL • Nocturia • Hesitancy • Frequency • Difficulty urinating

NANDA-I Nursing Diagnoses	Nursing Outcomes Classifications (NOC)	Nursing Intervention Classifications (NIC)
Noncompliance: Behavior of person and/or caregiver that fails to coincide with a health-promoting or therapeutic plan agreed on by the person (and/or family and/or community) and healthcare professional. In the presence of an agreed-upon, health-promoting or therapeutic plan, the person's or caregiver's behavior is fully or partly nonadherent and might lead to clinically ineffective or partially effective outcomes.	• Compliance Behavior Prescribed Diet • Compliance Behavior Prescribed Medications	• Case Management • Health System Guidance • Mutual Goal Setting
Obesity: A condition in which an individual accumulates abnormal or excessive fat for age and gender that exceeds overweight.	• Nutrient intake • Weight Loss Behavior	• Weight Management • Nutrition Management
Urinary Retention: Incomplete emptying of the bladder.	• Urinary Elimination	• Urinary Catheterization: Intermittent • Urinary Retention Care • Medication Management
Impaired Urinary Elimination: Dysfunction in urine elimination.	• Urinary Elimination	• Urinary Elimination Management

continues

TABLE 11.1   DOMAINS, CLASSES (NANDA-I TAXONOMY II), PATIENT CUES/PROBLEMS, NURSING DIAGNOSES, AND NOC AND NIC LABELS   (CONTINUED)

Domain	Classes	Identified Patient Problems
		• Due to pathophysiologic changes of detrusor muscle instability
		• Impaired bladder contractility
		• Irritation from infectious agents, involuntary sphincter muscle relaxation
Comfort: Freedom from danger, physical injury, or immune system damage; preservation from loss; and protection of safety and security	**Physical Comfort:** Sense of well-being or ease and/or freedom from pain	• Costovertebral angle (CVA) tenderness
		• Pain level 3/10 in low back and low abdomen
		• Feeling nauseated
		• No appetite the last 2 days
		• Limiting fluid intake to decrease urinary symptoms
Safety/Protection: Principles underlying conduct, thought, and behavior about acts, customs, or institutions viewed as being true or having intrinsic worth	**Infection:** Host responses following pathogenic invasion	• Incomplete bladder emptying and distention
		• UA results cloudy urine, positive for nitrites, leukocyte esterase, foul smelling
		• WBC 13,000
		• Temperature 100.6° F
	Thermoregulation	• Temperature 100.6° F
		• Skin very warm to touch, dry
		• Mucous membranes dry
		• Limiting fluid intake

*Butcher, H., Bulechek, G., Dochterman, J., & Wagner, C. M. (in press).
Herdman, T. H., & Kamitsuru, S. (Eds.). (2014).
Moorhead, S., Johnson, M., Maas, M. O., & Swanson, E. (Eds.). (2013).

NANDA-I Nursing Diagnoses	Nursing Outcomes Classifications (NOC)	Nursing Intervention Classifications (NIC)
Risk for Urge Urinary Incontinence: Vulnerable to involuntary passage of urine occurring soon after a strong sensation or urgency to void, which may compromise health.	• Urinary Continence	• Medication Management • Urinary Habit Training • Fluid Management
Acute Pain: Unpleasant sensory and emotional experience arising from actual or potential tissue damage or described in terms of such damage; sudden or slow onset of any intensity from mild to severe with an anticipated or predictable end.	• Pain level	• Pain management • Analgesic administration
Nausea: A subjective phenomenon of an unpleasant feeling in the back of the throat and stomach, which may or may not result in vomiting.	• Nausea and Vomiting Control • Nausea and Vomiting Disruptive Effect	• Nausea Management • Distraction • Fluid/Electrolyte Monitoring • Infection Control
Risk for Infection: At increased risk for being invaded by pathogenic organisms.	• Infection Severity	• Infection Control
Hyperthermia: Core body temperature above the normal diurnal range due to failure of thermoregulation.	• Thermoregulation • Vital Signs	• Fever Treatment • Temperature Regulation • Vital Signs Monitoring • Infection Control

CREATING A CLINICAL REASONING WEB

The *Clinical Reasoning Web* is a means by which the nurse analyzes and reasons through complex patient stories for the purpose of finding and prioritizing key healthcare issues. Using the web, the nurse defines problems based on patient cues in the data, identifies nursing diagnoses to address and define the various problems, and determines relationships among these diagnoses (Kuiper, Pesut, & Kautz, 2009). The web is a visual representation and iterative analysis of the functional relationships among diagnostic hypotheses and results in a keystone issue that requires nursing care. In other words, the Clinical Reasoning Web represents a graphic illustration of how the elements of the patient's story and issues relate to one another and is depicted by sketching lines of association among the nursing diagnoses (Kuiper, Pesut, & Arms, 2016). Whereas medical diagnoses are consistent labels for a cluster of symptoms, patient stories vary; and each Clinical Reasoning Web is written to reflect the patient's unique story and the human response to actual or potential health problems that are best represented in nursing diagnoses. For example, given two patients with identical medical diagnoses, the nurse might determine that different nursing diagnoses and keystone issues are the priority for each based on thinking strategies and diagnostic hypotheses associated with each case.

Constructing the Clinical Reasoning Web

After the problems are identified from the assessment data, evidence, and cues and the nursing diagnoses are chosen, the Clinical Reasoning Web is constructed using the following steps:

1. Place a general description of the patient in the central oval with the primary medical diagnoses. In this case study, the patient is a 61-year-old Native American male with benign prostatic hyperplasia and rule out pyelonephritis. He is currently being evaluated at the clinic.

2. Place each NANDA-I nursing diagnosis generated from the patient cues in the ovals surrounding the middle circle.

3. Under each nursing diagnosis, list supporting data that was gathered from the patient's story and assessment.

4. Because each nursing diagnosis is directly related to the center oval containing a brief description of the patient's situation, the nurse draws a line from the central oval to each of the outlying nursing diagnosis ovals. Figure 11.1 displays the beginning steps of constructing the Clinical Reasoning Web for this case study.

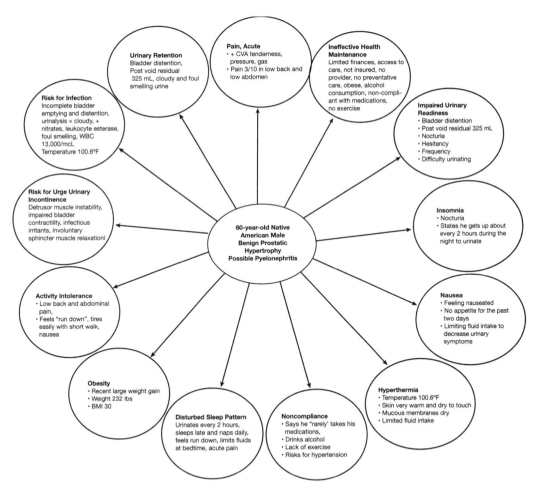

Figure 11.1   Clinical Reasoning Web: Older Adult Male With Benign Prostatic Hyperplasia: Connections from Medical Diagnosis to Nursing Diagnoses.

Spinning and Weaving the Reasoning Web

In spinning and weaving the Clinical Reasoning Web, the nurse must analyze and explain the relationships among the nursing diagnoses. This process involves thinking out loud; using self-talk; schema search; hypothesizing; if-then, how-so thinking; and comparative analysis, as described in Chapter 3 of this book. In doing so, the nurse determines possible connections and relationships among the nursing diagnoses contained in the outlying ovals.

The nurse continues to spin and weave using the following steps.

1. Consider how each of the nursing diagnoses and related healthcare issues it defines relates to all the other diagnoses. If there is a functional relationship between two diagnoses, then a line with a one-directional arrow is drawn to indicate a one-way connection; lines with two-directional arrows are drawn to indicate two-way connections. For example, what is the relationship between Impaired Urinary Elimination and Ineffective Health Management? How are these two diagnoses related? How do they influence one another? In the case of Mr. Freeman, the nurse would consider whether Impaired Urinary Elimination would cause Ineffective Health Management, or in a reciprocal fashion whether Ineffective Health Management would contribute to his Impaired Urinary Readiness. In this case, there is a one-way connection between Ineffective Health Management and Impaired Urinary Elimination. Another example would be to consider how the nursing diagnosis Activity Intolerance relates to the issue of Urinary Retention. In this case, there is a one-way connection between them with Activity Intolerance contributing to Urinary Retention, but no relationship between Urinary Retention and Activity Intolerance. Therefore, a one-way connection is made from Activity Intolerance to Urinary Retention.

2. The first step is repeated with each of the other ovals to determine relationships for connections. If there are functional relationships, connections are drawn until the process is exhausted; visually, the web emerges.

3. When all connections are made, the lines leading to and from each oval with nursing diagnoses are counted and recorded. The numbers can be recorded

on the Clinical Reasoning Web Worksheet. The hierarchy of priorities of Mr. Freeman's problems based on the number of connections is displayed in Table 11.2.

4. The nursing diagnosis with the most connecting lines radiating to and from that oval becomes the *keystone issue*. Figure 11.2 displays a completed Clinical Reasoning Web for this case.

TABLE 11.2 NURSING DOMAINS, NURSING DIAGNOSES, AND CONNECTIONS

Domain	Class	Nursing Diagnoses	Web Connections
Health Promotion	Health Management	Ineffective Health Maintenance	11
Activity/Rest	Sleep/Rest	Disturbed Sleep Pattern	10
Activity/Rest	Cardiovascular/Pulmonary Responses	Activity Intolerance	9
Elimination and Exchange	Urinary Function	Impaired Urinary Readiness	8
Comfort	Physical Comfort	Nausea	7
Activity/Rest	Sleep/Rest	Insomnia	7
Elimination and Exchange	Urinary Function	Urinary Retention	7
Comfort	Physical Comfort	Acute Pain	6
Nutrition	Ingestion	Obesity	5
Safety/Protection	Infection	Risk for Infection	5
Elimination and Exchange	Urinary Function	Risk for Urge Urinary Incontinence	4
Safety/Protection	Thermoregulation	Hyperthermia	4
Health Promotion	Health Management	Noncompliance	3

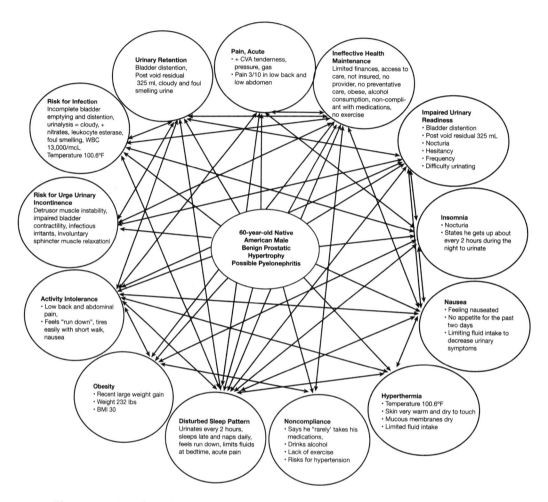

Figure 11.2 Clinical Reasoning Web: Older Adult Male with Benign Prostatic
Hyperplasia: Connections Among Nursing Diagnoses.

The keystone issue, the nursing diagnosis with the most connections, emerges as a priority problem. It is the basis for defining the patient's present state, and this in turn is contrasted with a desired outcome state (Kuiper et al., 2009). Identifying the keystone issue guides clinical reasoning by identifying the central NANDA-I diagnosis that needs to be addressed first and enables the nurse to focus on subsequent care planning (Butcher & Johnson, 2012). After a keystone issue is identified, there is continued knowledge work to identify the complementary nature of the problems ~ outcomes using the juxtaposing thinking strategy. The keystone issue in this case is Ineffective Health Maintenance. Interventions are chosen to assist Mr. Freeman with coping and resolving his barriers to managing his health problems. In doing so, these interventions are likely to influence other issues that are identified on the web.

STOP AND THINK

1. What are the relationships between and among the identified problems (diagnoses)?

2. What keystone issue(s) emerge?

COMPLETING THE OPT MODEL OF CLINICAL REASONING

After the Reasoning Web has been completed with identification of the keystone and cue logic, the OPT Model of Clinical Reasoning can be completed. All sections of the OPT Model are completed with the case study described in this chapter.

Patient-in-Context Story

Exhibit 11.1 displays the patient-in-context story for the adult male patient Adam Freeman. On the far-right side of the OPT Model in Figure 11.3, the patient-in-context story is recorded. This story underscores the patient demographics, medical diagnoses, and current situation. The information placed in this box is presented in a brief format with some relevant facts that support the rest of the model.

EXHIBIT 11.1

Patient-in-Context Story

Mr. Freeman is a 61-year-old Native American male with difficulty urinating, urinary hesitancy, and nocturia for a year. Feeling run down, low back pain, and nauseated. No insurance or regular health-care provider. No regular health checks or preventative measures.

Medical History: Hypertension, chronic lung disease.

Physical Assessment: Cardiovascular reveals irregular heartbeat with premature ventricular beats. Genitourinary reveals distended bladder, costovertebral tenderness, and urine issues (cloudy, amber, foul smelling). Digital rectal exam reveals a uniformly enlarged, non-tender prostate. Height is 6'2" and weight is 232 lb. BMI is 30 (obese).

Psychosocial Assessment: Widowed, lives with three sons and daughter-in-law in a trailer in rural area. Disabled and does not work. 70 pack/year smoking history. Drinks 3–4 beers per day. Active in tribal activities. He is adopted.

Vital Signs: Temperature 100.6°F; pulse 98 bpm, irregular; respiration 18 bpm; O2 saturation 96% on room air; blood pressure 146/94 mmHg; pain 3/10 in low abdomen and low back.

Laboratory Tests: Urinalysis positive for white blood cells, and protein. PSA (prostate specific antigen) 3.1 ng/mL BUN 27 mg/dL Cr 2.4 mg/dL CBC: WBC 13,000/mL.

Diagnostic Cluster/Cue Logic

The next step in the care planning process is completing the *diagnostic cluster/cue logic*. The keystone issue is placed at the bottom of the column with all the other identified nursing diagnoses and listed above it, in priority order. At this point, the nurse reflects on this list to ask if there is evidence to support these nursing diagnoses, and whether the keystone issue is correctly identified. *Cue logic* is the deliberate structuring of patient-in-context data to discern the meaning for nursing care (Butcher & Johnson, 2012). In this case study, the nursing diagnoses depicted in the outlying ovals on the Reasoning Web are recorded under diagnostic cluster/cue logic on the OPT Model of Clinical Reasoning Worksheet along with the number of arrows radiating to/from each diagnosis. Exhibit 11.2 displays the identified keystone issue—in this case, Ineffective Health Maintenance—and is listed directly below the other nursing diagnoses.

Framing

In the center and top of the worksheet is a box to indicate the *frame* or theme that best represents the background issue(s) regarding the patient-in-context story. The frame of this case is a 61-year-old Native American man with limited resources, who presents to the clinic with urinary complaints for the last year that have worsened, and he now has a suspected urinary tract infection. He is noncompliant and needs assistance obtaining care. He lives with family, and there are uncertain social dynamics. This frame helps to organize the present state and outcome state, and it illustrates the gaps between them to provide insights about essential care needs. The frame is the lens or background view to help the nurse differentiate this patient schema and prototype from others the nurse may have dealt with in the past. The interventions and tests that will be used in this care plan are specific to the frame that is identified. Exhibit 11.3 displays the frame in the case of Mr. Freeman.

EXHIBIT 11.2

Diagnostic Cluster/Cue Logic

1. Disturbed Sleep Pattern (10)
2. Activity Intolerance (7)
3. Nausea (7)
4. Urinary Retention (6)
5. Insomnia (6)
6. Impaired Urinary Readiness (5)
7. Pain, Acute (5)
8. Risk for Infection (4)
9. Obese (4)
10. Risk for Urge Urinary Incontinence (3)
11. Hyperthermia (3)
12. Noncompliance (2)

Keystone Issue
Ineffective Health Maintenance (11)

EXHIBIT 11.3

Frame

A 61-year-old Native American man with limited resources, urinary complaints that progressed to a urinary tract infection. Noncompliant, needs assistance with care. Lives with a family of uncertain dynamics.

Present State

The *present state* is a description of the patient-in-context story or the initial condition of the patient (Butcher & Johnson, 2012). The items listed in this section change over time as a result of nursing actions and the patient's situation. The cues and problems identified for the patient listed under the keystone issue capture the present state of the patient. These are the problems in which the care of the patient will be planned, implemented, and evaluated. The present-state items are listed in the oval of the identified keystone issue and, in this case, there are five primary issues related to the keystone issue, including: 1) he does not obtain basic preventative screenings or immunization; 2) he does not follow healthcare provider recommendations for disease management; 3) he admits to not taking his medications as prescribed by his provider; 4) he has no health insurance; and 5) he has limited financial resources. Exhibit 11.4 displays the list of present-state issues that relate to the keystone issue and will be subjected to selected tests to determine whether the identified outcomes are achieved.

Outcome State

Given a defined present state, consideration must be given to desired outcomes that will be achieved to resolve the keystone issue. In other words, one outcome state or goal is listed for each present-state item, and each can be tested and achieved through nursing and collaborative interventions. Exhibit 11.5 displays the outcome

EXHIBIT 11.4

Present State

1. Does not obtain basic preventive screenings or immunizations.

2. Does not follow health recommendations for disease management.

3. Does not take medications as prescribed.

4. No health insurance.

5. Limited financial resources.

EXHIBIT 11.5

Outcome State

1. **Health-Seeking Behavior:** Obtains vaccinations and screenings by follow up.

2. **Health Beliefs:** Perceived Control: Has personal goals and mutually agreed upon disease management strategies by discharge.

3. **Compliance Behavior:** Prescribed Medication: Follows medication regimen by follow up.

4. **Client Satisfaction:** Access to Care Resources: Engage case manager, social worker to obtain benefits (Medicaid etc.)

5. **Health Beliefs:** Perceived Resources: At least two community resources, services for healthcare goals.

states for this case study. In this case study, the outcome states with NOC labels (in bold) aim to assist Mr. Freeman to 1) demonstrate healthcare behaviors, such as obtaining health screenings and immunizations by his follow-up visit; 2) state his personal goals and steps he will take to follow mutually agreed upon disease management strategies such as exercise by discharge; 3) follow medication regimen as mutually agreed upon with provider by follow up; 4) discuss barriers to implementing healthcare regimen with case manager or social worker to obtain benefits (Medicaid, etc.); and 5) identify two community resources or services to assist in meeting healthcare goals.

Since each present state and its corresponding outcome state directly relate to each other, they are placed next to each other for juxtaposition. This placement will assist the nurse with comparative analysis and reflection while exercising clinical reasoning in this care situation.

Tests

The differences or gaps between the present state and outcome state become the foci of concern in the next step of care planning. The nurse must consider what tests and related interventions are most appropriate to fill the gap between the present state and the desired outcomes. Based on these clinical decisions, the nurse considers evidence that might indicate whether the gaps have been filled. The tests for Mr. Freeman are displayed in Exhibit 11.6. In collaboration with other healthcare providers and the patient, tests are conducted to measure changes and gather data. The nurse asks what and if clinical indicators are available for each desired outcome state—that is, what to consider as to whether the desired outcome is achieved. The tests chosen in this case include 1) completes health-related tasks such as immunization records and screenings; 2) exercise diary, verbal report of alcohol intake, and

EXHIBIT 11.6

Tests

1. Completes immunizations and screenings

2. Exercise, alcohol intake, blood alcohol content log

3. Prescription refills, blood pressure assessment

4. Case management reports of insurance benefits

5. Uses community resources, support group attendance

blood alcohol content; 3) prescription refills and blood pressure assessment; 4) case management reports of access to insurance benefits; and 5) utilization of community resources and support group attendance.

STOP AND THINK

1. Is the patient-in-context story complete?

2. How am I framing the situation?

3. How is the *present state* defined?

4. What is/are the desired outcomes?

5. What outcomes do I have in mind given the diagnoses?

6. What is/are the gaps or complementary pairs (~) of outcomes and present states?

7. What are the clinical indicators of the desired outcomes?

8. On what scales or tests will the desired outcome be measured?

9. How will I know when the desired targeted outcomes are achieved?

Interventions

At the bottom of the OPT Model of Clinical Reasoning Worksheet, there is a box that indicates *Patient Care Interventions* (NIC), which are the evidence-based nursing care activities that will assist the patient to reach the outcome states. The nurse must make clinical decisions or choices about interventions that will help the patient transition from present state to the desired outcome state. As interventions are implemented, the nurse evaluates the degree to which outcomes are being achieved. Interventions are evidence-based and gathered from current resources, such as literature, recognized textbooks, and prototype examples. Rationales are listed and cited in a separate page column next to interventions. Listing the rationales for each intervention enhances understanding and justification for nursing activities. The interventions and the rationales for this case study are listed in Table 11.3 and include the measures of noninvasive pain relief methods and assessment, encouraging verbalization of feelings and reflection on life achievements, and facilitating resources to support spiritual care.

STOP AND THINK

1. What clinical decisions or interventions help to achieve the outcomes?

2. What specific intervention activities will I implement?

3. Why am I considering these activities?

TABLE 11.3   INTERVENTIONS AND RATIONALES

Interventions	Rationales

1. Self-Efficacy Enhancement
 	
  a. Explore his perception of his ability to perform the required health behaviors
 	
  b. Identify his perceptions of the risk of not carrying out the health behaviors
 	
  c. Identify barriers to changing behavior and offer strategies to overcome the barriers
 	
  d. Provide an environment supportive to learning and skills needed to carry out the behaviors
 	
  e. Model or demonstrate the desired behaviors and have him role play or rehearse the behavior
 	
2. Decision-Making Support
 	
  a. Determine if there are differences in the way the individual and the way healthcare providers view the condition and how the patient feels, their values and reasons for not following the treatment plan; establish a collaborative goal for treatment
 	
  b. Inform the patient about alternative views
 	
  c. Respect patient's right to receive or not receive information and provide it accordingly
 	
  d. Refer to support groups
 	
3. Teaching Prescribed Medication; Mutual Goal Setting
 	
  a. Help him to determine how to manage his medication schedule
 	
  b. Identify alternative, complementary, and adjunctive therapies that will help him manage his disease processes
 	
  c. Encourage a regular routine for health-related behaviors
	1. Older women were amenable to interventions for negative beliefs about managing symptoms, perceived negative attitudes of healthcare providers, and difficulties in communicating about symptoms (Yeom & Heidrich, 2009). In nursing and other discipline studies, self-efficacy was shown to improve with education (Frank-Bader, Beltran, & Dojlidko, 2011). Individualized instruction, such as how to use a peak flow meter, improved clinical markers for asthma and control (Janson, McGrath, Covington, Cheng, & Boushey, 2009). Patients often want more influence on decision-making than they are afforded (Tariman, Berry, Cochrane, Doorenbox, & Schepp, 2010).
	
	2. Respect for an individual is a necessary condition for the experience of participation in healthcare decisions (Eldh, Ekman, & Ehnfors, 2006). Factors such as faith in health professionals and belief in the local health system affected self-care practices in a qualitative study (Clark et al., 2009). Results of a study on a videoconferencing healthcare support program showed that participants appreciated the information shared by others about self-care and responded positively to the professional and peer support (Marziali, 2009). A patient must be able to understand the information given, evaluate the consequences of the options presented, decide on the options based on their values, and communicate the choice (Soriano & Lagman, 2012).
	
	3. A mutual goal-setting intervention helped to promote receptivity to health promotion behaviors (Meyerson & Kline, 2009). Tailored decision-support information was effective in supporting adults with low levels of education in making informed choices and increased involvement in decisions about treatments (Smith et al., 2010). Individuals who establish a regular routine for exercise are more likely to be compliant over time (Hines, Seng, & Messer, 2007).

Interventions	Rationales

4. Case Management
 	
  a. Explain the role of case manager to him as well as social worker if involved in care
 	
  b. Assess his physical and mental status, functional capability, formal and informal support systems, financial resources, and environmental conditions
 	
  c. Identify resources and/or services needed
 	
  d. Identify health and social services available within his own community and facilitate his access to these services, such as senior resource center, health department, and free clinics closer to home
 	
5. Financial Resource Assistance; Support System Enhancement
 	
  a. Assess for economic issues and cultural patterns that influence compliance with a given regimen
 	
  b. Facilitate the client and family to obtain health insurance and drug payment plans whenever needed and possible
	4. When appropriate referrals are missed or delayed, clients often experience poor outcomes, including complications and hospital readmissions (Lebecque et al., 2009). Individuals who attend support groups demonstrate improved disease management and enhanced quality of life (Song, Lindquist, Windenberg, Cairns, & Thakur, 2011). Encouraging independence and enhancing social networks can enhance client autonomy (Rosland, Heisler, & Choi, 2010). Developing partnerships with community-based programs, health providers, and family fosters ongoing relationships toward enhanced self-health promotion (Peterson, Dolan, & Hanft, 2010).
	
	5. Cultural beliefs play an important role in attitudes towards diabetes among people of South Asian origin and therefore understanding these beliefs assists in promoting self-management. A culturally based adaptation of a program to promote physical activity significantly improved self-reported readiness to engage in physical activity (Coleman et al., 2012). Adherence to medications and self-health regimes is facilitated by payers' knowledge and use of value-based insurance designs (Cohen, Christensen, & Feldman, 2012).

Judgments

The final step in constructing the OPT Model of Clinical Reasoning Worksheet is to reflect on the tests and interventions to determine whether the outcomes were achieved. The consequences of the tests are data one uses to make clinical judgments (Pesut, 2008). In the far-left column on the OPT Model of Clinical Reasoning Worksheet, judgments are listed for each outcome. *Judgments* are conclusions about outcome achievements. Each judgment requires four elements: 1) a contrast between present and desired state; 2) criteria associated with a desired outcome

EXHIBIT 11.7

Judgments

1. Consented to having a flu and pneumonia vaccine after education.

2. Identified three goals related to managing hypertension and exercise plan at senior center.

3. Agreed to take medications as ordered when financial aid available for the cost.

4. Identified lack of healthcare due to no financial resources, obtaining Medicaid.

5. Identified community resources: health department, senior center, free clinic at a local church.

(i.e., test); 3) consideration of the effects and influence of nurse interventions; and 4) a conclusion as to whether the intervention has been effective in the outcome achievement (Kuiper et al., 2009). Based on the analysis of tests, judgments are made as to whether the problem has been resolved. The nurse may have to reframe or attribute a different meaning to the facts in the patient-in-context story. Table 11.4 depicts the outcome states and judgments for this case study. A third column has been added within the table to provide the clinical reasoning used to guide each judgment statement. Exhibit 11.7 displays the judgments in this case.

TABLE 11.4   TABLE OF OUTCOME STATES, JUDGMENTS, AND RATIONALES

Outcome State	Judgment	Clinical Reasoning
Health-Seeking Behavior: Demonstrate health behavior changes—i.e., getting vaccinations and screenings by follow up.	He consented to having a flu and pneumonia vaccine after education session on risks of getting the disease from vaccine.	While Mr. Freeman has consented to receiving the flu vaccine today, whether he will continue to seek preventive care will depend upon his financial situation and ability to obtain insurance benefits. Understanding the motivators and barriers are essential to this outcome being met.

Outcome State	Judgment	Clinical Reasoning
Health Beliefs: Perceived Control: States personal goals and steps to follow mutually agreed upon disease management strategies, such as exercise by discharge.	He can identify three goals he wants to achieve related to managing his hypertension and an exercise group he will attend at the senior center.	Mr. Freeman needs to be part of a group to be more successful in his health behaviors. Because of his rural dwelling, he does not have access to sidewalks, parks, and safe places to ride a bike, so the senior center is a realistic option. He will also need financial resources to be successful in his other goals.
Compliance Behavior: Prescribed Medication: Will follow medication regimen as prescribed by follow up.	He agreed to take medications as ordered if he is able to get financial assistance in obtaining them.	The social worker is working with him to get Medicaid due to his disability. In the meantime, case managers worked to get his prescriptions filled at the local Walmart, which has his diuretic and antihypertensive on the $4 list. Depending on the treatment of his BPH, his urologist will be asked about medications that are on the list for him.
Client Satisfaction: Access to Care Resources: Discuss barriers to implementing healthcare regimen with case manager/social worker to obtain benefits (Medicaid etc.).	He identified having no healthcare insurance and has started the process of obtaining Medicaid.	He is eligible for Medicaid and should receive approval for benefits. At that time, he can continue with the public health department or establish himself with a primary care provider.
Health Beliefs: Perceived Resources: Identify two community resources/services to assist in meeting healthcare goals.	He identified the county health department, senior center, and free clinic at a church in town to obtain care as needed in the future.	Mr. Freeman agreed that the senior center and free clinic are easier for him to access than the health department, but for some health needs he might have to go to the health department and will need his family to take him on days when they are not working, so it will require advanced planning.

STOP AND THINK

1. Given the tests that have been chosen, what is my clinical judgment of the evidence regarding reaching the outcome state?

2. Based on my judgment, have I achieved the outcome or do I need to reframe the situation?

3. How can I specifically take this experience and learning with me into the future as schema to reason about similar cases?

The Completed OPT Model of Clinical Reasoning

The completed OPT Model of Clinical Reasoning for an older adult male experiencing men's health problems is displayed in Figure 11.3.

SUMMARY

Clinical reasoning for older men experiencing male health problems who have difficulty accessing healthcare resources and who may encounter complications of delaying care-seeking begins with an understanding of who the patient is and his story given the context of his abilities and understanding. Using the OPT Model of Clinical Reasoning as a conceptual framework and the Clinical Reasoning Web as a tool helps develop the clinical reasoning associated with a particular case.

The OPT Model of Clinical Reasoning provides a visual illustration of where the patient is (present state). Five present-state items were identified: does not obtain basic preventive screenings and immunizations; does not follow health recommendations for disease management; does not take medications as prescribed; does not have health insurance; and has limited financial resources. From these present states, the nurse was able to establish where he or she hoped the patient to be (outcome states). In this case study the nurse was able to determine the following outcomes (using NOC terminology): health-seeking behavior; health beliefs: perceived control; compliance behavior: prescribed medication; client satisfaction: access to care resources; and health beliefs: perceived resources. All considerations for present state and outcome state are framed through identification of background issues of the patient's story (framing).

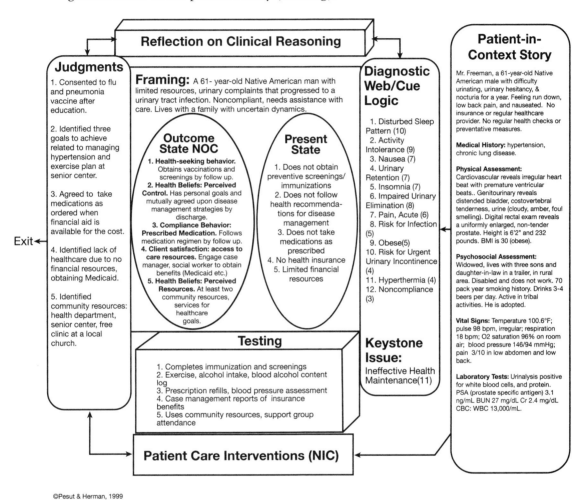

Reflection on Clinical Reasoning

Patient-in-Context Story

Mr. Freeman, a 61-year-old Native American male with difficulty urinating, urinary hesitancy, & nocturia for a year. Feeling run down, low back pain, and nauseated. No insurance or regular healthcare provider. No regular health checks or preventative measures.

Medical History: hypertension, chronic lung disease.

Physical Assessment: Cardiovascular reveals irregular heart beat with premature ventricular beats.. Genitourinary reveals distended bladder, costovertebral tenderness, urine (cloudy, amber, foul smelling). Digital rectal exam reveals a uniformly enlarged, non-tender prostate. Height is 6'2" and 232 pounds. BMI is 30 (obese).

Psychosocial Assessment: Widowed, lives with three sons and daughter-in-law in a trailer, in rural area. Disabled and does not work. 70 pack year smoking history. Drinks 3-4 beers per day. Active in tribal activities. He is adopted.

Vital Signs: Temperature 100.6°F; pulse 98 bpm, irregular; respiration 18 bpm; O2 saturation 96% on room air; blood pressure 146/94 mmHg; pain 3/10 in low abdomen and low back.

Laboratory Tests: Urinalysis positive for white blood cells, and protein. PSA (prostate specific antigen) 3.1 ng/mL BUN 27 mg/dL Cr 2.4 mg/dL CBC: WBC 13,000/mL.

Judgments

1. Consented to flu and pneumonia vaccine after education.

2. Identified three goals to achieve related to managing hypertension and exercise plan at senior center.

3. Agreed to take medications as ordered when financial aid is available for the cost.

Exit ◄—

4. Identified lack of healthcare due to no financial resources, obtaining Medicaid.

5. Identified community resources: health department, senior center, free clinic at a local church.

Framing: A 61- year-old Native American man with limited resources, urinary complaints that progressed to a urinary tract infection. Noncompliant, needs assistance with care. Lives with a family with uncertain dynamics.

Outcome State NOC

1. **Health-seeking behavior.** Obtains vaccinations and screenings by follow up.
2. **Health Beliefs: Perceived Control.** Has personal goals and mutually agreed upon disease management strategies by discharge.
3. **Compliance Behavior: Prescribed Medication.** Follows medication regimen by follow up.
4. **Client satisfaction: access to care resources.** Engage case manager, social worker to obtain benefits (Medicaid etc.)
5. **Health Beliefs: Perceived Resources.** At least two community resources, services for healthcare goals.

Present State

1. Does not obtain preventive screenings/ immunizations
2. Does not follow health recommendations for disease management
3. Does not take medications as prescribed
4. No health insurance
5. Limited financial resources

Diagnostic Web/Cue Logic

1. Disturbed Sleep Pattern (10)
2. Activity Intolerance (9)
3. Nausea (7)
4. Urinary Retention (7)
5. Insomnia (7)
6. Impaired Urinary Elimination (8)
7. Pain, Acute (6)
8. Risk for Infection (5)
9. Obese(5)
10. Risk for Urgent Urinary Incontinence (4)
11. Hyperthermia (4)
12. Noncompliance (3)

Testing

1. Completes immunization and screenings
2. Exercise, alcohol intake, blood alcohol content log
3. Prescription refills, blood pressure assessment
4. Case management reports of insurance benefits
5. Uses community resources, support group attendance

Keystone Issue:

Ineffective Health Maintenance(11)

Patient Care Interventions (NIC)

©Pesut & Herman, 1999

Figure 11.3   OPT Model of Clinical Reasoning for an Older Adult Male with Benign Prostatic Hypertrophy.

The nurse framed this patient situation as a 61-year-old Native American man with limited resources who presents to the clinic with urinary complaints that have worsened and now has a suspected urinary tract infection. He is noncompliant with treatment regimens and needs assistance obtaining care. He lives with family, and there is an uncertain social dynamic. Ultimately the nurse must determine what evidence supports evaluations (tests) that bridge the gap between the two states and make decisions (judgments) of patient progress in meeting the outcomes. The nurse identified these tests to consider: 1) completes health-related tasks, such as immunization records and screenings; 2) exercise diary, verbal report of alcohol intake, and blood alcohol content; 3) prescription refills and blood pressure assessment; 4) case management reports of access to insurance benefits; and 5) utilization of community resources and support group attendance. Experience with case studies of this nature augments the nurse's experience and adds to her clinical reasoning skill set that can be activated with future cases of a similar nature.

KEY POINTS

- Clinical reasoning for an older adult male who is experiencing physical, developmental, and psychosocial challenges can be promoted with the OPT Model of Clinical Reasoning.

- Various thinking and reflection strategies are used throughout the clinical reasoning process to complete the Clinical Reasoning Web and OPT Model of Clinical Reasoning.

- A step-by-step approach is used in this case study involving an older adult man who has delayed care-seeking due to financial limitations and barriers to accessing care who will need assistance in obtaining services. This approach can be used for similar schema and prototypes of men in other health settings.

STUDY QUESTIONS AND ACTIVITIES

1. Describe the benefits of using the OPT Clinical Reasoning Model to plan and evaluate patient care.

2. How does this model differ from other nursing plans of care models?

3. What thinking strategies would you use in spinning and weaving the Clinical Reasoning Web?

4. Are there other nursing diagnoses you would assign to this case study involving an older adult male patient? If so and given the patient data presented in the case study, what would you suggest?

5. Are there other priorities you would give to this case study? In other words, is there a different keystone issue you would recommend in planning care?

6. What other tests would you consider appropriate to bridge the gap between present state and outcome state in this patient scenario?

References

Ackley, B., & Ladwig, G. (2017). *Nursing diagnosis handbook: An evidence-based guide to planning care* (11th ed.). St. Louis, MO: Mosby Elsevier.

Butcher, H., & Johnson, M. (2012). Use of linkages for clinical reasoning and quality improvement. In M. Johnson, S. Moorhead, G. Bulechek, H. Butcher, M. Maas, & E. Swanson (Eds.), *NOC and NIC linkages to NANDA-I and clinical conditions* (3rd ed.), pp. 11–23. Maryland Heights, MO: Elsevier.

Carpenito, L. J. (2016). *Nursing diagnosis: Application to clinical practice* (15th ed.). Philadelphia, PA: Wolters Kluwer Health.

Clark, A., Freydberg, N., McAlister, F., Tsuyuki, R., Armstrong, P., & Strain, L. (2009). Patient and informal caregiver's knowledge of heart failure: Necessary but insufficient for effective self-care. *European Journal of Heart Failure, 11*(6), 617–621.

Cohen, J., Christensen, K., & Feldman, L. (2012). Disease management and medication compliance. *Population Health Management, 15*(1), 20–28.

Coleman, K. J., Farrell, M. A., Rocha, D. A., Hayashi, T., Hernandez, M., Wolf, J., & Lindsay, S. (2012). Readiness to be physically active and self-reported physical activity in low-income Latinas, California WISEWOMAN, 2006–2007. *Preventing Chronic Disease, 9*, E87.

Doenges, M. E., Moorhouse, M. F., & Murr, A. C. (2016). *Nursing diagnosis manual: Planning, individualizing and documenting client care* (5th ed.). Philadelphia, PA: F. A. Davis Company.

Eldh, A., Ekman, I., & Ehnfors, M. (2006). Conditions for patient participation and non-participation in health care. *Nursing Ethics, 13*(5), 503–514.

Frank-Bader, M., Beltran, K., & Dojlidko, D. (2011). Improving transplant discharge education using a structured teaching approach. *Progress in Transplantation, 21*(4), 332–339.

Gulanick, M., & Myers, J. L. (2014). *Nursing care plans: Diagnoses, interventions, and outcomes.* Philadelphia, PA: Mosby Elsevier.

Herdman, T. H., & Kamitsuru, S. (Eds.). (2014). *NANDA International nursing diagnoses: Definition and classifications, 2015-2017.* Oxford, England: Wiley Blackwell.

Hines, S., Seng, J., & Messer, K. (2007). Adherence to a behavioral program to prevent incontinence. *Western Journal of Nursing Research, 29*(1), 36–56.

Janson, S., McGrath, K., Covington, J., Cheng, S. C., & Boushey, H. (2009). Individualized asthma self-management improves medication adherence and markers of asthma control. *Journal of Allergy and Clinical Immunology, 123*(4), 840–846.

Johnson, M., Moorhead, S., Bulechek, G., Butcher, H., Maas, M., & Swanson, E. (Eds.). (2012). *NOC and NIC linkages to NANDA-I and clinical conditions* (3rd ed.). Maryland Heights, MO: Elsevier.

Kuiper, R. A., Pesut, D. J., & Arms, T. (2016). *Clinical reasoning and care coordination in advanced practice nursing.* New York, NY: Springer Publishing Company.

Kuiper, R., Pesut, D., & Kautz, D. (2009). Promoting the self-regulation of clinical reasoning skills in nursing students. *The Open Nursing Journal, 3,* 76–85. Retrieved from http://doi.org/10.2174/1874434600903010076

Lebecque, P., Leonard, A., DeBoeck, K., DeBaets, F., Malfroot, A., Casimir, G., . . . Leal, T. (2009). Early referral to cystic fibrosis specialist centre impacts on respiratory outcome. *Journal of Cystic Fibrosis, 8*(1), 26–30.

Marziali, E. (2009). E-health program for patients with disease. *Telemedicine and eHealth, 15,* 176–181.

Meyerson, K., & Kline, K. (2009). Qualitative analysis of a mutual goal-setting intervention in participants with heart failure. *Heart & Lung, 38*(1), 1–9.

Miller, O., & Hemphill, R. R. (2001). Urinary tract infection and pyelonephritis. *Emergency Medicine Clinics of North America, 19*(3), 655–674.

Moorhead, S., Johnson, M., Maas, M. O., & Swanson, E. (Eds.). (2013). *Nursing Outcomes Classification (NOC): Measurement of health outcomes* (5th ed.). St. Louis, MO: Elsevier.

Pesut, D. (2008). Thoughts on thinking with complexity in mind. In C. Lindberg, S. Nash, & C. Lindberg (Eds.), *On the edge: Nursing in the age of complexity* (pp. 211–238). Bordentown, NJ: PlexusPress.

Peterson, T., Dolan, T., & Hanft, S. (2010). Partnering with youth organizers to prevent violence: An analysis of relationships, power, and change. *Progress in Community Health Partnerships, 4*(3), 235–242.

Ralph, S. S., & Taylor, C. M. (2014). *Nursing diagnosis reference manual* (9th ed.). Philadelphia, PA: Wolters Kluwer/Lippincott Williams & Wilkins.

Roberts, R. G., & Hartlaub, P. P. (1999). Evaluation of dysuria in men. *American Family Physician, 60*(3), 865–872.

Rosland, A. M., Heisler, M., & Choi, H. J. (2010). Family influence on self-management among functionally independent adults with diabetes or heart failure: Do family members hinder as much as they help? *Chronic Illness, 6*(1), 22–33.

Smith, S., Trevena, L., Simpson, J., Barratt, A., Nutbeam, D., & McCaffery, K. (2010). A decision aid to support informed choices about bowel cancer screening among adults with low education: Randomized controlled trial. *Bioorganic & Medicinal Chemistry, 341*, c5370.

Song, Y., Lindquist, R., Windenberg, D., Cairns, B., & Thakur, A. (2011). Review of outcomes of cardiac support groups after cardiac events. *Western Journal of Nursing Research, 33*(2), 224–246.

Soriano, M., & Lagman, R. (2012). When the patient says no. *American Journal of Hospice and Palliative Medicine, 29*(5), 401–404.

Tariman, J. D., Berry, D. L., Cochrane, B., Doorenbos, A., & Schepp, K. (2010). Preferred and actual participation roles during health care decision making in persons with cancer: A systematic review. *Annals of Oncology, 21*(6), 1145–1151.

Teichman, J. M. (2001). *20 Common Problems in Urology.* New York, NY: McGraw Hill Professional.

Yeom, H., & Heidrich, S. (2009). Effect of perceived barriers to symptom management on quality of life in older breast cancer survivors. *Cancer Nursing, 32*(4), 309–316.

CHAPTER 12

CLINICAL REASONING AND GERIATRIC HEALTH ISSUES

LEARNING OUTCOMES

- Explain the components of the OPT Model essential to reflective clinical reasoning to manage the problems, interventions, and outcomes of a patient who has recently experienced a stroke.

- Identify relevant nursing diagnoses specific to the health issues of the gerontology patient with a stroke.

- Identify outcomes appropriate for the health problems assessed in a stroke scenario.

- Describe relevant tests and clinical judgments used to reason about present-state to outcome-state changes for an individual who has had a stroke.

- Describe the different thinking processes that support clinical reasoning skills and strategies to determine priorities and desired outcomes for a patient with a stroke.

This chapter presents a case study involving an active 78-year-old African-American woman who lost consciousness and collapsed at home. The Emergency Medical Service (EMS) was called and responded. It was determined that the woman had suffered a stroke, and she was transferred to a stroke center.

Stroke occurs when the blood supply to part of the brain is suddenly interrupted or when a blood vessel in the brain bursts, spilling blood into the spaces surrounding brain cells (National Institutes of Health [NIH], 2004). Approximately 87% of strokes result from blood clots that have formed in arteries narrowed or clogged with plaque (Yew and Cheng, 2015). A clot (or thrombus) develops and thereby blocks blood flow, which leads to an ischemic stroke. At times a clot may form elsewhere in the body, such as within the heart or a neck artery, and is embolized to the brain. Yet another cause of stroke that occurs in the remaining percentage of the population and carries a higher mortality rate than ischemic stroke is a hemorrhagic stroke (Yew and Cheng, 2015). A hemorrhagic stroke results from a rupture of a blood vessel within the brain, causing blood to spread into or around the brain. In both ischemic and hemorrhagic strokes, blood flow to the brain has been disrupted, and brain cells within the surrounding areas die due to the lack of oxygen and nutrients needed for the cells to function.

A transient ischemic attack (TIA) is a brief episode of an ischemic stroke. It is considered to be a warning sign. A TIA results from a brief interruption in cerebral blood flow causing temporary neurologic dysfunction (Ignatavicius & Workman, 2016). Due to the short duration of symptoms (i.e., resolution typically resolves within 30 to 60 minutes), TIAs often go unreported or are not acted upon by the victims. There are nearly 800,000 strokes in the United States annually (American Heart Association, 2016). Stroke is the fifth-leading cause of death in this country, preceded by heart disease, cancer, lower respiratory tract disease, and accidents (Centers for Disease Control [CDC], 2015). However, stroke causes more serious long-term disabilities than any other disease (NIH, 2004).

The symptoms of a stroke include sudden numbness or weakness, especially on one side of the body; sudden confusion or trouble speaking or understanding speech; sudden trouble seeing in one or both eyes; sudden trouble with walking, dizziness, or loss of balance or coordination; or sudden severe headache with no known cause.

Several risk factors are associated with the development of a stroke. Unmodifiable risk factors are 1) age (increased age correlates to a greater risk); 2) gender (strokes are more prevalent in males); and 3) family history of stroke. Race is a fourth unmodifiable risk factor. African Americans have nearly twice the risk for a first-ever stroke than Caucasians and a much higher death rate from stroke (American Heart Association, 2016). This is most likely due to Blacks having a greater burden of stroke risk factors rather than there being any substantial racial differences in the associations between risk factors and stroke outcomes (Huxley, 2014).

Treatable risk factors include high blood pressure, smoking, heart disease (such as coronary artery disease, valve defects, atrial fibrillation, and enlargement of one of the heart's chambers resulting in clots), a history of stroke or TIA, diabetes, low-density lipoprotein cholesterol, physical inactivity, and obesity (NINDS, 2004).

The only Food and Drug Administration (FDA)–approved treatment for ischemic strokes is tissue plasminogen activator or tPA (Stroke Association, 2013). Given intravenously, tPA dissolves ischemic clots and thereby improves blood circulation to the part of the brain being deprived of blood flow. This treatment is designed to improve functional outcomes for patients younger than the age of 80 and leads to patient improvements that are sustained for at least 18 months (Hughes, 2013). Unfortunately, tPA has a very limited window of time for its initiation in order for it to be effective because tissue that is irreversibly injured in an acute ischemic stroke expands very rapidly over time (Wardlaw et al., 2012). The benefit from thrombolysis declines with delays in initiating treatment while the mortality rate of an intracranial hemorrhage increases (Saver, 2013). The FDA recommends administration within 3 hours of stroke occurrence.

THE PATIENT STORY

Meet Mrs. Jane Tillis, an active 78-year-old African-American woman who lost consciousness and collapsed at home. Her son made the discovery while he was visiting her at the time. He did not witness the collapse but found his mother on the floor, awake, confused, with slurred speech and numbness on her right side. The son immediately called EMS within 5 minutes after the collapse. EMS responded within 10 minutes, evaluated Mrs. Tillis, and suggested that she may have had a stroke. She was transferred to a stroke center within 15 minutes. On presentation in the emergency department, Mrs. Tillis was confused, and her health history was obtained from her son. The son reported that his mother had had an episode a few days ago of sudden onset numbness and tingling in the right lower extremity with slight confusion and slurred speech. The episode lasted only 5 minutes, and her primary care physician was not notified.

Medical History

Mrs. Tillis has a history of Type 2 diabetes mellitus, hypertension, hyperlipidemia, and a mild ischemic stroke 2 years ago that resulted in a full recovery. She has never smoked or used illicit drugs. Occasionally she drinks wine (three to five glasses per week).

Physical Assessment

Mrs. Tillis is lethargic and oriented to person and place. Her speech is slurred. She exhibits no signs of distress but reports a slight headache (a 2 on a pain scale of 0 to 10). Auscultation of the left carotid artery indicates bruits. There is evidence of right hemiparesis and right visual-spatial neglect. Mrs. Tillis's height is 5'6" and she weighs 175 pounds. Her body mass index (BMI) is 28.3, which denotes that she is overweight. Her blood pressure is 164/105 mmHg in her left arm, temperature is 98.4° Fahrenheit, heart rate is 80 beats per minute and irregular, and respirations are 18 breaths per minute. The blood pressure of 164/105 mmHg denotes hypertension.

Laboratory Test Results

The following laboratory tests were performed: complete blood count (CBC), pro-thrombin time, serum electrolyte levels, and cardiac and renal function studies. The results were all within normal limits. Abnormal laboratory values were blood glu-cose of 142 mg/dL and hemoglobin A1C at 7.5%.

Other Diagnostic Tests

The results of a computed tomography (CT) scan reveal a thrombus in a branch of the left internal carotid artery with approximately 50% occlusion of the vessel due to atherosclerosis. There is an area of infarction in the left anterior hemisphere of the brain. The diagnosis of ischemic stroke was made 2 hours after Mrs. Tillis's arrival in the emergency department. The National Institutes of Health Stroke Scale was administered in the emergency department, resulting in a score of 28 out of 42. This score is indicative of a severe stroke.

Nutrition

Dysphagia was assessed after Mrs. Tillis was admitted to the step-down unit in the hospital. A percutaneous endoscopic gastrostomy (PEG) tube has been placed with intermittent feedings of Glucerna® 1.2 at a frequency of four times a day.

Medications

Her medications include metformin 500 mg twice a day, metoprolol 50 mg daily, atorvastatin 80 mg daily, aspirin 81 mg daily, and docusate sodium 100 mg twice a day. She has no drug allergies.

Psychosocial Assessment

Mrs. Tillis exhibits confusion, fatigue, and a flat psychological affect. She verbal-izes to the night nurse that she is feeling despondent and saddened by the recent changes in her health and ability to care for herself. She relies on her children for her social support even though her children both work full time and have children living at home. She also reports that she doesn't always take her home medications and does not check her blood sugar on a regular basis unless she has an upcoming doctor's appointment.

Current Physical Condition

Mrs. Tillis has been treated with intravenous tPA at a dose of 0.9 mg/kg. Aspirin antiplatelet therapy has been started at an initial dose of 325 mg, 24 hours after thrombolytic therapy, and a maintenance dose of 75 mg per day. She has been admitted to the step-down unit and her condition has stabilized. Although strength in her right-sided extremities has increased since her arrival in the emergency department, she is unable to bathe and dress herself without assistance. She also requires assistance in transferring to and from the bedside commode. Muscle weakness and physical disabilities are expected to improve over the next 3 months. She is expected to be discharged to a stroke rehabilitation unit within 24 hours.

PATIENT-CENTERED PLAN OF CARE USING THE OPT MODEL OF CLINICAL REASONING

The patient story in this case study has been obtained from all possible sources, including a physical examination, a current list of medications, and care conferences. The lists of patient problems and relevant nursing diagnoses support the creation of the Clinical Reasoning Web Worksheet and the OPT Model of Clinical Reasoning that help the nurse begin to filter the assessment data and information, frame the context of the story, and focus on the priority care needs and outcomes (Butcher & Johnson, 2012).

PATIENT PROBLEMS AND NURSING DIAGNOSES IDENTIFICATION

The first step of care planning is to identify the various problems and cues presented by the patient and select the nursing diagnoses whose defining characteristics capture these cues and problems. The medical diagnosis for this patient is ischemic stroke affecting the left side of the brain.

Nursing Care Priority Identification

The nurse identifies the cues and problems collected from the physiologic assessment, psychosocial assessment, and the medical record. The similar problems and cues are clustered for interpretation and meaning. Then relevant nursing diagnoses that "fit" the cluster of cues and problems are identified based on definitions and defining characteristics of each nursing diagnosis.

An assessment worksheet listing the major taxonomy domains, classes of each domain, patient cues and problems, relevant NANDA-I diagnoses with definitions (Herdman & Kamitsuru, 2014), Nursing Outcomes Classification (NOC) (Moorhead, Johnson, Maas, & Swanson, 2013), and Nursing Interventions Classification (NIC) (Butcher, Bulechek, Dochterman, & Walker [in press]) labels has been created. This worksheet is designed to assist the nurse in organizing patient care issues and to generate appropriate nursing diagnoses. An example of a completed table of the taxonomy domains, classes, patient cues and problems, relevant nursing diagnoses, and suggested NOC and NIC labels for this case study is presented in Table 12.1.

STOP AND THINK

1. What taxonomy domains are affected, and which diagnoses have I generated?

2. What cues/evidence/data from the patient and evidence from the patient assessment support the diagnoses?

TABLE 12.1 DOMAINS, CLASSES (NANDA-I TAXONOMY II), PATIENT CUES/PROBLEMS, NURSING DIAGNOSES, NOC AND NIC LABELS

Domain	Classes	Identified Patient Problems
Nutrition: The activities of taking in, assimilating, and using nutrients for the purposes of tissue maintenance, tissue repair, and the production of energy	**Ingestion:** Taking food or nutrients into the body	• Dysphagia
Activity/Rest: The production, conservation, expenditure, or balance of energy resources	**Activity/Exercise:** Moving parts of the body (mobility), doing work, or performing actions often (but not always) against resistance	• Right-sided weakness, fatigue, decrease in gross motor skills, confusion
	Energy Balance: A dynamic state of harmony between intake and expenditure of resources	• Fatigue and lethargy
	Self-Care: Ability to perform activities to care for one's body and bodily functions	• Inability to dress self
		• Inability to bathe self
Perception/Cognition: The human information processing system including attention, orientation, sensation, perception, cognition, and communication	**Cognition:** Use of memory, learning, thinking, problem-solving, abstraction, judgment, insight, intellectual capacity, calculation, and language	• Confusion and orientation to place and self only due to ischemic stroke

NANDA-I Nursing Diagnoses	Nursing Outcomes Classifications (NOC)	Nursing Intervention Classifications (NIC)
Impaired Swallowing: Abnormal functioning of the swallowing mechanism associated with deficits in oral, pharyngeal, or esophageal structure of function	Aspiration Prevention	Aspiration Precautions
Impaired Physical Mobility: Limitation in independent, purposeful physical movement of the body or of one or more extremities	Ambulation Mobility Transfer Performance	Exercise Promotion: Strength Training Exercise Therapy: Ambulation Exercise Therapy: Joint Mobility Self-Care Assistance: Transfer
Fatigue: An overwhelming sustained sense of exhaustion and decreased capacity for physical and mental work at usual level	Endurance Energy Conservation	Energy Management Environmental Management
Self-Care Deficit (Bathing): Impaired ability to perform or complete bathing/hygiene activities for self	Self-Care: Bathing	Self-Care Assistance: Bathing
Self-Care Deficit (Dressing): An impaired ability to perform or complete dressing and grooming activities for self	Self-Care: Dressing	Self-Care Assistance: Dressing
Acute Confusion: Abrupt onset of reversible disturbances of consciousness, attention, cognition, and perception that develops over a short period of time	Information Processing Reality Orientation	Cognitive Stimulation Memory Training

continues

TABLE 12.1 DOMAINS, CLASSES (NANDA-I TAXONOMY II), PATIENT CUES/PROBLEMS, NURSING DIAGNOSES, NOC AND NIC LABELS (CONTINUED)

Domain	Classes	Identified Patient Problems
Role Relationship: The positive and negative connections or associations between people or groups of people and the means by which those connections are demonstrated	**Family Relationships:** Associations of people who are biologically related or related by choice	• Impaired physical abilities that affect usual family functions • Impaired communication that impacts family relationships
Coping/Stress Tolerance: Contending with life events/life processes	**Coping Responses:** The process of managing environmental stress	• Verbal reports of despondency over physical/cognitive disabilities
Safety/Protection: Principles underlying conduct, thought, and behavior about acts, customs, or institutions viewed as being true or having intrinsic worth	**Physical Injury:** Bodily harm or hurt	• Dysphagia • Difficulty with mobility and turning self • Impaired mobility and confusion

*Butcher, H., Bulechek, G., Dochterman, J., & Wagner, C. M. (in press).
Herdman, T. H., & Kamitsuru, S. (Eds.). (2014).
Moorhead, S., Johnson, M., Maas, M. O., & Swanson, E. (Eds.). (2013).

NANDA-I Nursing Diagnoses	Nursing Outcomes Classifications (NOC)	Nursing Intervention Classifications (NIC)
Interrupted Family Processes: Change in family relationships and/or functioning	Family Coping Family functioning	Coping Enhancement Family Integrity Promotion
Ineffective Coping: Inability to form a valid appraisal of the stressors, inadequate choices of practices responses, and/or inability to use available resources	Adaptions to Physical Disability Coping	Behavior Modification Coping Enhancement Decision-Making Support
Risk for Aspiration: At risk for entry of gastrointestinal secretions, oropharyngeal secretions, solids, or fluids, into tracheobronchial passages	Respiratory Status	Aspiration Prevention
Risk for Impaired Skin Integrity: At risk for skin being adversely altered	Tissue Integrity: Skin and Mucous Membranes	Pressure Ulcer Prevention
Risk for Injury (Falls): At risk of injury as a result of environmental conditions interacting with the individual's adaptive and defensive resources	Falls Occurrence	Fall Prevention

CREATING A CLINICAL REASONING WEB

The *Clinical Reasoning Web* is a means by which the nurse analyzes and reasons through complex patient stories for the purpose of finding and prioritizing key healthcare issues. Using the web, the nurse defines problems based on patient cues in the data, identifies nursing diagnoses to address and define the various problems, and determines relationships among these diagnoses (Kuiper, Pesut, & Kautz, 2009). The web is a visual representation and iterative, concurrent analysis of the functional relationships between and among diagnostic hypotheses results in a keystone issue that requires nursing care. In other words, the Clinical Reasoning Web represents a graphic illustration of how the elements of the patient's story and issues relate to one another and is depicted by sketching lines of association among the nursing diagnoses (Kuiper, Pesut, & Arms, 2016).

Whereas medical diagnoses are consistent labels for a cluster of symptoms, patient stories vary. Each Clinical Reasoning Web is written to reflect the patient's unique story and the human response to actual or potential health problems that are best represented in nursing diagnoses. For example, given two patients with identical medical diagnoses, the nurse might determine that different nursing diagnoses and keystone issues are the priority for each based on thinking strategies and diagnostic hypotheses associated with each case.

Constructing the Clinical Reasoning Web

After the problems are identified from the assessment data, evidence, and cues and the nursing diagnoses are chosen, the Clinical Reasoning Web is constructed using the following steps:

1. Place a general description of the patient in the central oval with the primary medical diagnoses. In this case study it is a 78-year-old African-American female who has recently suffered an ischemic stroke and been treated with tissue plasminogen activator (tPA). She is currently hospitalized on a step-down unit in the hospital.

2. Place each NANDA-I nursing diagnosis generated from the patient cues in the ovals surrounding the middle circle.

3. Under each nursing diagnosis, list supporting data that was gathered from the patient's story and assessment.

4. Because each nursing diagnosis is directly related to the center oval containing a brief description of the patient's situation, the nurse draws a line from the central oval to each of the outlying nursing diagnosis ovals. Figure 12.1 displays the beginning steps of constructing the Clinical Reasoning Web for this case study.

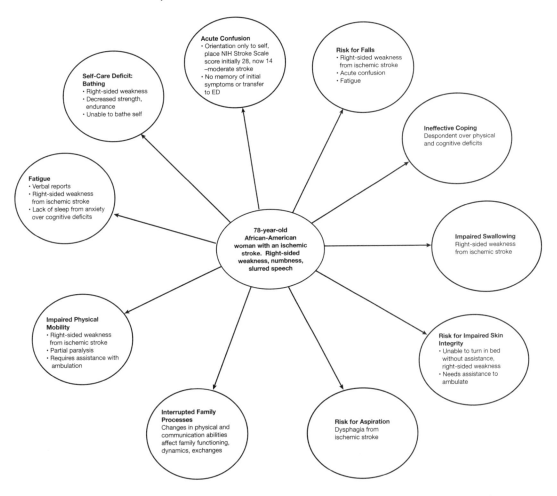

Figure 12.1 Clinical Reasoning Web: Gerontology Patient with a Stroke: Connections from Medical Diagnosis to Nursing Diagnoses.

Spinning and Weaving the Reasoning Web

In spinning and weaving the Clinical Reasoning Web, the nurse must analyze and explain the relationships among the nursing diagnoses. This process involves thinking out loud; using self-talk; schema search; hypothesizing; if-then, how-so thinking; and comparative analysis, as described in Chapter 3 of this book. In doing so, the nurse determines possible connections and relationships among the nursing diagnoses contained in the outlying ovals.

The nurse continues to spin and weave using the following steps:

1. Consider how each of the nursing diagnoses and related healthcare issues it defines relates to all the other diagnoses. If there is a functional relationship between two diagnoses, then a line with a one-directional arrow is drawn to indicate a one-way connection; lines with two-directional arrows are drawn to indicate two-way connections. For example, what is the relationship between Impaired Physical Mobility and Fatigue? How are these two diagnoses related? How do they influence one another? In the case of Mrs. Tillis, the nurse would consider whether Impaired Physical Mobility would cause Fatigue, or in a reciprocal fashion whether the feeling of Fatigue would contribute to Impaired Physical Mobility. In this case, there are two-way connections between Impaired Physical Mobility and Fatigue. Another example would be to consider how the nursing diagnosis Interrupted Family Processes relates to the issue of Risk for Aspiration. In this case, there is no relationship. Therefore, no connection is made between these two diagnoses.

2. The first step is repeated with each of the other ovals to determine relationships for connections. If there are functional relationships, connections are drawn until the process is exhausted, and visually, the web emerges.

3. When all connections are made, the lines leading to and from each oval with nursing diagnoses are counted and recorded. The numbers can be recorded on the Clinical Reasoning Web Worksheet. The hierarchy of priorities of Mrs. Tillis's problems based on the number of connections is displayed in Table 12.2.

4. The nursing diagnosis with the most connecting lines radiating to and from that oval becomes the *keystone issue*. Figure 12.2 displays a completed Clinical Reasoning Web for this case.

TABLE 12.2 NURSING DOMAINS, NURSING DIAGNOSES, AND CONNECTIONS

Domain	Class	Nursing Diagnoses	Web Connections
Activity/Rest	Activity/Exercise	Impaired Physical Mobility	9
	Energy Balance	Fatigue	7
	Self-Care	Self-Care Deficit: Bathing	5
Perception/Cognition	Cognition	Acute Confusion	4
Role Relationships	Family Relationships	Interrupted Family Processes	4
Coping/Stress Tolerance	Coping Response	Ineffective Coping	4
Safety/Protection	Physical Injury	Risk for Falls	4
	Physical Injury	Risk for Aspiration	2
	Physical Injury	Risk for Impaired Skin Integrity	2
Nutrition	Ingestion	Impaired Swallowing	2

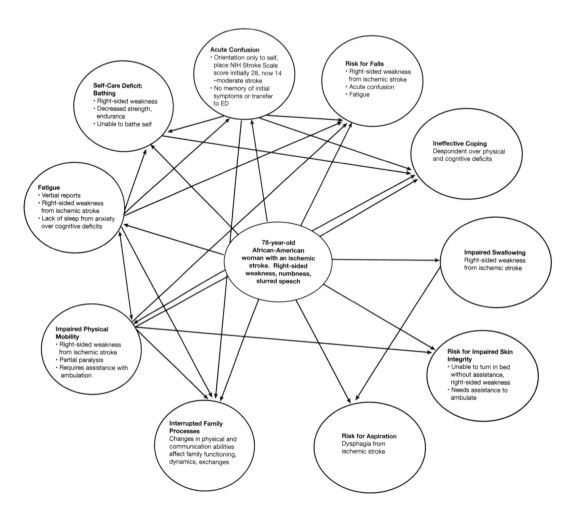

Figure 12.2   Clinical Reasoning Web: Gerontology Patient With a Stroke:
Connections Among Nursing Diagnoses.

The keystone issue, the nursing diagnosis with the most connections, emerges as a
priority problem. It is the basis for defining the patient's present state, and this in
turn is contrasted with a desired outcome state (Kuiper et al., 2009). Identifying
the keystone issue guides clinical reasoning by identifying the central NANDA-I
diagnosis that needs to be addressed first and enables the nurse to focus on

subsequent care planning (Butcher & Johnson, 2012). After a keystone issue is identified, there is continued knowledge work to identify the complementary nature of the problems ~ outcomes using the juxtaposing thinking strategy. The keystone issue in this case is Impaired Physical Mobility.

Interventions are chosen to assist Mrs. Tillis with coping and resolving her physical mobility issues. In doing so, these interventions are likely to influence other issues that are identified on the web.

STOP AND THINK

1. What are the relationships between and among the identified problems (diagnoses)?

2. What keystone issue(s) emerge?

COMPLETING THE OPT CLINICAL REASONING MODEL

After the Reasoning Web has been completed with identification of the keystone and cue logic, the OPT Model of Clinical Reasoning can be completed. All sections of the OPT Model are completed with the case study described in this chapter.

Patient-in-Context Story

Exhibit 12.1 displays the patient-in-context story for the elderly patient Jane Tillis. On the far-right side of the OPT Model in Figure 12.3, the patient-in-context story is recorded. This story underscores the patient demographics, medical diagnoses, and the current situation. The information placed in this box is presented in a brief format with some relevant facts that support the rest of the model.

EXHIBIT 12.1

Patient-in-Context Story

Mrs. Tillis is an active 78-year-old woman, who lost consciousness and collapsed at home. She presented to the emergency department where a CT scan revealed an ischemic stroke. Her son reported an episode of tingling in the right lower extremity with slight confusion and slurred speech a few days ago. This resolved after 5 minutes and was not reported.

Medical History: Type 2 diabetes mellitus, hypertension, and hyperlipidemia.

Social History: Occasional glass of wine (3–5 glasses/week). Relies on children for her social support even though her children both work full time.

Vital Signs: Height 5'6", weight: 175; BMI 28.3 (overweight).

Treatment: Intravenous tissue plasminogen activator (tPA).

Current Condition: Stable, awake but lethargic, oriented to person and place. Speech is slurred with difficulty swallowing. Slight facial drooping on the right. Unable to bathe, dress, transfer from commode without assistance. Confusion, fatigue, flat affect, despondent and saddened by health status.

Nutrition: Percutaneous endoscopic gastrostomy tube.

Diagnostic Cluster/Cue Logic

The next step in the care planning process is completing the *diagnostic cluster/cue logic*. The keystone issue is placed at the bottom of the column with all the other identified nursing diagnoses listed above it, in priority order. At this point, the nurse reflects on this list to ask if there is evidence to support these nursing diagnoses and whether the keystone issue is correctly identified. *Cue logic* is the deliberate structuring of patient-in-context data to discern the meaning for nursing care (Butcher & Johnson, 2012). In this case study, the nursing diagnoses depicted in the outlying ovals on the Reasoning Web are recorded under diagnostic cluster/cue logic on the OPT Model Clinical Reasoning Worksheet along with the number of arrows radiating to/from each diagnosis. Exhibit 12.2 displays the identified keystone issue—in this case, Impaired Physical Mobility—and it is listed directly below the other nursing diagnoses.

Framing

In the center and top of the worksheet is a box to indicate the *frame* or theme that best represents the background issue(s) regarding the patient-in-context story. The frame of this case is a 78-year-old woman who suffered an ischemic stroke, was treated with tPA, and is currently in stable condition. She exhibits partial paralysis and numbness, confusion, and fatigue and is expected to be transferred to a stroke rehabilitation unit. This frame helps to organize the present state and outcome state, and it illustrates the gaps between them to provide insights about essential care needs. The frame is the lens or background view to help the nurse differentiate this patient schema and prototype from others the nurse might have dealt with in the past. The interventions and tests that will be used in this care plan are specific to the frame that is identified. Exhibit 12.3 displays the frame in the case of Mrs. Tillis.

> **EXHIBIT 12.2**
>
> **Diagnostic Cluster/Cue Logic**
>
> 1. Fatigue (7)
> 2. Acute Confusion (6)
> 3. Self-Care Deficit (5)
> 4. Ineffective Coping (4)
> 5. Risk for Falls (4)
> 6. Interrupted Family Processes (4)
> 7. Impaired Swallowing (2)
> 8. Risk for Impaired Skin Integrity (2)
>
> **Keystone Issue/Theme**
> Impaired Physical Mobility (8)

> **EXHIBIT 12.3**
>
> **Frame**
>
> A 78-year-old woman who suffered an ischemic stroke, was treated with tPA, and is currently in stable condition. She exhibits partial paralysis and numbness, confusion, and fatigue; she is expected to be transferred to a stroke rehabilitation unit.

Present State

The *present state* is a description of the patient-in-context story or the initial condition of the patient (Butcher & Johnson, 2012). The items listed in this section change over time as a result of nursing actions and the patient's situation. The cues and problems identified for the patient listed under the keystone issue capture the present state of the patient. These are the problems in which the care of the patient will be planned, implemented, and evaluated. The present-state items are listed in the oval of the identified keystone issue and, in this case, there are five primary issues related to the keystone issue: 1) right-sided muscle weakness due to ischemic stroke, 2) slowed and uncoordinated movement affecting safety, 3) decreased motivation and depressed state, 4) fatigue, and 5) cognitive impairment, namely confusion. Exhibit 12.4 displays the list of present-state issues that relate to the keystone issue and will be subjected to tests to determine if the identified outcomes are achieved.

EXHIBIT 12.4

Present State

1. Right-sided muscle weakness due to ischemic stroke

2. Slowed and uncoordinated movement affecting safety

3. Decreased motivation and depressed state

4. Fatigue

5. Cognitive impairment (confusion)

EXHIBIT 12.5

Outcome State

1. **Ambulation:** Patient will demonstrate the use of an assistive device to increase mobility and lessen the risk of falls.

2. **Mobility:** Patient will demonstrate safety measures to minimize potential for injury.

3. **Coping and Adaption:** Patient will identify present strengths and means in which to alleviate or improve upon weaknesses.

4. **Energy Conservation:** Patient will verbalize her priorities for daily activities.

5. **Information Processing:** Patient will participate in activities of daily living at her maximum level of functioning ability in a therapeutic environment (stroke rehabilitation facility).

Outcome State

Given a defined present state, consideration must be given to desired outcomes that will be achieved to resolve the keystone issue. In other words, one outcome state or goal is listed for each present-state item, and each can be tested and achieved through nursing and collaborative interventions. Exhibit 12.5 displays the outcome states for this case study. The outcome states with NOC labels (in bold) aim to assist Mrs. Tillis to 1) demonstrate the use of an assistive device to increase mobility and lessen the risk of fall; 2) demonstrate safety measures to minimize potential for injury; 3) identify present strengths and means in which to alleviate or improve upon weaknesses, 4) verbalize her priorities for daily activities; and 5) participate in activities of daily living at her maximum level of functioning ability in a therapeutic environment (stroke rehabilitation facility).

Because each present state and its corresponding outcome state directly relate to each other, they are placed next to each other for juxtaposition. This placement assists the nurse with comparative analysis and reflection while exercising clinical reasoning in this care situation.

Tests

The differences or gaps between the present state and outcome state become the foci of concern in the next step of care planning. The nurse must consider what tests and related interventions are most appropriate to fill the gap between the present state and the desired outcomes. Based on these clinical decisions, the nurse considers evidence that might indicate whether the gaps have been filled. In collaboration with other healthcare providers and the patient, tests are conducted to measure changes and gather data. The nurse asks what and if clinical indicators are available for each desired outcome state—that is, what to consider as to whether the desired outcome is achieved. The tests chosen in this case include 1) the Morse Fall Risk Scale, 2) Elderly Mobility Scale, 3) NIH Stroke Scale, 4) Katz Activities of Daily Living Scale; Bristol Activities of Daily Living Scale, and 5) Stroke Rehabilitation Assessment of Movement. The tests for Mrs. Tillis are displayed in Exhibit 12.6.

> **EXHIBIT 12.6**
>
> **Tests**
>
> 1. Morse Fall Risk Scale
> 2. Elderly Mobility Scale
> 3. NIH Stroke Scale
> 4. Katz Activities of Daily Living Scale; Bristol Activities of Daily Living Scale
> 5. Stroke Rehabilitation Assessment of Movement

STOP AND THINK

1. Is the patient-in-context story complete?

2. How am I framing the situation?

3. How is the *present state* defined?

4. What is/are the desired outcomes?

5. What outcomes do I have in mind given the diagnoses?

6. What is/are the gaps or complementary pairs (~) of outcomes and present states?

7. What are the clinical indicators of the desired outcomes?

8. On what scales or tests will the desired outcome be measured?

9. How will I know when the desired targeted outcomes are achieved?

Interventions

At the bottom of the OPT Model of Clinical Reasoning Worksheet, there is a box that indicates *Patient Care Interventions* (NIC), which are the evidence-based nursing care activities that will assist the patient to reach the outcome states. The nurse must make clinical decisions or choices about interventions that will help the patient transition from the present state to the desired outcome state. As interventions are implemented, the nurse evaluates the degree to which outcomes are being achieved or not. Interventions are evidence-based and gathered from current resources such as literature, recognized textbooks, and prototype examples. Rationales are listed and cited in a separate page column next to interventions. Listing the rationales for each intervention enhances understanding and justification for nursing activities. The interventions and the rationales for this case study are listed in Table 12.3.

STOP AND THINK

1. What clinical decisions or interventions help to achieve the outcomes?

2. What specific intervention activities will I implement?

3. Why am I considering these activities?

TABLE 12.3 INTERVENTIONS AND RATIONALES

Interventions	Rationales
1. If the client has had a cerebrovascular accident (CVA), recognize that balance and mobility are likely impaired and engage client in fall prevention strategies and protect from falling (Ackley & Ladwig, 2017).	1. A randomized controlled trial studied the effect of a 6-month treadmill-training program versus a stretching program for stroke survivors. Both groups experienced increased self-efficacy for exercise and a significant increase in outcome expectations for exercise and ADLs on the Stroke Impact Scale (Shaughnessy et al., 2012, as cited in Ackley & Ladwig, 2017, p. 591).
2. If client has had a cerebrovascular accident (CVA) with hemiparesis, consider use of constraint-induced movement therapy, wherein the functional extremity is purposely constrained and the client is forced to use the involved extremity (Ackley & Ladwig, 2017).	2. The plasticity of the brain allows the brain to rewire and reroute neural connections to take up the work of the injured area of the brain. Constrain therapy was effective with improved motor function and health-related quality of life (Wu et al., 2007, as cited in Ackley & Ladwig, 2017, p. 591).
3. a. Consult with a physical therapist to assess present level of participation and for a plan to determine areas for potentially increased participation in each self-care activity (Carpenito, 2016). b. Promote patient's independence by allowing time to complete activities without help (Carpenito, 2016).	3. Offering choice and including the individual in planning care reduces feelings or powerlessness, promotes feeling of freedom, control, and self-worth, and increases his or her willingness to comply with therapeutic regimen (Carpenito, 2016, p. 674).
4. Specifically address daily stressors (i.e., self-care inability, housekeeping, medication schedule) and review possible options to reduce the daily stressors, such as weekly pill boxes, assistance with home and household care (Carpenito, 2016, p. 240).	4. Older adults who experience daily stressors more frequently reported their memory to be significantly worse and overall psychological functioning is affected (Stawski, Mogle, & Sliwinski, 2013, as cited in Carpenito, 2016, p. 240).
5. Increase independence in ADLs encouraging self-efficacy and discouraging helplessness as the client gets stronger. Providing unnecessary assistance with transfers and bathing activities might promote dependence and a loss of mobility (Ackley & Ladwig, 2017, p. 591).	5. A function-focused care intervention (designed to optimize physical activity and function in clients with Parkinson's disease) demonstrated a significant effect on increasing outcome expectations for exercise, improving functional performance, and increasing time spent in exercise and physical activity (Pretzer-Abhoff, Galik, & Resnick, 2011, p. 591).

EXHIBIT 12.7

Judgments

1. Patient is able to ambulate 25 feet with a "rollator" walker. A fall prevention program is in place because the patient is at a high risk for falls based on the Morse Fall Risk Scale.

2. Patient is able to apply brakes effectively with her rollator walker while ambulating. She is able to verbalize safety precautions required to prevent a fall.

3. Physical mobility and speech deficits continue to improve. NIH Stroke Scale score has improved from 24 out of a possible 42 to 14 (the lower the score the less the impact of the stroke).

4. Patient is able to identify which activities should be undertaken earlier in the day when her strength is at its peak. Patient verbalizes the importance of rest periods.

5. Patient is currently receiving physical and speech therapies. Based on her STREAM test score, she continues to improve upon her upper and lower limb movements and mobility. She is expected to be discharged to a stroke rehabilitation facility.

Judgments

The final step in constructing the OPT Model Worksheet is to reflect on the tests and interventions to determine whether the outcomes were achieved. The consequences of the tests are data one uses to make clinical judgments (Pesut, 2008). In the far-left column on the OPT Model of Clinical Reasoning Worksheet, judgments are listed for each outcome. *Judgments* are conclusions about outcome achievements. Each judgment requires four elements: 1) a contrast between present and desired state, 2) criteria associated with a desired outcome (i.e., test), 3) consideration of the effects and influence of nurse interventions, and 4) a conclusion as to whether the intervention has been effective in the outcome achievement (Kuiper et al., 2009). Based on the analysis of tests, judgments are made as to whether the problem has been resolved. The nurse may have to reframe or attribute a different meaning to the facts in the patient-in-context story. Table 12.4 depicts the outcome states and judgments for this case study. A third column has been added within the table to provide the clinical reasoning used to guide each judgment statement. Exhibit 12.7 displays the judgments in this case.

STOP AND THINK

1. Given the tests that have been chosen, what is my clinical judgment of the evidence regarding reaching the outcome state?

2. Based on my judgment, have I achieved the outcome or do I need to reframe the situation?

3. How can I specifically remember this experience and take the schema into the future when I reason about similar cases?

TABLE 12.4   TABLE OF OUTCOME STATES, JUDGMENTS, AND RATIONALES

Outcome State	Judgment	Clinical Reasoning
Ambulation: Patient will demonstrate the use of an assistive device to increase mobility and lessen the risk of falls.	Patient is able to ambulate 25 feet with assistance using a rollator walker. Morse Fall Risk Scale score: 90 (high risk for falls).	Currently participating in a physical therapy program that is designed to facilitate use of assistive devices and strengthen muscle groups. Fall risk prevention program in place.
Mobility: Patient will demonstrate safety measures to minimize potential for injury.	Patient is able to apply "brakes" with her rollator walker. Patient verbalizes safety precautions that are essential to prevent a fall. Elderly Mobility Scale score: 12 out of 20.	Elderly Mobility Scale score indicates borderline for safe mobility and independence in ADLs. This means that help is needed for mobility maneuvers.
Coping and Adaption: Patient will identify present strengths and means in which to alleviate or improve upon weaknesses.	Patient verbalizes areas in which her strength has not been affected by the stroke. Patient continues to work with a physical therapist to regain muscle strength and endurance. Initial NIH Stroke Scale score: 24 out of 42 (severe stroke).	NIH Stroke Scale score continues to improve with time (post treatment). Current score of 14 indicates a moderate stroke. (Earlier scores were higher.)

continues

TABLE 12.4 TABLE OF OUTCOME STATES, JUDGMENTS, AND RATIONALES (CONTINUED)

Outcome State	Judgment	Clinical Reasoning
Energy Conservation: Patient will verbalize her priorities for daily activities.	Patient is able to list activities that she hopes to accomplish by the end of the day. She is able to identify which activities should be undertaken earlier in the day when her strength is at its peak. Katz Activities of Daily Living Scale score: 3 out 6.	The score of 3 indicates that the patient requires assistance. Scoring ranges from 0 (patient is dependent) to 6 (patient is independent).
Information Processing: Patient will participate in activities of daily living at her maximum level of functioning ability in a therapeutic environment.	Patient is expected to be transferred to a stroke rehabilitation facility. Stroke Rehabilitation Assessment of Movement (STREAM) score: 28 out of 70, which is an improvement over initial score.	The score of 28 indicates less independence and marked deviation from the normal pattern or only partial movement. Scoring ranges from 0 (minimal active participation) to 70 (maximum participation).

The Completed OPT Model of Clinical Reasoning

The completed OPT Model of Clinical Reasoning for a gerontology patient with a stroke is displayed in Figure 12.3.

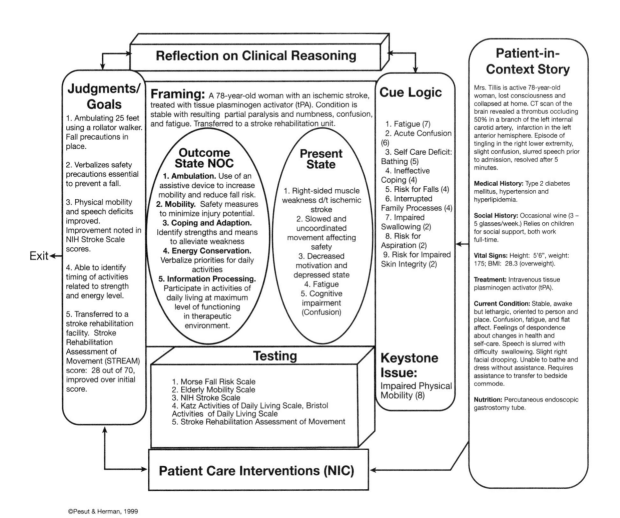

Reflection on Clinical Reasoning

Patient-in-Context Story

Mrs. Tillis is active 78-year-old woman, lost consciousness and collapsed at home. CT scan of the brain revealed a thrombus occluding 50% in a branch of the left internal carotid artery, infarction in the left anterior hemisphere. Episode of tingling in the right lower extremity, slight confusion, slurred speech prior to admission, resolved after 5 minutes.

Medical History: Type 2 diabetes mellitus, hypertension and hyperlipidemia.

Social History: Occasional wine (3 – 5 glasses/week.) Relies on children for social support, both work full-time.

Vital Signs: Height: 5'6", weight: 175; BMI: 28.3 (overweight).

Treatment: Intravenous tissue plasminogen activator (tPA).

Current Condition: Stable, awake but lethargic, oriented to person and place. Confusion, fatigue, and flat affect. Feelings of despondence about changes in health and self-care. Speech is slurred with difficulty swallowing. Slight right facial drooping. Unable to bathe and dress without assistance. Requires assistance to transfer to bedside commode.

Nutrition: Percutaneous endoscopic gastrostomy tube.

Judgments/ Goals

1. Ambulating 25 feet using a rollator walker. Fall precautions in place.

2. Verbalizes safety precautions essential to prevent a fall.

3. Physical mobility and speech deficits improved. Improvement noted in NIH Stroke Scale scores.

4. Able to identify timing of activities related to strength and energy level.

5. Transferred to a stroke rehabilitation facility. Stroke Rehabilitation Assessment of Movement (STREAM) score: 28 out of 70, improved over initial score.

Framing: A 78-year-old woman with an ischemic stroke, treated with tissue plasminogen activator (tPA). Condition is stable with resulting partial paralysis and numbness, confusion, and fatigue. Transferred to a stroke rehabilitation unit.

Cue Logic

1. Fatigue (7)
2. Acute Confusion (6)
3. Self Care Deficit: Bathing (5)
4. Ineffective Coping (4)
5. Risk for Falls (4)
6. Interrupted Family Processes (4)
7. Impaired Swallowing (2)
8. Risk for Aspiration (2)
9. Risk for Impaired Skin Integrity (2)

Outcome State NOC

1. **Ambulation.** Use of an assistive device to increase mobility and reduce fall risk.
2. **Mobility.** Safety measures to minimize injury potential.
3. **Coping and Adaption.** Identify strengths and means to alleviate weakness
4. **Energy Conservation.** Verbalize priorities for daily activities
5. **Information Processing.** Participate in activities of daily living at maximum level of functioning in therapeutic environment.

Present State

1. Right-sided muscle weakness d/t ischemic stroke
2. Slowed and uncoordinated movement affecting safety
3. Decreased motivation and depressed state
4. Fatigue
5. Cognitive impairment (Confusion)

Exit

Testing

1. Morse Fall Risk Scale
2. Elderly Mobility Scale
3. NIH Stroke Scale
4. Katz Activities of Daily Living Scale, Bristol Activities of Daily Living Scale
5. Stroke Rehabilitation Assessment of Movement

Keystone Issue:

Impaired Physical Mobility (8)

Patient Care Interventions (NIC)

©Pesut & Herman, 1999

Figure 12.3   OPT Model of Clinical Reasoning for Gerontology Patient With a Stroke.

SUMMARY

Clinical reasoning for a geriatric patient who has experienced an ischemic stroke and has been treated with tissue plasminogen activator begins with an understanding of who the patient is and what her story entails given the context of residual effects of the stroke and the treatment. Using the OPT Model as a conceptual framework and the Clinical Reasoning Web as a tool helps develop the clinical reasoning associated with a particular case. The OPT Clinical Reasoning Model provides a visual illustration of where the patient is (present state) and where the nurse hopes the patient to be (outcome state), all of which is framed through identification of background issues of the patient's story (framing). Through "spinning and weaving" of the web, the nurse can determine the priority of care through the generation of hypotheses and thinking out loud (self-talk) to make explicit functional relationships between and among competing nursing care needs. Once the priority issue (the keystone) is identified, planning can begin. In this case study the identified keystone issue is Impaired Physical Mobility.

The OPT Clinical Reasoning Model provides a visual illustration of where the patient is (present state). Five present-state items were identified: right-sided muscle weakness, slowed and uncoordinated movement, decreased motivation and depressed state, fatigue, and cognitive impairment (confusion). From this point the nurse was able to establish where he or she hoped the patient to be (outcome state). In this case study the nurse was able to determine the following outcomes (using NOC terminology): ambulation, mobility, coping and adaption, energy conservation, and information processing. All considerations for present state and outcome state are framed through identification of background issues of the patient's story (framing). The nurse framed this patient situation as a 78-year-old African-American woman with an ischemic stroke and treated with tissue plasminogen activator. She has been transferred to a stroke rehabilitation unit, where her condition is stable, and she is experiencing partial paralysis and numbness, confusion, and fatigue.

Ultimately the nurse must determine what evidence supports evaluations (tests) that bridge the gap between the two states and make decisions (judgments) of patient progress in meeting the outcomes. The nurse identified these tests to consider: 1) Morse Fall Risk Scale, 2) Elderly Mobility Scale, 3) NIH Stroke Scale, 4) Katz Activities of Daily Living Scale and the Bristol Activities of Daily Living Scale, and 5) Stroke Rehabilitation Assessment of Movement. Experience with case studies of this nature augments the nurse's experience and adds to her clinical reasoning skill set that can be activated with future cases of a similar nature.

KEY POINTS

- Clinical reasoning for a stroke victim who is experiencing physical, cognitive, and speech impediments can be promoted with the OPT Model.

- A step-by-step approach is used in this case study involving a patient who has recently experienced an ischemic stroke and has received recommended medical treatment. This approach can be used for similar schema and prototypes of a gerontology patient in other health settings.

- Various thinking and reflection strategies are used throughout the clinical reasoning process to complete the Clinical Reasoning Web and OPT Model of Clinical Reasoning.

STUDY QUESTIONS AND ACTIVITIES

1. Describe the benefits of using the OPT Clinical Reasoning Model to plan and evaluate patient care given the case study presented in this chapter.

2. How does this model differ from other nursing plans of care models?

3. What thinking strategies would you use in spinning and weaving the Reasoning Web?

4. Are there other nursing diagnoses you would assign to this case study involving a stroke victim? If so and given the patient data presented in the case study, what would you suggest?

5. Are there other priorities you would give to this case study? In other words, is there a different keystone issue you would recommend in planning care?

6. What other tests would you consider appropriate to bridge the gap between present state and outcome state in this patient scenario?

References

Ackley, B., & Ladwig, G. (2017). *Nursing diagnosis handbook: An evidence-based guide to planning care* (11th ed.). St. Louis, MO: Mosby Elsevier.

Ahmed, S., Mayo, N. E., Higgins, J., Salbach, N. M., Finch, L., & Wood-Dauphinée, S. L. (2003). The Stroke Rehabilitation Assessment of Movement (STREAM): A comparison with other measures used to evaluate effects of stroke and rehabilitation. *Journal of the American Physical Therapy Association*, 83(7), 617–630.

American Heart Association. (2016). Heart and stroke statistics. Retrieved from http://www.heart.org/HEARTORG/General/Heart-and-Stroke-Association-Statistics_UCM_319064_SubHomePage.jsp

American Stroke Association. (2013). Spot a stroke: Stroke warning signs and symptoms. Retrieved from http://www.strokeassociation.org/STROKEORG/WarningSigns/Stroke-Warning-Signs-and-Symptoms_UCM_308528_SubHomePage.jsp

American Stroke Association. (2016). Impact of stroke. Retrieved from http://www.strokeassociation.org/STROKEORG/AboutStroke/Impact-of-Stroke-Stroke-statistics_UCM_310728_Article.jsp#.V-QaQ2cVBet

Butcher, H. K., Bulechek, G. M., Dochterman, J. M., & Wagner, C. M. (in press). *Nursing Interventions Classification (NIC)* (7th ed.). St. Louis, MO: Mosby Elsevier.

Butcher, H., & Johnson, M. (2012). Use of linkages for clinical reasoning and quality improvement. In M. Johnson, S. Moorhead, G. Bulechek, H. Butcher, M. Maas, & E. Swanson (Eds.), *NOC and NIC linkages to NANDA-I and clinical conditions* (3rd ed.), pp. 11–23. Maryland Heights, MO: Elsevier.

Carpenito, L. J. (2016). *Nursing diagnosis: Application to clinical practice* (15th ed.). Philadelphia, PA: Wolters Kluwer Health.

Centers for Disease Control. (2015). Stroke in the United States. Retrieved from http://www.cdc.gov/stroke/facts.htm

Herdman, T. H., & Kamitsuru, S. (Eds.). (2014). *NANDA International nursing diagnoses: Definition and classifications, 2015–2017*. Oxford, England: Wiley Blackwell.

Hughes, S. (2013). IST-3: tPA benefits sustained out to 18 months. *Medscape*. June 21, 2013. Retrieved from http://www.medscape.com/viewarticle/806690#vp_1

Huxley, R. R. (2014). A comparative analysis of risk factors for stroke in blacks and whites: The Atherosclerosis Risk in Communities study. *Ethnicity and Health*, *19*(6), 601–616. Retrieved from http://dx.doi.org/10.1080/13557858.2013.857765

Ignatavicius, D., & Workman, L. (2016). *Medical-surgical nursing: Patient-centered collaborative care* (8th ed.). St. Louis, MO: Elsevier.

Johnson, M., Moorhead, S., Bulechek, G., Butcher, H., Maas, M., & Swanson, E. (Eds.). (2012). *NOC and NIC linkages to NANDA-I and clinical conditions* (3rd ed.), pp. 17–20. Maryland Heights, MO: Elsevier.

Kuiper, R. A., Pesut, D. J., & Arms, T. (2016). *Clinical reasoning and care coordination in advanced practice nursing*. New York, NY: Springer Publishing Company.

Kuiper, R., Pesut, D., & Kautz, D. (2009). Promoting the self-regulation of clinical reasoning skills in nursing students. *The Open Nursing Journal*, *3*, 76–85. Retrieved from http://doi.org/10.2174/1874434600903010076

Moorhead, S., Johnson, M., Maas, M. O., & Swanson, E. (Eds.). (2013). *Nursing Outcomes Classification (NOC): Measurement of health outcomes* (5th ed.). St. Louis, MO: Elsevier.

National Institutes of Health/National Institute of Neurological Disorders and Stroke (NINDS). (2004). Stroke information page. Retrieved from http://www.ninds.nih.gov/disorders/stroke/stroke.htm

Pesut, D. (2008). Thoughts on thinking with complexity in mind. In C. Lindberg, S. Nash, & C. Lindberg (Eds.), *On the edge: Nursing in the age of complexity* (pp. 211–238). Bordentown, NJ: PlexusPress.

Pike, E., & Landers, M. (2010). Responsiveness of the Physical Mobility Scale in long-term care facility residents. *Journal of Geriatric Physical Therapy*, *33*(2), 92–97.

Pretzer-Aboff, I., Galik, E., & Resnick, G. (2011). Feasibility and impact of a function focused care intervention for Parkinson's disease in the community. *Nursing Research, 60*(4), 276–283.

Saver, J. L. (2013). Time to treatment with intravenous tissue plasminogen activator and outcome from acute ischemic stroke. *JAMA, 309*(23), 2480–2488. doi:10.1001/jama.2013.6959

Wardlaw, J. M., Murray, V., Berge, E., del Zoppo, G., Sandercock, P., Lindley, R., & Cohen, G. (2012). Recombinant tissue plasminogen activator for acute ischemic stroke: An updated systematic review and meta-analysis. *Lancet*, *379*, 2364–2372. doi:10.1016/S0140-6736(12)60738

Yew, K., & Cheng, E. M. (2015). Diagnosis of acute stroke. *American Family Physician*, *91*(8), 528–536.

13

CLINICAL REASONING AND HOSPICE AND PALLIATIVE CARE

LEARNING OUTCOMES

- Explain the components of the OPT Model that are essential to the reflective clinical reasoning to manage the problems, interventions, and outcomes of a patient receiving palliative and hospice care.

- Identify relevant nursing diagnoses specific to the health issues of palliative care and hospice care patients.

- Identify outcomes appropriate for the health problems assessed in a palliative and hospice care scenario.

- Describe relevant tests and clinical judgments used to reason about present-state to outcome-state changes for a palliative and hospice care patient.

- Describe the different thinking processes that support clinical reasoning skills and strategies to determine priorities and desired outcomes for a palliative and hospice care patient.

This chapter presents a case study involving a terminally ill female with end-stage ovarian cancer who has been receiving palliative care. She recently enrolled in a hospice care program that offers, at her discretion, the use of a hospice care center. *Palliative care* is an approach to care designed to address problems of patients (adults and children) and their families who face a life-threatening illness with the goal of improving the quality of life (World Health Organization, 2015). Further, palliative care is intended to support patient autonomy, access to information, and choice. Frequently the term *palliative care* is referred to as *comfort care, supportive care,* and *symptom management*. Often palliative care is associated with end-of-life care, but palliative care is recommended *throughout* the chronically ill patient's experience, beginning with the initial diagnosis of the disease. Improved quality of life, more positive attitudes, and improvement in one-year survival rates form the basis for recommendations of early palliative care for cancer patients with metastasis and high symptom burden (Bakitas et al., 2015).

Palliative care goals are not focused on cure; rather, palliative care is focused on the prevention and treatment of disease symptoms and side effects of treatment to promote quality of life. Palliative care is the focus when successful curative treatment appears unlikely because further treatment will not result in a cure or the patient chooses not to seek further curative treatments. Palliative care is an adjunct with chronic illness treatment.

The term *hospice care* is a form of palliative care. Similar to palliative care, hospice is a system of care using an interdisciplinary approach with a focus on symptom management, meeting psychosocial needs, and promoting quality end-of-life care. Its main focus is to assess and address holistic needs of end-of-life patients and their families to facilitate a peaceful death. According to the National Hospice and Palliative Care Organization (2015), the number of hospice programs nationwide continues to grow from the first program that opened in 1974 to approximately 6,100 programs today. Although routine hospice home care comprises the majority of hospice patient care, many patients receive care in inpatient facilities for pain control and complex symptom management that cannot be managed in other settings (NHPCO, 2015).

Hospice care and benefits require a prognosis of 6 months or less. For those patients with chronic, serious illness whose prognosis may be longer than 6 months, palliative care has developed. Palliative care is not limited by specific time periods, and it begins earlier in the disease process as treatments are initiated. The benefits of both palliative care and hospice care are well documented. A review of the most common hospice enrollment periods (Kelley, Deb, Du, Aldridge Carlson, & Morrison, 2013) suggests hospice enrollment had significantly lower rates of hospital and critical care use, hospital readmissions, and in-hospital death when compared with those not enrolled. It was recommended by Healthy People 2020 (Office of Disease Prevention and Health Promotion, 2014) that increases and measured access for safe long-term and palliative care services be monitored over the next decade.

THE PATIENT STORY

Meet Mrs. Page, a 53-year-old divorced mother who was diagnosed in 2015 with stage IV ovarian cancer. Up until 6 months ago, she was receiving curative treatment that consisted of surgery, chemotherapy, and radiation. Palliative care was presented to assist Mrs. Page with improved symptom management related to treatment. Three months ago, Mrs. Page was informed curative treatment for her cancer was not possible, and she was advised to receive hospice care at home. Meetings with hospice staff and a social worker offered support for the expected trajectory of her disease, including illness treatments, death preparation, and dying. Advanced directives are in place.

During the meeting with the social worker, Mrs. Page voiced concerns regarding her children, ages 26, 15, and 13 years. She completed a statement confirming that she wanted her oldest daughter to have guardianship for the younger children. A full family assessment was conducted to identify other guardianship issues. Her 26-year-old daughter willingly agreed to assume the custodial and financial responsibilities of her younger siblings. This daughter is currently working full time at a local bank and is the primary caregiver of her mother at home.

Last week Mrs. Page phoned her hospice nurse to report that she felt very weak, tired, and was experiencing an increase in pain. She indicated that she would like to come to the hospice care center as she thought she might be dying. She was admitted to the center that same day. Currently, Mrs. Page appears depressed. Her verbal responses regarding the presence of pain indicate that it is being controlled through a continuous infusion of morphine. She is not able to move independently and needs repositioning at least every 2 hours. Mrs. Page's children make regular visits to the care center while the social worker and nurses offer support and answer questions regarding their mother's deteriorating condition.

Physical Assessment

The physical examination reveals that Mrs. Page is 5'6" tall, weighs 102 pounds, and has a body mass index (BMI) of 16.5. These measurements signify that she is underweight. Her other vital signs include a blood pressure of 102/64 mmHg, heart rate of 68 beats per minute, respiratory rate of 22 breaths per minute (shallow, unlabored with rhonchi and crackles in the lower lobes), and a temperature of 97.8° Fahrenheit. Her oxygen saturation level is 96% on room air. Pulses are irregular and faint with 2+ edema in lower extremities. Her abdomen is rounded with hypoactive bowel sounds in all four quadrants. Her skin is pale with a gray-bluish hue on the nailbeds. Mrs. Page has no voluntary muscle movement. Her urine output is scant and dark in color. Her last bowel movement is unknown.

PATIENT-CENTERED PLAN OF CARE USING THE OPT MODEL OF CLINICAL REASONING

The patient story in this case study has been obtained from all possible sources, including relevant laboratory values, vital signs, pain assessment, current medications list, and various care conferences. The OPT Model of Clinical Reasoning Patient Problems and Nursing Diagnosis list support the creation of the Clinical Reasoning Web Worksheet that helps the nurse begin to filter the assessment data and information, frame the context of the story, and focus on the priority care needs (Butcher & Johnson, 2012).

PATIENT PROBLEMS AND NURSING DIAGNOSES IDENTIFICATION

The first step of care planning is to identify the various problems and cues presented by the patient and select the nursing diagnoses whose defining characteristics capture these cues and problems. The medical diagnosis for this patient is end-stage ovarian cancer.

Nursing Care Priority Identification

The first step of the care planning is to identify the various problems and cues presented by the patient and select the nursing diagnoses whose defining characteristics capture these cues and problems. The medical diagnosis for Mrs. Page is stage IV ovarian cancer. The nurse identifies the cues and problems collected from the physiologic assessment, psychosocial assessment, and the medical record. The similar problems and cues are clustered for interpretation and meaning. Then relevant nursing diagnoses that "fit" the cluster of cues and problems are identified based on definitions and defining characteristics of each nursing diagnosis.

An assessment worksheet listing the major taxonomy domains, classes of each domain, patient cues and problems, relevant NANDA-I diagnoses with definitions (Herdman & Kamitsuru, 2014), Nursing Outcomes Classification (NOC) (Moorhead, Johnson, Maas, & Swanson, 2013), and Nursing Interventions Classification (NIC) (Butcher, Bulechek, Dochterman, & Walker [in press]) labels has been created. This worksheet is designed to assist the nurse in organizing patient care issues and to generate appropriate nursing diagnoses. An example of a completed table of the taxonomy domains, subcategories, patient cues and problems, relevant nursing diagnoses, and suggested NOC and NIC labels for this case study is presented in Table 13.1.

STOP AND THINK

1. What taxonomy domains are affected, and which diagnoses have I generated?

2. What cues/evidence/data from the patient assessment support the diagnoses?

TABLE 13.1 DOMAINS, CLASSES (NANDA-I TAXONOMY II), PATIENT CUES/PROBLEMS, NURSING DIAGNOSES, NOC, AND NIC LABELS

Domain	Classes	Identified Patient Problems
Activity/Rest: The production, conservation, expenditure, or balance of energy resources	**Activity/Exercise:** Moving parts of the body (mobility), doing work, or performing actions often (but not always) against resistance	• Chronic fatigue • Weakness • Treatment related activity intolerance • Decrease in gross motor skills • Chronic pain
	Cardiovascular/Pulmonary responses: Cardiopulmonary mechanisms that support activity/rest	• Bradycardia • Fatigue • Peripheral cyanosis
Role Relationship: The positive and negative connections or associations between people or groups of people and the means by which those connections are demonstrated	**Role Performance:** Quality of functioning in socially expected behavior patterns	• Unable to assist others and complete activities of daily living • Lethargy
Coping/Stress Tolerance: Contending with life events/life processes	**Coping Responses:** The process of managing environmental stress	• Fatigue and lethargy • Impending death • Dependency on others for care • Concern over children's welfare • Chronic pain

NANDA-I Nursing Diagnoses	Nursing Outcomes Classifications (NOC)	Nursing Intervention Classifications (NIC)
Fatigue: An overwhelming sustained sense of exhaustion and decreased capacity for physical and mental work at the usual level	• Fatigue Level	• Coping Enhancement
Impaired Physical Mobility: Limitation in independent, purposeful physical movement of the body or of one or more extremities	• Activity Tolerance • Immobility Consequences: Physiological • Pain Level	• Positioning • Self-Care Assistance
Decreased Cardiac Output: Inadequate blood pumped by the heart to meet metabolic demands of the body	• Tissue Perfusion: Cellular	• Vital Signs Monitoring
Ineffective Role Performance: Patterns of behavior and self-expression that do not match the environmental context, norms, and expectations	• Acceptance: Health Status • Adaption to Physical Disability • Family Functioning	• Role Enhancement
Powerlessness: The lived experience of lack of control over a situation, including a perception that one's actions do not significantly affect an outcome	• Acceptance: Health Status • Fatigue Control • Knowledge: Perceived Resources • Health Beliefs: Perceived Control • Spiritual Health • Client Satisfaction: Pain	• Self-Esteem Enhancement • Mutual Goal Setting • Pain Management

continues

TABLE 13.1 DOMAINS, CLASSES (NANDA-I TAXONOMY II), PATIENT CUES/PROBLEMS, NURSING DIAGNOSES, NOC, AND NIC LABELS (CONTINUED)

Domain	Classes	Identified Patient Problems
Safety/Protection: Principles underlying conduct, thought, and behavior about acts, customs, or institutions viewed as being true or having intrinsic worth	**Physical Injury:** Bodily harm or hurt	• Impaired mucous membranes from treatment
		• Difficulty with swallowing • Ineffective cough
		• Immobility • Immunodeficiency • Cachexia
Comfort: Freedom from danger, physical injury, or immune system damage; preservation from loss; and protection of safety and security	**Physical Comfort:** Sense of well-being or ease and/or freedom from pain	• Pain related to cancer

Butcher, H., Bulechek, G., Dochterman, J., & Wagner, C. M. (in press).
Herdman, T. H., & Kamitsuru, S. (Eds.). (2014).
Moorhead, S., Johnson, M., Maas, M. O., & Swanson, E. (Eds.). (2013).

NANDA-I Nursing Diagnoses	Nursing Outcomes Classifications (NOC)	Nursing Intervention Classifications (NIC)
Impaired Oral Mucous Membranes: Damage to mucous membrane, corneal, integumentary, or subcutaneous tissues	• Tissue Integrity: Skin & Mucous Membranes	• Oral Health Restoration
Risk for Aspiration: At risk for entry of gastrointestinal secretions, oropharyngeal secretions, solids, or fluids into tracheobronchial passages	• Aspiration Prevention	• Aspiration Precautions
Risk for Impaired Skin Integrity: At risk for alteration in epidermis and/or dermis	• Tissue Integrity: Skin & Mucous Membranes	• Positioning: Pressure Management • Pressure Ulcer Prevention, Skin Surveillance
Chronic Pain: Unpleasant sensory and emotional experience arising from actual or potential tissue damage or described in terms of such damage; sudden or slow onset of any intensity from mild to severe, constant or recurring without an anticipated or predictable end and a duration of > 6 months.	• Client Satisfaction: Pain	• Pain Management

CREATING A CLINICAL REASONING WEB

The Clinical Reasoning Web is a means by which the nurse analyzes and reasons through complex patient stories for the purpose of finding and prioritizing key healthcare issues. Using the web, the nurse defines problems based on patient cues in the data, identifies nursing diagnoses to address and define the various problems, and determines relationships among these diagnoses (Kuiper, Pesut, & Kautz, 2009). The web is a visual representation and iterative analysis of the functional relationships among diagnostic hypotheses and results in a *keystone* issue that requires nursing care. In other words, the Clinical Reasoning Web represents a graphic illustration of how the elements of the patient's story and issues relate to one another and is depicted by sketching lines of association among the nursing diagnoses (Kuiper, Pesut, & Arms, 2016).

Whereas medical diagnoses are consistent labels for a cluster of symptoms, patient stories vary; each Clinical Reasoning Web is written to reflect the patient's unique story and the human response to actual or potential health problems that are best represented in nursing diagnoses. For example, given two patients with identical medical diagnoses, the nurse might determine that different nursing diagnoses and keystone issues are the priority for each based on thinking strategies and diagnostic hypotheses associated with each case.

Constructing the Clinical Reasoning Web

After the problems are identified from the assessment data, evidence, and cues, and the nursing diagnoses are chosen, the Clinical Reasoning Web is constructed using the following steps.

1. Place a general description of the patient in the central oval with the primary medical diagnoses. In this case study, it is a 53-year-old white female with end-stage ovarian cancer.

2. Place each NANDA-I nursing diagnosis generated from the patient cues in the ovals surrounding the middle circle.

3. Under each nursing diagnosis, list supporting data that was gathered from the patient's story and assessment.

4. Because each nursing diagnosis is directly related to the center oval containing the description of the patient and the medical diagnosis, the nurse draws a line from the central oval to each of the outlying nursing diagnosis ovals. Figure 13.1 displays the beginning steps of constructing the Clinical Reasoning Web for this case study.

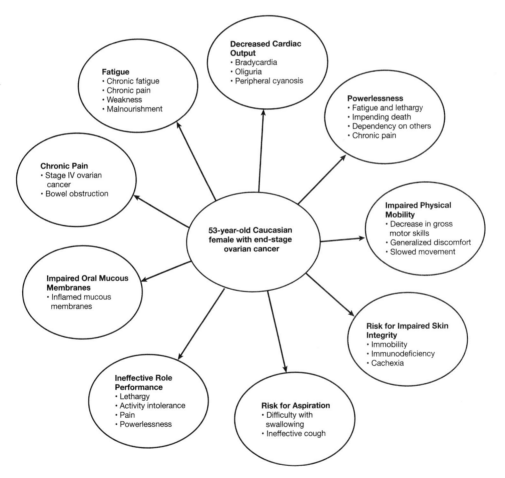

Figure 13.1 Clinical Reasoning Web—Palliative Care: Connections from Medical Diagnosis to Nursing Diagnoses.

Spinning and Weaving the Reasoning Web

In spinning and weaving the Clinical Reasoning Web, the nurse must analyze and explain the relationships among the nursing diagnoses. This process begins with drawing lines from the central oval to each of the outlying nursing diagnoses ovals. Then thinking out loud, using self-talk, schema search, hypothesizing, if-then, how-so thinking, and comparative analysis, as described in Chapter 3 of this book, the nurse determines the connections and relationships among the nursing diagnoses.

The nurse continues to spin and weave using the following steps.

1. Consider how each of the nursing diagnoses and related healthcare issues it defines relates to all the other diagnoses. If there is a functional relationship between two diagnoses, then a line with a one-directional arrow is drawn to indicate a one-way connection and a line with two-directional arrows is drawn to indicate a two-way connection. For example, what is the relationship between decreased cardiac output and activity intolerance? How are these two diagnoses related? How do they influence one another? In the case of Mrs. Page, the nurse would consider if the Decreased Cardiac Output would cause Activity Intolerance or if in a reciprocal fashion, the activity also further decreases cardiac output. In her case, there is a one-way connection between Decreased Cardiac Output to the oval with Activity Intolerance. Another example would be to consider how the nursing diagnosis Impaired Physical Mobility relates to the issue of Impaired Mucous Membranes. In this case, there is no relationship, so no connection is made between these two diagnoses.

2. The first step is repeated with each of the other ovals to determine relationships for connections. If there are functional relationships, connections are drawn until the process is exhausted; visually, the web emerges.

3. When all connections are made, the lines leading to and from each oval with nursing diagnoses are counted and recorded. The numbers can be recorded on the Clinical Reasoning Web Worksheet. A table showing the hierarchy of

priorities of Mrs. Page's problems based on the number of connections is displayed in Table 13.2.

4. The nursing diagnosis with the most connecting lines radiating to and from that oval becomes the *keystone* issue. Figure 13.2 displays a completed Clinical Reasoning Web for this case.

TABLE 13.2 NURSING DOMAINS, NURSING DIAGNOSES, AND CONNECTIONS

Nursing Domain	Class	Nursing Diagnoses	Web Connections
Psychosocial Domain	Emotional	Powerlessness	7
	Roles/Relationships	Ineffective Role Performance	6
Functional Domain	Activity/Exercise	Impaired Physical Mobility	5
		Activity Intolerance	5
	Comfort	Chronic Pain	5
	Self-Care	Activity Intolerance	5
	Nutrition	Impaired Mucous Membranes	3
Physiological Domain	Cardiac Function	Decreased Cardiac Output	4
Environmental Domain	Risk Management	Risk for Impaired Skin Integrity	5
		Risk for Aspiration	2

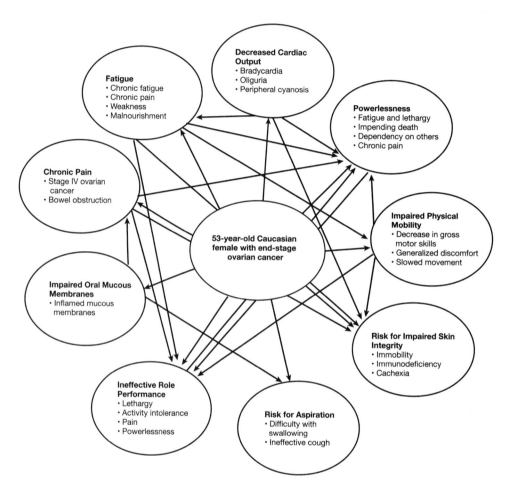

Figure 13.2 Clinical Reasoning Web—Palliative Care: Connections Among Nursing Diagnoses.

The *keystone* issue, the nursing diagnosis with the most connections, emerges as a priority problem. It is the basis for defining the patient's present state, which is contrasted with a desired outcome state (Kuiper et al., 2009). Identifying the keystone issue enables the nurse to focus on subsequent care planning (Butcher & Johnson, 2012; Herdman & Kamitsuru, 2014). After a keystone issue is identified, there is continued knowledge work to identify the complementary nature of the problems ~ outcomes using the juxtaposing thinking strategy. The keystone issue and nursing diagnosis in this case is Powerlessness. Interventions are chosen to assist Mrs. Page with coping and resolving mental conflicts related to her failing health, and they are likely to influence other issues that are identified on the web.

STOP AND THINK

1. What are the relationships between and among the identified problems (diagnoses)?

2. What *keystone* issue(s) emerge?

COMPLETING THE OPT CLINICAL REASONING MODEL

After the Reasoning Web has been completed with identification of the keystone and cue logic, the OPT Model of Clinical Reasoning can be completed. All sections of the OPT Model are completed with the case study described in this chapter.

Patient-in-Context Story

Exhibit 13.1 displays the patient-in-context story for the adult female Julia Page. On the far-right side of the OPT Model in Figure 13.3, the patient-in-context story is recorded. This story underscores the patient demographics, medical diagnoses, and current situation. The information placed in this box is presented in a brief format with some relevant facts that support the rest of the model.

EXHIBIT 13.1

Patient-in-Context Story

53-year-old female with stage IV ovarian cancer since 2011 is admitted to a hospice care center to receive palliative care. Do not resuscitate orders are in place.

Social: Divorced (twice) with three children ages 26, 15, and 13. Guardianship of the two minor children has been transferred to eldest daughter.

Vital Signs: Temperature 97.2° F, heart rate 96 bpm, blood pressure 102/64 mmHg, respiratory rate 22 bpm.

Laboratory Values: O2 saturation 97% on room air.

Status: Verbalization of "tolerable" pain with morphine infusing via PCU pump. Respirations are shallow and uneven. She has weak pulses with +2 edema in lower extremities. She is lethargic and has difficult speech due to dry mouth. Her skin is pale with gray-blue nailbeds and cool lower extremities.

Medications: Morphine 5 mg every hour; lorazepam PRN for agitation.

Diagnostic Cluster/Cue Logic

The next step in the care planning process is completing the web diagnostic cluster/cue logic. The keystone issue is placed at the bottom of the column with all the other identified nursing diagnoses listed above it, in priority order. At this point, the nurse reflects on this list to ask whether there is evidence to support these nursing diagnoses and whether the keystone issue is correctly identified. Cue logic is the deliberate structuring of patient-in-context data to discern the meaning for nursing care (Butcher & Johnson, 2012). In this case study, the nursing diagnoses depicted in the outlying ovals on the reasoning web are recorded under Diagnostic Cluster/Cue Logic on the OPT Model Clinical Reasoning Worksheet along with the number of arrows radiating to/from each diagnosis. Exhibit 13.2 displays the identified keystone issue—in this case, Powerlessness—and it is listed directly below the other nursing diagnoses.

Framing

In the center and top of the worksheet is a box to indicate the *frame* or theme that best represents the background issue(s) regarding the patient-in-context story. The frame of this case is a 53-year-old female with stage IV ovarian cancer receiving inpatient hospice care to facilitate comfort and a peaceful death. The patient's eldest daughter will be assuming custody of her younger siblings. This frame helps to organize the present state and outcome state, and it illustrates the gaps between them to provide insights about essential care needs. The frame is the lens or background view to help the nurse differentiate this patient schema and prototype from others the nurse might have dealt with in the past. The interventions and tests that will be used in this care plan are specific to the frame that is identified. Exhibit 13.3 displays the frame in the case of Mrs. Page and her family.

Present State

The *present state* is a description of the patient-in-context story or the initial condition of the patient (Butcher & Johnson, 2012). The items listed in this section change over time as a result of nursing actions. The cues and problems identified for the patient listed under the keystone issue capture the present state of the patient. These are the problems in which the care of the patient will be planned, implemented, and evaluated. The present-state items are listed in an oval in the

EXHIBIT 13.2

Diagnostic Cluster/Cue Logic

1. Ineffective Role Performance (6)
2. Impaired Physical Mobility (6)
3. Activity Intolerance (5)
4. Risk for Impaired Skin Integrity (5)
5. Chronic Pain (5)
6. Decreased Cardiac Output (4)
7. Impaired Oral Mucous Membranes (3)
8. Risk for Aspiration

Keystone Issue/Theme
Powerlessness (7)

EXHIBIT 13.3

Frame

53-year-old female with stage IV ovarian cancer receiving palliative care at a hospice care center to facilitate comfort and a peaceful death. The divorced mother of three children, ages 26, 15, and 13, has transferred custodial responsibilities to her oldest daughter.

EXHIBIT 13.4

Present State

1. Fatigue and lethargy due to impending death

2. Feelings of powerlessness related to disease process and dependency on others

3. Desire to reconnect with religious beliefs

4. Concern about children's welfare

5. Chronic pain

EXHIBIT 13.5

Outcome State

1. **Rest and Energy Conservation:** Patient will recognize energy limitations and balance activity and rest.

2. **Health Beliefs:** Perceived Control: Pain levels and physical/emotional needs are being met through hospice care.

3. **Spiritual Health:** Verbalization of feelings of peacefulness and finding meaning in a higher power.

4. **Knowledge:** Health Resources: Acknowledgment of agreeable custodial arrangements and available resources for children.

5. **Client Satisfaction:** Pain Management: Self-report of achieving a mutually set comfort goal.

center of the worksheet, and, in this case, there are five primary health issues related to the keystone issue: 1) fatigue and lethargy, 2) expressed feelings of powerlessness, 3) expressed a desire to reconnect with religious beliefs, 4) concern for children's welfare, and 5) chronic pain. Exhibit 13.4 displays the list of present-state issues that relate to the keystone issue and will be subjected to tests to determine whether the identified outcomes are achieved.

Outcome State

Given a defined present state, consideration must be given to desired outcomes that will be achieved to resolve the keystone issue. In other words, one outcome state or goal is listed for each present-state item, and each can be tested and achieved through nursing and collaborative interventions. In this case study, the outcome states with NOC labels (in bold in Exhibit 13.5) aim to assist Mrs. Page to 1) recognize energy limitations and balance activity and rest, 2) acknowledge that pain control and physical/emotional needs are being met through hospice care, 3) verbalize feelings of peacefulness and finding meaning in a higher power, 4) acknowledge custodial arrangements and resources for her children, and 5) report the achievement of a mutually set comfort goal.

Because each present state and its corresponding outcome state directly relate to each other, they are placed next to each other for juxtaposition. This placement will assist the nurse with comparative analysis and reflection while exercising clinical reasoning in this care situation.

Tests

The differences or gaps between the present state and outcome state become the foci of concern in the next step of care planning. The nurse must consider what tests and related interventions are most appropriate to fill the gap between the present state and the desired outcomes. Based on these clinical decisions, the nurse considers evidence that might indicate whether the gaps have been filled. In collaboration with other healthcare providers and the patient, tests are conducted to measure changes and gather data. The nurse asks what and if clinical indicators are available for each desired outcome state; that is, what to consider as to whether the desired outcome is achieved. The tests chosen in this case include 1) vital signs and patient observations, 2) patient verbalization of comfort, 3) patient verbalization of spiritual well-being, 4) case management reports involving the availability of community resources for the support and well-being of the patient's children, and 5) a pain scale. The tests for Mrs. Page are displayed in Exhibit 13.6.

> **EXHIBIT 13.6**
>
> **Tests**
>
> 1. Vital signs and patient observations
>
> 2. Patient verbalization of comfort
>
> 3. Patient verbalization of spiritual well-being
>
> 4. Case management reports: community resource availability for children's support and well-being
>
> 5. Pain scale

STOP AND THINK

1. Is the patient-in-context story complete?

2. How am I framing the situation?

3. How is the *present state* defined?

4. What is/are the desired outcomes?

5. What outcomes do I have in mind given the diagnoses?

6. What is/are the gaps or complementary pairs (~) of outcomes and present states?

7. What are the clinical indicators of the desired outcomes?

8. On what scales or *tests* will the desired outcome be measured?

9. How will I know when the desired targeted outcomes are achieved?

Interventions

At the bottom of the OPT Model of Clinical Reasoning Worksheet, there is a box that indicates Patient Care Interventions (NIC), which are the evidence-based nursing care activities that will assist the patient to reach the outcome states. The nurse must make clinical decisions or choices about interventions that will help the patient transition from present state to the desired outcome state. As interventions are implemented, the nurse evaluates the degree to which outcomes are being achieved. Interventions are evidence-based and gathered from current resources such as literature, recognized textbooks, and prototype examples. Rationales are listed and cited in a separate page column next to interventions. Listing the rationales for each intervention enhances understanding and justification for nursing activities. The interventions and the rationales for this case study are listed in Table 13.3 and include the measures of noninvasive pain relief methods and assessment, encouraging verbalization of feelings and reflection on life achievements, and facilitating resources to support spiritual care.

STOP AND THINK

1. What clinical decisions or interventions help to achieve the outcomes?

2. What specific intervention activities will I implement?

3. Why am I considering these activities?

TABLE 13.3 INTERVENTIONS AND RATIONALES

Intervention	Rationales
1. Provide various noninvasive pain-relief methods to the client and family and explain why they are effective, such as music therapy (Carpenito, 2016).	1. Evidence suggests that music-based interventions can have a positive impact on pain, anxiety, mood disturbance, and quality of life in cancer patients (Archer, Bruera, & Cohen, 2012; Beebe & Wyatt, 2009, as cited in Carpenito, 2016, p. 163).
2. a. Encourage patient to verbalize her feelings, perceptions, and fears concerning her disease (Gulanick & Myers, 2014, p. 156).	2. a. This approach creates a supportive climate and sends a message of caring. The verbalization of feelings and perceptions helps the patient develop a more realistic appraisal of the stressful situation (Gulanick & Myers, 2014, p. 157).
b. Encourage the patient to reflect on past achievements (Ralph & Taylor, 2014, p. 636).	b. This fosters a sense of satisfaction and promotes acceptance of the current status (Ralph & Taylor, 2014, p. 636).
3. Facilitate access to resources to support spiritual well-being (Ackley & Ladwig, 2017, p. 467).	3. Health-promoting conversations about hope and suffering with couples in palliative care has potential for improving hope (Benzein & Savemant, 2008, as cited in Ackley & Ladwig, 2017, p. 467).
4. Make necessary referrals to social services regarding custodial and financial arrangements (Ralph & Taylor, 2014, p. 454).	4. This will ensure social support, resources, and continuity of care for younger children (Ralph & Taylor, 2014, p. 454).
5. Provide comprehensive assessment of pain problem, noting its duration, who has been consulted, and what therapies (including alternative/complementary) have been used (Doenges, Moorhouse & Murr, 2016, p. 599).	5. The pathophysiology of chronic pain is multifactorial. If the condition causing the persistent pain is physiological and incurable (e.g., terminal cancer), all diagnostics and treatments might have been exhausted and pain management becomes the primary goal (Stopper, 2014, as cited in Doenges, Moorhouse, & Murr, 2016, p. 599).

STOP AND THINK

1. What clinical decisions or interventions help to achieve the outcomes?

2. What specific intervention activities will I implement?

3. Why am I considering these activities?

Judgments

The final step in constructing the OPT Model Worksheet is to reflect on the tests and interventions to determine whether the outcomes were achieved. The consequences of the tests are data one uses to make clinical judgments (Pesut, 2008). In the far-left column on the OPT Model of Clinical Reasoning Worksheet, judgments are listed for each outcome. Judgments are conclusions about outcome achievements. Each judgment requires four elements: 1) a contrast between present and desired state, 2) criteria associated with a desired outcome (i.e., test), 3) consideration of the effects and influence of nursing interventions, and 4) a conclusion as to whether the intervention has been effective in the outcome achievement (Kuiper et al., 2009). Based on the analysis of tests, judgments are made as to whether the problem has been resolved. The nurse might have to reframe or attribute a different meaning to the facts in the patient-in-context story. Table 13.4 depicts the outcome states and judgments for this case study. The third column provides the rationales for making the specific judgments regarding whether an outcome state was achieved. Exhibit 13.7 displays the judgments made in this case.

EXHIBIT 13.7

Judgments

1. Resting without signs of distress, all needs met, and emotional support through hospice care.

2. Content, nutrition held for comfort measures.

3. Met with religious leader and verbalizes spiritual peace.

4. Custodial arrangements according to wishes and approval of children, community resources in place with follow-up strategies.

5. Pain is managed, 2 out of 10 on the pain scale (10 is highest level of pain).

STOP AND THINK

1. Given the *tests* that I choose, what is my clinical judgment of the evidence regarding reaching the *outcome state*?

2. Based on my judgment, have I achieved the outcome or do I need to reframe the situation?

3. How can I specifically remember this experience and take the schema into the future when I reason about similar cases?

TABLE 13.4 TABLE OF OUTCOME STATES, JUDGMENTS, AND RATIONALES

Outcome State	Judgment	Rationale
Rest and Energy Conservation: Patient will recognize energy limitations and balance activity and rest.	Patient is resting without signs of distress; physical needs are being met and emotional support provided through palliation and hospice care.	Patient's vital signs are monitored with evidence of impending death (decreased BP, temperature, and heart rate and uneven respirations). Comfort is being maintained and emotional support given.
Health Beliefs: Perceived Control: Pain levels and physical/emotional needs are being met through hospice care.	Patient exhibits contentment; basic needs (safety, hygiene, warmth, and hydration) are being met. (Nutrition has been withheld for comfort measures.)	No physical evidence or verbal report of uncontrolled pain. Patient's basic needs are met. (Nutrition has been withheld for comfort measures.)
Spiritual Health: Verbalization of feelings of peacefulness and finding meaning in a higher power.	Patient has met with religious leader and verbalizes finding peace with spiritual self.	Patient has met with religious leader. Patient expresses her personal perception of spiritual well-being.
Knowledge: Health Resources: Acknowledgment of agreeable custodial arrangements and available resources for children.	Custodial arrangements have been planned in accordance with patient's wishes and with the approval of her children. Community resources have been provided. Follow-up strategies are being developed for implementation at a later date.	Custodial arrangements have been planned and community resources in place. Follow-up strategies are being developed with implementation expected prior to mother's death.
Client Satisfaction: Pain Management: Self-report of achieving a mutually set pain goal.	Pain is being successfully managed. Patient is comfortable.	Pain is successfully managed with a reported pain score of 2 out of 10 (on a scale of 0 to 10 with 10 being the highest level of pain).

The Completed OPT Model of Clinical Reasoning

The completed OPT Model of Clinical Reasoning for a hospice and palliative care patient is displayed in Figure 13.3.

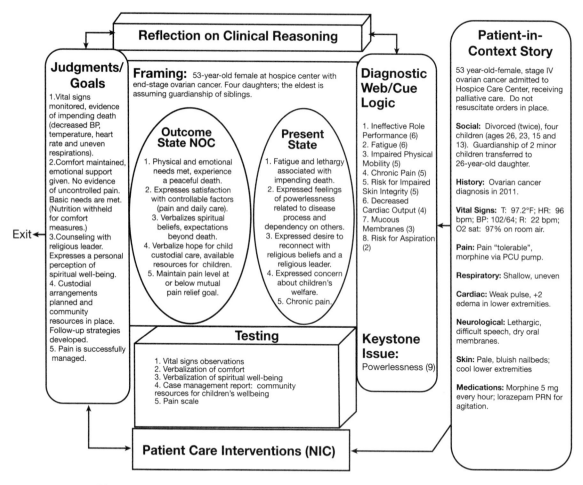

Reflection on Clinical Reasoning

Patient-in-Context Story

53 year-old-female, stage IV ovarian cancer admitted to Hospice Care Center, receiving palliative care. Do not resuscitate orders in place.

Judgments/ Goals

1. Vital signs monitored, evidence of impending death (decreased BP, temperature, heart rate and uneven respirations).
2. Comfort maintained, emotional support given. No evidence of uncontrolled pain. Basic needs are met. (Nutrition withheld for comfort measures.)
3. Counseling with religious leader. Expresses a personal perception of spiritual well-being.
4. Custodial arrangements planned and community resources in place. Follow-up strategies developed.
5. Pain is successfully managed.

Exit ←

Framing: 53-year-old female at hospice center with end-stage ovarian cancer. Four daughters; the eldest is assuming guardianship of siblings.

Outcome State NOC

1. Physical and emotional needs met, experience a peaceful death.
2. Expresses satisfaction with controllable factors (pain and daily care).
3. Verbalizes spiritual beliefs, expectations beyond death.
4. Verbalize hope for child custodial care, available resources for children.
5. Maintain pain level at or below mutual pain relief goal.

Present State

1. Fatigue and lethargy associated with impending death.
2. Expressed feelings of powerlessness related to disease process and dependency on others.
3. Expressed desire to reconnect with religious beliefs and a religious leader.
4. Expressed concern about children's welfare.
5. Chronic pain.

Diagnostic Web/Cue Logic

1. Ineffective Role Performance (6)
2. Fatigue (6)
3. Impaired Physical Mobility (5)
4. Chronic Pain (5)
5. Risk for Impaired Skin Integrity (5)
6. Decreased Cardiac Output (4)
7. Mucous Membranes (3)
8. Risk for Aspiration (2)

Testing

1. Vital signs observations
2. Verbalization of comfort
3. Verbalization of spiritual well-being
4. Case management report: community resources for children's wellbeing
5. Pain scale

Keystone Issue:

Powerlessness (9)

Social: Divorced (twice), four children (ages 26, 23, 15 and 13). Guardianship of 2 minor children transferred to 26-year-old daughter.

History: Ovarian cancer diagnosis in 2011.

Vital Signs: T: 97.2°F; HR: 96 bpm; BP: 102/64; R: 22 bpm; O2 sat: 97% on room air.

Pain: Pain "tolerable", morphine via PCU pump.

Respiratory: Shallow, uneven

Cardiac: Weak pulse, +2 edema in lower extremities.

Neurological: Lethargic, difficult speech, dry oral membranes.

Skin: Pale, bluish nailbeds; cool lower extremities

Medications: Morphine 5 mg every hour; lorazepam PRN for agitation.

Patient Care Interventions (NIC)

Figure 13.3 OPT Model of Clinical Reasoning for Palliative Care Patient.

SUMMARY

Clinical reasoning for the terminally ill patient receiving palliative care begins with an understanding of the patient's story and with consideration of family issues. Using the OPT Model as a conceptual framework and the Clinical Reasoning Web as a tool helps develop the clinical reasoning associated with a particular case. The OPT Clinical Reasoning Model provides a visual illustration of where the patient is (present state) and where the nurse hopes the patient to be (outcome state), all of which is framed through identification of background issues of the patient's story (framing). The Clinical Reasoning Web is a graphic representation of the patient's medical diagnosis (placed in the center oval on the web) with outlying ovals containing relevant nursing diagnoses that reflect the patient's health and psychosocial issues and risks. Through "spinning and weaving" of the web, the nurse can determine the priority of care through the generation of hypotheses and thinking out loud (self-talk) to make explicit functional relationships between and among competing nursing care needs. Once the priority issue (the keystone) is identified, planning can begin. In this case study the keystone issue is Powerlessness.

The OPT Clinical Reasoning Model provides a visual illustration of where the patient is (present state). Five present-state items were identified: 1) fatigue and lethargy, 2) expressed feelings of powerlessness, 3) expressed desire to reconnect with religious beliefs and a religious leader, 4) expressed concern about the children's welfare, and 5) chronic pain. From here the nurse was able to establish where he or she hoped the patient to be (outcome state).

In this case study, the nurse was able to determine these outcomes (using NOC terminology) to be Rest and Energy Conservation, Health Beliefs, Spiritual Health, Knowledge: Health Resources, and Client Satisfaction: Pain Management. The present-state and outcome-state items are framed through identification of background issues of the patient's story (framing). The nurse framed this patient and family situation as a 53-year-old female at the hospice center with end-stage ovarian cancer. Patient is the mother of three daughters, the eldest of whom is assuming guardianship of her siblings.

Ultimately the nurse must determine what evaluation tools (tests) bridge the gap between the two states and make decisions (judgments) of patient progress in meeting the outcomes. The nurse identified these tests to consider: 1) vital sign observations, 2) patient verbalization of comfort, 3) patient verbalization of spiritual well-being, 4) case management reports relating to community resources for children's well-being, and 5) a pain scale. Experience with case studies with these types of health issues augments the nurse's experience and adds to the clinical reasoning skill set that can be activated with future cases of a similar nature.

KEY POINTS

- Clinical reasoning for a patient receiving hospice and palliative care can be promoted with the OPT Model.

- A step-by-step approach is used in this case study involving a patient receiving palliative and hospice care. This approach can be used for similar schema and prototypes of end-of-life care in other health settings.

- Various thinking and reflection strategies are used throughout the clinical-reasoning process to complete the Clinical Reasoning Web and OPT Model of Clinical Reasoning.

STUDY QUESTIONS AND ACTIVITIES

1. Describe in your own words the benefits of using the OPT Clinical Reasoning Model to plan and evaluate patient care given the case study presented in this chapter.

2. How does this model differ from other nursing plans of care models?

3. What thinking strategies would you use in spinning and weaving the Reasoning Web?

4. Are there other nursing diagnoses you would assign to this case study involving palliative/hospice care? If so and given the patient data presented in the case study, what would you suggest?

5. Are there other priorities you would give to this case study? In other words, is there a different keystone issue you would recommend in planning care?

6. What other tests would you consider appropriate to bridge the gap between the present state and outcome state in this patient scenario?

References

Ackley, B., & Ladwig, G. (2017). *Nursing diagnosis handbook: An evidence-based guide to planning care* (11th ed.). St. Louis, MO: Mosby Elsevier.

Bakitas, M. A., Tosteson, T. D., Li, Z., Lyons, K. D., Hull, J. G., Li, Z, . . . Ahles, T. A. (2015). Early versus delayed initiation of concurrent palliative oncology care: Patient outcomes in the ENABLE III randomized controlled trial. *Journal of Clinical Oncology, 33*(13), 1420–1421. doi:10.1200/JCO.2014.60.5386

Butcher, H. K., Bulechek, G. M., Dochterman, J. M., & Wagner, C. M. (in press). *Nursing Interventions Classification (NIC)* (7th ed.). St. Louis, MO: Mosby Elsevier.

Butcher, H., & Johnson, M. (2012). Use of linkages for clinical reasoning and quality improvement. In M. Johnson, S. Moorhead, G. Bulechek, H. Butcher, M. Maas, & E. Swanson (Eds.), *NOC and NIC linkages to NANDA-I and clinical conditions* (3rd ed.), pp. 11–23. Maryland Heights, MO: Elsevier.

Carpenito, L. J. (2016). *Nursing diagnosis: Application to clinical practice* (15th ed.). Philadelphia, PA: Wolters Kluwer Health.

Doenges, M. E., Moorhouse, M. F., & Murr, A. C. (2016). *Nursing diagnosis manual: Planning, individualizing and documenting client care* (5th ed.). Philadelphia, PA: F. A. Davis Company.

Gulanick, M., & Myers, J. L. (2014). *Nursing care plans: Diagnoses, interventions, and outcomes.* Philadelphia, PA: Mosby Elsevier.

Healthy People 2020. (2014). Access to health services. Washington, DC: U.S. Department of Health and Human Services, Office of Disease Prevention and Health Promotion. Retrieved from https://www.healthypeople.gov/2020/topics-objectives/topic/Access-to-Health-Services

Herdman, T. H., & Kamitsuru, S. (Eds.). (2014). *NANDA International nursing diagnoses: Definition and classifications, 2015–2017.* Oxford, England: Wiley Blackwell.

Ignatavicius, D. D., & Workman, M. L. (2016). *Medical surgical nursing: Patient centered collaborative care* (8th ed.). St. Louis, MO: Elsevier.

Kelley, A. S., Deb, P., Du, Q., Aldridge Carlson, M. C., & Morrison, R. S. (2013). Hospice enrollment saves money for Medicare and improves care quality across a number of different lengths of stay. *Health Affairs, 32*(3), 552–561.

Kuiper, R. A., Pesut, D. J., & Arms, T. (2016). *Clinical reasoning and care coordination in advanced practice nursing.* New York, NY: Springer Publishing.

Kuiper, R., Pesut, D., & Kautz, D. (2009). Promoting the self-regulation of clinical reasoning skills in nursing students. *The Open Nursing Journal, 3,* 76–85. http://doi.org/10.2174/1874434600903010076

Moorhead, S., Johnson, M., Maas, M. O., & Swanson, E. (2013). *Nursing Outcomes Classification (NOC): Measurement of health outcomes* (5th ed.). St. Louis, MO: Elsevier.

National Hospice and Palliative Care Organization. (2015). NHPCO facts and figures on hospice care. Retrieved from http://www.nhpco.org/sites/default/files/public/Statistics_Research/2015_Facts_Figures.pdf

Pesut, D. (2008). Thoughts on thinking with complexity in mind. In C. Lindberg, S. Nash, & C. Lindberg (Eds.), *On the edge: Nursing in the age of complexity* (pp. 211–238). Bordentown, NJ: PlexusPress.

Ralph, S. S., & Taylor, C. M. (2014). *Nursing diagnosis reference manual* (9th ed.). Philadelphia, PA: Wolters Kluwer/Lippincott Williams & Wilkins.

World Health Organization. (2015). Palliative care fact sheet No. 402. Retrieved from http://www.who.int/mediacentre/factsheets/fs402/en/

Zimmerman, C. (May 2014). Early palliative care for patients with advanced cancer: A cluster-randomized controlled trial. *The Lancet, 383*(9930), 1721–1730. doi:10.1016/S0140-6736(13)62416-2

INNOVATIVE APPLICATIONS OF THE OPT MODEL OF CLINICAL REASONING

14

USING THE OPT MODEL WITH THE OMAHA SYSTEM*

The authors appreciate and are grateful to Dr. Karen Monsen for her contributions and consultation on the material developed for this chapter.

LEARNING OUTCOMES

- Use the OPT Model and the Omaha System for structuring the case study content and clinical reasoning given a community health context.

- Explain how the OPT Model and the Omaha System Problem Classification Scheme, Intervention Scheme, and Problem Rating Scale for Outcomes support clinical reasoning in community contexts.

- Create a Clinical Reasoning Web using information about Ms. Bessie Lee, a patient with type 2 diabetes who is visually impaired and homebound.

- Explain the clinical reasoning and the thinking strategies associated with reasoning about Ms. Bessie Lee's case study.

- Evaluate the usefulness of the Omaha System of standardized terminologies as a support for reasoning in community health contexts.

This chapter uses the Omaha System to support reasoning about a patient needing care in the home. As you work through this example, compare and contrast the Problem Classification Scheme, Intervention Scheme, and Problem Rating Scale for Outcomes of the Omaha System with the other standardized nursing terminologies that are used in this text. After reading the chapter and studying the case example, consider the usefulness of the Omaha System for generating and organizing community healthcare (Martin, Monsen, & Bowles, 2011; Monsen, Peters, Schlesner, Vanderboom, & Holland, 2015; Monsen, Banerjee, & Das, 2010).

COMMUNITY CARE AND CLINICAL REASONING

Healthcare is moving from acute care hospitals to community settings. Community care is a venue for practice that allows for autonomous nursing practice. In a community context, nursing practice values support patient values for disease prevention, health promotion, and maintenance or recovery from illness. In the community, clinicians learn from patients who maintain health in the context of their homes. Community health nurses appreciate how systems interact in order to achieve health outcomes. Community care often focuses on issues related to environmental health. Community care also highlights psychosocial, physiological, and health-behavior-related issues.

Categories of interventions in the community consist of health teaching, guidance and counseling, and disease prevention. Interventions include administration of treatments and procedures, case management, and surveillance. In some cases, care planning and resource acquisition for patients and communities require political action. When thinking and reasoning in a community context, one needs to consider how patients fit into the big picture of public policy, resource allocation, and health programming efforts. A special nursing knowledge classification system called the *Omaha System* has been developed within the community context and is successfully being used nationally and internationally.

STANDARDIZED TERMINOLOGIES FOR COMMUNITY CARE: THE OMAHA SYSTEM

The Omaha System is an example of a practice-based effort to name activities involved in community nursing practice (Bowles, 2000; Martin & Scheet, 1992, 2005). The Omaha System consists of standardized terms for multidisciplinary problems (diagnoses), interventions, and measures of problem-specific outcomes. The Problem Classification Scheme consists of more than 42 health concepts (problems) organized around four areas of concern: the environment, psychosocial issues, physiological issues, and health-related behaviors. Definitions of each area of concern and examples of patient problems within each are listed in Table 14.1.

TABLE 14.1   OMAHA SYSTEM DOMAINS AND PROBLEMS

Environmental Domain: The material resources, physical surroundings, substances both internal and external to client, home, neighborhood, and broader community	
Income	
Sanitation	
Residence	
Neighborhood/workplace safety	
Psychosocial Domain: Patterns of behavior, communication, relationship, and development	
Communication with community resources	Mental health
Social contact	Sexuality
Role change	Caretaking/parenting
Interpersonal relationship	Neglect
Spirituality	Abuse
Grief	Growth and development

continues

TABLE 14.1 OMAHA SYSTEM DOMAINS AND PROBLEMS (CONTINUED)

Physiological Domain: Functional status of processes that maintain life	
Vision	Circulation
Speech and language	Digestion-hydration
Oral health	Bowel function
Cognition	Urinary function
Pain	Reproductive function
Consciousness	Pregnancy
Skin	Postpartum
Neuro-musculoskeletal function	Communicable/infectious condition
Respiration	
Health-Related Behaviors Domain: Activities that maintain or promote wellness, promote recovery, or maximize rehabilitation potential	
Nutrition	Substance use
Sleep and rest patterns	Family planning
Physical activity	Healthcare supervision
Personal care	Medication regimen

Omaha System. Retrieved from http://www.omahasystem.org/

Each of the 42 problems is defined and has a unique set of signs/symptoms. The problems are taxonomic and represent a holistic, comprehensive view of health consistent with community health nursing practice. One of the unique aspects of the Omaha System is the relationship between the Problems Classification Scheme (problems) with the Intervention Scheme and the Problem Rating Scale for Outcomes. *Outcomes* in this knowledge system are defined as changes in knowledge, behavior, and status of a given problem. The Problem Rating Scale for Outcomes helps one judge if outcomes have been achieved. Parts of the Omaha System are described in the following sections.

Omaha System: Problem Domains

The Omaha System supports a problem identification approach to nursing care. Patient problems are organized in four areas. The areas of nursing care concern are called *domains*. The four domains are the environment, psychosocial, physiological, and health-related behaviors. The domains and examples of problems in each category are described in the next four paragraphs and displayed in Table 14.1.

- The *Environmental Domain* consists of concerns about the physical surroundings, including the home, the neighborhood, and community in which the patient resides. Material and natural resources are also considered a part of the environmental domain. Examples of problems in the environmental domain relate to financial, sanitation, residential, and safety issues.

- The *Psychosocial Domain* involves behavioral patterns, communication issues, relationships, and issues of growth and development. Examples of problems contained in the psychosocial domain are availability and access of community resources, social contact, role changes, interpersonal relationships, spirituality, grief, mental health, and sexuality. Other issues such as caretaking, parenting, neglect, and abuse are classified within this domain.

- The *Physiological Domain* is defined by those processes that maintain life. Problems classified in this area include issues with hearing, vision, speech and language, oral health, cognition, and pain. Problems associated with consciousness, skin, neuro-musculoskeletal function, respiration, circulation, digestion, communicable/infections conditions, and urinary, bowel, and reproductive function are included in this domain. For example, a specific problem associated with circulation, such as "irregular heart rate," would be included in this domain.

- The fourth and final area of the Omaha System is the *Health-Related Behaviors Domain*. It includes behaviors and activities that maintain or promote wellness, recovery, or maximize rehabilitation. Problems within this domain relate to nutrition, sleep and rest patterns, physical activity, personal care, substance use, family planning, healthcare supervision, and medication regimen. Specific signs/symptoms for problems in this domain include issues such as "sedentary lifestyle" under the problem of physical activity and "abuses alcohol" under the problem of substance use.

Interventions and definitions are used to specify and qualify the problems and are displayed in Table 14.2. There are two types of modifiers: one that specifies the level at which the problem is identified—individual, family, and community—and one that specifies the severity of the problem—health promotion, potential, and actual. For example, a problem may be substance use and the sign/symptom is "smokes/uses tobacco." If an individual patient does not smoke but a close friend does and encourages the patient to participate, the first modifier would be "individual" for the patient, and the second modifier would be "potential" for substance use.

STOP AND THINK

1. To what degree do you think the problems in the Omaha System capture the scope of nursing care problems in community health contexts?

2. How are the Omaha System problems similar and different from NANDA-I diagnoses?

3. Do you believe practice in a community health context is significantly different to warrant a unique nursing knowledge classification system? Why or why not?

Omaha System: Interventions and Targets

The second level of the Omaha System is a description of four categories of action. Seventy-five target actions further specify the intervention. Nursing interventions are defined as 1) teaching, guidance, and counseling, 2) treatments and procedures, 3) case management, and 4) surveillance. *Targets,* defined as objects of nursing interventions or nursing activities, are used to further specify the intervention. One intervention in the Omaha System consists of a combination of three defined terms and one customizable field. For example, a wound care intervention description would include skin problem, the treatments and procedures category, and the dressing change/wound care target, with a care description that may describe a wound care protocol. The definitions of the interventions and a list of targets within the intervention scheme are contained in Tables 14.2 and 14.3.

TABLE 14.2   INTERVENTION DEFINITIONS IN THE OMAHA SYSTEM

Interventions	Definitions
Teaching, Guidance, and Counseling	Activities designed to provide information and materials, encourage action and responsibility for self-care and coping, and assist the individual/family/community to make decisions and solve problems.
Treatments and Procedures	Technical activities such as wound care, specimen collection, resistive exercises, and medication prescriptions that are designed to prevent, decrease, or alleviate signs and symptoms of the individual/family/community.
Case Management	Activities such as coordination, advocacy, and referral that facilitate service delivery, improve communication among health and human service providers, promote assertiveness, and guide the individual/family/community toward use of appropriate resources.
Surveillance	Activities such as detection, measurement, critical analysis, and monitoring intended to identify the individual/family/community's status in relation to a given condition or phenomenon.

Omaha System. Retrieved from http://www.omahasystem.org/

TABLE 14.3 TARGET ACTIONS FOR INTERVENTIONS IN THE OMAHA SYSTEM

Target Actions	
Anatomy/physiology	Medication action/side effects
Anger management	Medication administration
Behavior modification	Medication coordination/ordering
Bladder care	Medication prescription
Bonding/attachment	Medication set-up
Bowel care	Mobility/transfers
Cardiac care	Nursing care
Caretaking/parenting skills	Nutritionist care
Cast care	Occupational therapy care
Communication	Ostomy care
Community outreach worker services	Other community resource
Continuity of care	Paraprofessional/aide care
Coping skills	Positioning
Day care/respite	Recreational therapy care
Dietary management	Relaxation/breathing techniques
Discipline	Respiratory care
Dressing change/wound care	Respiratory therapy care
Durable medical equipment	Rest/sleep
Education	Safety
Employment	Screening procedures
Environment	Sickness/injury care
Exercises	Signs/symptoms-mental/emotional
Family planning care	Signs/symptoms-physical
Feeding procedures	Skin care
Finances	Social work/counseling care
Gait training	Specimen collections
Genetics	Speech and language pathology care
Growth/development	Spiritual care
Home	Stimulation/nurturance
Homemaking/housekeeping	Stress management
Infection precautions	Substance use cessation
Interaction	Supplies
Interpreter/translator services	Support group
Laboratory findings	Support system
Legal system	Transportation
Medical/dental care	Wellness

Omaha System. Retrieved from http://www.omahasystem.org/

Omaha System: Problem Rating Scale for Outcomes

The individuals who developed the Omaha System realized the importance of outcome measurement. Outcomes in the Omaha System are evaluated in three areas: knowledge, behavior, and status. The Problem Rating Scale for Outcomes, designed for use throughout the time of patient service, is intended to measure progress in relation to specific problems and to provide both a guide for practice and a method of documentation. When initially assessing patient problems, the nurse observes and documents a baseline score, capturing the condition and circumstances of the patient at a given point in time. This admission baseline score(s) for one or more problems is used to compare and contrast the patient's condition and circumstances over time. The comparison or change in ratings over time is used to assess the patient progress in relation to nursing intervention and thus to evaluate the effectiveness of the plan of care. This documentation system also enables the nurse to communicate patient progress to others (Martin, 2005).

The Problem Rating Scale for Outcomes consists of five-point Likert-type ordinal scales with definitions shown in Table 14.4. For example, for Knowledge the scale is 1 = no knowledge to 5 = superior knowledge. The Problem Rating Scale for Outcomes does not include a formal set of questions that can be scored and summed to produce a final numeric rating. Instead, nurses are expected to have a knowledge base and the clinical-judgment skills that allow them to assign a score or rating based on these definitions (Martin, 2005). The Omaha System book provides examples of ratings for each problem at the individual, family, and community levels (Martin, 2005). Using the Problem Rating Scale for Outcomes enables comparison of needs and health outcomes across problems, populations, and practice settings.

TABLE 14.4 PROBLEM RATING SCALE FOR OUTCOMES DEFINITIONS

Outcome / Concept	1	2	3	4	5
Knowledge: The ability of the client to remember and interpret information	No Knowledge	Minimal Knowledge	Basic Knowledge	Adequate Knowledge	Superior Knowledge
Behavior: The observable responses, actions, or activities of the client fitting the occasion	Not appropriate behavior	Rarely appropriate behavior	Inconsistently appropriate behavior	Usually appropriate behavior	Consistently appropriate behavior
Status: Condition of the client in relation to objective and subjective defining characteristics	Extreme signs and symptoms	Severe signs and symptoms	Moderate signs and symptoms	Minimal signs and symptoms	No signs and symptoms

Omaha System. Retrieved from http://www.omahasystem.org/

An advantage of the Omaha System is that it provides standardization of the framework and structure for documenting care in many community contexts. Standard language provides useful information for clinical decision-making and facilitates continuity of care among and across agencies. The Omaha System facilitates management of clinical data in the areas of public health, home health, colleges of nursing, ambulatory care centers, and, more recently, acute care settings (Monsen et al., 2010; Monsen et al., 2015; Monsen, Schenk, Schleyer, & Schiavenato, 2015). The major strengths of the system are the relevant labels for problems and interventions, the taxonomic structure with definitions and signs/symptoms, and the ability to relate problems, interventions, and outcomes. It is simple, holistic, and comprehensive and has been used by many healthcare clinicians, as well as social workers, chaplains, police, and others (Martin, 2005).

Some of the limitations of the Omaha System are its problem-oriented focus, although terminology researchers are exploring the use of Omaha System terms as strengths as well as problems (Monsen et al., 2010; Monsen et al., 2015). The Problem Classification Scheme relies on a body-system structure especially within the Physiological Domain. The knowledge, behavior, and status outcomes relate to general problem terms rather than specific signs/symptoms or situation.

THE PATIENT STORY

Consider the Bessie Lee story and use the structure of the OPT Model of Clinical Reasoning and the Omaha System to reason about Bessie Lee's nursing care needs. Bessie Lee is a 77-year-old African-American woman who has glaucoma in both eyes and is legally blind in the left eye. She has type 2 diabetes that is controlled with insulin and oral hypoglycemic agents. She has a nurse that comes in and prepares her insulin injections, which Ms. Lee gives to herself. Ms. Lee has a neighbor who comes to take her vital signs and make her breakfast every morning. Ms. Lee is unable to see well enough to prepare her meals. Because she has trouble preparing meals, she eats very little, and the visiting nurse is concerned about her calorie intake.

STOP AND THINK

1. How do I reason about Ms. Lee's needs and care?

2. Based on the information in the clinical vignette and a review of the problem classifications listed in Table 14.1, what problems do Ms. Lee and the nurse have to deal with?

3. Based on data from the story, what outcomes are important in terms of knowledge, behavior, and status?

4. How might the OPT Model of Clinical Reasoning assist me in structuring and reasoning about outcomes that would be important in this case?

5. How does the Omaha System help me reason about the problems, interventions, and outcomes important to this case?

SPINNING AND WEAVING THE CLINICAL REASONING WEB

Relying on the standardized terminology of the Omaha System, the nurse uses the terms to give meaning to the facts and cues as he or she reasons, spins, and weaves a Clinical Reasoning Web. Remember, clinical reasoning presupposes that you have done the reading, memorizing, drilling, writing, and practicing necessary to gain the clinical vocabulary of the classification system in order to interpret data from the patient story. In this case, such knowledge work includes being familiar with the Omaha System, and problem, category, and target actions. Fundamental knowledge needed to plan care for Bessie Lee includes knowledge about the pathophysiology of type 2 diabetes, glaucoma, and the physiological, psychological, and sociological sequela of aging. Fundamental knowledge in these areas helps support clinical reasoning. Spinning and weaving the web involves the use of several thinking strategies in order to determine the *keystone issue* that is likely to benefit from intervention and influence many of the healthcare issues and concerns that have been identified. The thinking strategies of self-talk, prototype identification, schema search, hypothesizing, and if-then, how-so thinking support the nurse as relationships in the Clinical Reasoning Web are established. Figure 14.1 displays the Omaha System domains and patient problems with the case of Ms. Bessie Lee.

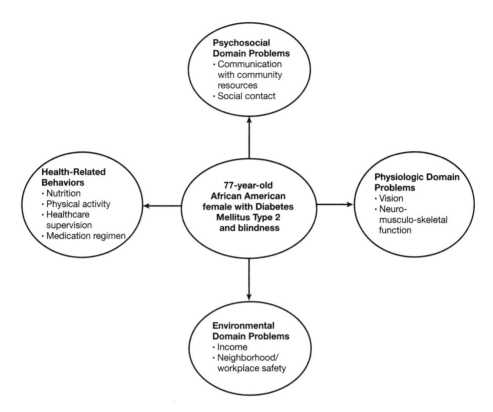

Figure 14.1 Beginning Clinical Reasoning Web: Type 2 Diabetes with Blindness Using the Omaha System Domains and Problems.

STOP AND THINK

1. What are some of the functional relationships among the vision problems, meal preparation, medication administration, dietary intake, and Ms. Lee's nutritional status?

2. How will representing these issues in a Clinical Reasoning Web make the relationships more explicit?

3. What thinking strategies are needed during this process?

4. What keystone issue emerges from the reasoning activities?

THINKING STRATEGIES THAT SUPPORT CLINICAL REASONING

It is difficult to generate diagnostic hypotheses for Bessie Lee's case if one does not know the concepts and definitions of the Omaha System. The thinking strategies of self-talk, prototype identification, schema search, hypothesizing, and if-then, how-so thinking support the nurse while he or she is creating, spinning, and weaving relationships in the Clinical Reasoning Web.

Self-Talk

Self-talk answers the question, "What are the nursing diagnostic possibilities associated with the issue of an elderly person living alone who has type 2 diabetes and is legally blind in the left eye, and who has no healthcare supervision?" Given the Omaha System, problems in the domains are fairly well categorized. The answer to this question results in the identification of problems relevant to the case.

For example, Ms. Lee faces challenges with low income and lives alone (Environmental Domain: Income and Neighborhood/workplace safety). She relies on others for assistance with obtaining services and is homebound; thus, she lacks social interaction (Psychosocial Domain: Communication with community resources, Social contact). Her physical issues include her type 2 diabetes and visual impairment (Physiological Domain: Vision, Digestion/hydration, and Neuro-musculoskeletal function). Finally, she has several problems managing her chronic conditions and maintaining good health (Health-Related Behaviors Domain: Nutrition, Physical activity, Healthcare supervision, Medication regimen). These concepts provide a focus for the care planning around Ms. Lee's story. While spinning and weaving the Clinical Reasoning Web one has to think out loud to oneself and reason about the possible nursing diagnoses that are relevant to Ms. Lee's story.

Prototype Identification

Prototype identification is use of a model case as a reference point for comparative analysis. Bessie Lee's case is one instance of an elderly woman living alone with a chronic medical condition, in need of adherence to a medication regimen that requires healthcare supervision. With prototype identification, one considers the textbook descriptions and explanations of the care needs of patients with the medical condition of type 2 diabetes. The prototype is a reference point for comparative analysis. Using knowledge from the prototype helps in thinking about relationships among problems, interventions, and outcomes. The Omaha System provides the structure and terminology to categorize problems and organize the nursing care focus for an older adult with chronic illness (Monsen, Holland, Fung-Houger, & Vanderboom, 2014), in regard to knowledge, behavior, and status outcomes the nurse hopes to influence in Bessie Lee's case.

Schema Search

Public health nurses often see patients similar to Bessie Lee. Past clinical experiences are helpful in reasoning about this specific case. Schema search is the process of accessing general and/or specific patterns of past experiences that might apply to the current situation. Based on these clinical experiences, nurses collect repertoires of care patterns that help them add to their clinical reasoning knowledge base. The more experiences one has, the more associations one can make and the greater the understanding in complex cases.

Hypothesizing

Given Ms. Lee's story, explain the set of facts identified in the story. Using the Omaha System, the problems become the origins and insertion points for making associations as one develops a Reasoning Web. As one begins spinning and weaving the web, it is easy to see how the data from this case leads one to identify some hypotheses about the patient situation. Table 14.5 displays the diagnostic hypotheses generated for this case.

TABLE 14.5 DOMAIN, DATA, AND PROBLEMS FOR MS. BESSIE LEE

Domain	Data	Problem
Environmental	77-year-old lives alone	Income, Neighborhood/work-place safety
Psychosocial	Isolated at home because of visual impairment	Communication with community resources, Social contact
Physiological	Blind in left eye, secondary to type 2 diabetes	Vision, Neuro-musculoskeletal function
Health-Related Behavior	Does not eat regularly	Nutrition
	Needs supervision for medication administration	Physical activity
		Medication regimen
		Healthcare supervision

The lines indicate there are relationships among type 2 diabetes and problems across the four domains.

If-Then, How-So Thinking

In the Bessie Lee case, examples of if-then, how-so thinking are as follows: If Ms. Lee has significant Physiological Domain–Vision problems, then she will have difficulty with Health-Related Behaviors Domain problems of Nutrition and Physical activity because she is homebound, and the Psychosocial Domain problem of Social contact. The Environmental Domain problem of Income may limit her resources for care and nutrition assistance. Because of all of these relationships she needs Healthcare supervision. Figure 14.2 displays the Clinical Reasoning Web with these relationships connected by lines drawn to and from each domain and patient problems.

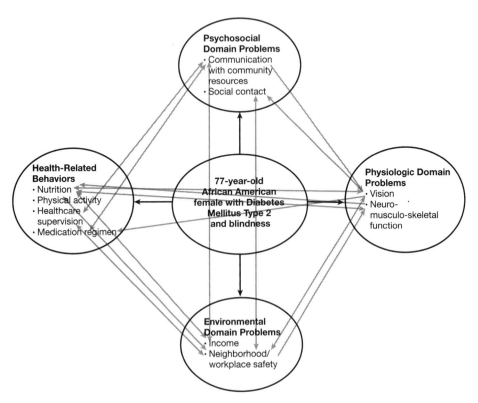

Figure 14.2 Clinical Reasoning Web: Type 2 Diabetes with Blindness Using the Omaha System Domains and Patient Problem Relationships.

Using knowledge from prototype identification of a patient with circumstances similar to those of Ms. Lee, the nurse will be alert to safety issues which may span the domains. For example, Environment Domain issues including Neighborhood/workplace could relate to safety because of living alone. Physiological Domain issues including Vision and Neuro-musculoskeletal function may cause sufficient risk that Ms. Lee might not be able to continue to live independently. Look at Figure 14.2 and see how these relationships continue to fill the web.

Figure 14.3 is a completed Clinical Reasoning Web for Ms. Lee. Here additional relationships have been identified. With Ms. Lee's low income, she may have difficulty with nutrition, which requires communication with community resources.

She lives alone and might have deficits with social contacts, which can cause problems in the psychosocial domain. As the nurse reasons about relationships and draws lines of association and connections on the web, there seems to be a convergence of functional relationships around the keystone issue of nutrition. Doesn't it make sense that if Ms. Lee maintains her nutrition and medication regimen, her diabetes will be better controlled, she will have more energy for activity, and safety will not be so compromised? There are a number of ways to frame the data from this case study. Because Ms. Lee has vision problems, lives alone, has safety issues, and has type 2 diabetes with a complicated medical regimen, it follows that her story presents the frame of healthcare supervision.

Comparative Analysis

Once diagnostic hypotheses and their relationships are made explicit using the web, comparative analysis determines which of these relationships is the keystone or the central supporting issues of Ms. Lee's nursing care focus. Identification of keystone issues enables one to clarify the problem, target, and intervention. For example, managing Ms. Lee's nutrition more effectively contributes to health maintenance in other areas of her life. Identification of these issues helps frame the reasoning tasks and determine the outcome present state and test that will fill the evidence gap needed to make clinical judgments.

STOP AND THINK

1. What theme emerges from creating the Clinical Reasoning Web?

2. What present state does the theme suggest?

3. Given the present state, what outcome is suggested?

4. How does concurrent consideration of outcome state, present state, and frame lead to specification of outcome criteria?

5. What is the gap between the present state and outcome state?

6. What evidence will fill the gap and move Ms. Lee from the defined present state to the desired outcome state?

7. What clinical decisions do I need to make in order to help Ms. Lee achieve the desired state?

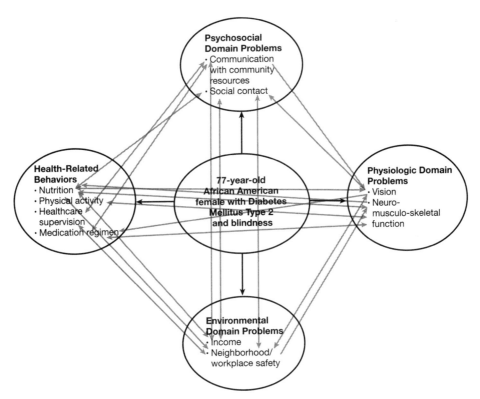

Figure 14.3   Completed Clinical Reasoning Web: Type 2 Diabetes with Blindness using the Omaha System Domains and Patient Problem Relationships.

Healthcare supervision is one possible frame for Ms. Lee's case. When a frame has been identified, the stage is set for clarification of the present state and outcome state. The gap between the outcome state and the present state sets up a test. Evidence that fills the gap stimulates decision-making or choices of nursing interventions that are targeted toward outcome achievement. Figure 14.4 displays the OPT Model of Clinical Reasoning Worksheet for Ms. Bessie Lee.

Because health-seeking behavior is the frame or backdrop of Ms. Lee's story, and given the fact that the Omaha System has three outcomes related to knowledge, behavior, and status, one can begin to generate clinical decision-making or specific interventions that will help Ms. Lee transition from poor nutrition to adequate intake. Using the thinking strategy of juxtaposition, one can contrast the present state (poor nutrition) with a desired outcome state of a 1200-calorie American Diabetic Association (ADA) diet.

Juxtaposing

The side-by-side contrast of one state with the other suggests the gap that needs to be filled to achieve the outcome. The differences or gaps evident from the present to desired state help establish the creation of a test. Given Ms. Lee's case, the nurse contrasts poor nutritional intake with the desired outcome of a 1200-calorie ADA diet for a person with type 2 diabetes. The side-by-side comparison of these two states or conditions creates a gap. The gap must be bridged from one state to the other. Bridging the gap is influenced by clinical decisions and nursing actions. In order to meet or match the desired outcome criteria of maintaining a daily 1200-calorie ADA diet, the nurse works with Ms. Lee and the home health aide to make arrangements for insulin injections and design a diet using the resources available to Ms. Lee in the community.

STOP AND THINK

1. What evidence do I use to know the gap has been filled?

2. What nursing care actions or clinical decisions need to be made to obtain the evidence?

3. Given the Omaha System, what outcomes need to be specified in terms of knowledge, behavior, and status of this problem?

Given the frame of healthcare supervision and juxtaposing of present state and outcomes state, a test between Ms. Lee's present state of nutrition and desired outcome state of 1200 calories per day is created. This outcome involves both knowledge and behavior. The outcome according to the Omaha System also includes some measure related to status of the problem so changes over time can be noted. These outcomes can then be scaled based on the five-point rating scales.

Decision-Making (Interventions)

To assist Ms. Lee in the transition from the present state of inadequate nutrition to the desired outcome of 1200 calories per day, the nurse used all four categories in the Omaha System: Teaching, guidance, and counseling; Treatments and procedures; Case management, and Surveillance. Clinical decision-making related to interventions that help the patient transition from present state to desired state is key. The Omaha System book and Omaha System Guidelines website (Omaha System, n.d.) provide guidance concerning activities and interventions nurses use to help patients transition from identified present states to specified outcomes states. How is the nurse going to assist Ms. Lee to move from present state to outcome state? The goal of this decision-making is to select the interventions and actions that will have the most influence on the outcome and eliminate interventions and actions that have little or no influence on the outcome. The nurse will know because of comparative analysis and use of the outcome rating scale. Conducting tests involves use of the thinking strategy of comparative analysis and reflexive comparison, and with the Omaha System use of the Problem Rating Scale for Outcomes as a measure of progress or change. Review the completed OPT Model of Clinical Reasoning Worksheet for Ms. Lee in Figure 14.4.

Reflexive Comparison

The next time the nurse comes to see Ms. Lee, the nurse will compare Ms. Lee's progress from one observation or visit to the next. In this way, the nurse is using both the identified outcome criteria and Ms. Lee as her own standard of progress or outcome achievement. The nurse will use reflexive comparison as a way to conduct a test. By juxtaposing the outcome-state criteria with a reflexive comparison of Bessie Lee's current state, the nurse will have data and evidence that can be used in making a clinical judgment. For example, if Ms. Lee achieved the outcome criteria of maintaining a 1200-calorie diet, she would have achieved the outcome. If, however, Ms. Lee's conditions deteriorated, reflection and reframing of the keystone issue or the present state would need to take place.

This situation would change the story and activate the diagnostic cluster/cue logic and result in a different present state, outcome state, and test. A third possibility is that Ms. Lee could improve but not achieve or meet the desired outcome. If this were the case, then reflection is likely to provide new data and insights resulting in another frame or set of clinical decisions or interventions to promote the transition to the outcome state. Data or evidence derived from these comparisons are the facts one uses to make clinical judgments.

On her next visit, Ms. Lee reports that the home health aide who gives her insulin also prepares her breakfast and visits with her while she eats. At noon she receives Meals-on-Wheels service and eats most of her lunch, saving some for her dinner. She has also started having a snack before bedtime to get additional calories for the day.

STOP AND THINK

1. Given what Ms. Lee reports, what judgments do I make about outcome achievement?

2. How would this judgment be documented using the Omaha System?

3. How did the OPT Model and the Omaha System help structure the reasoning and problem identification in this case?

4. Given Ms. Lee's report, is it necessary to reframe this situation?

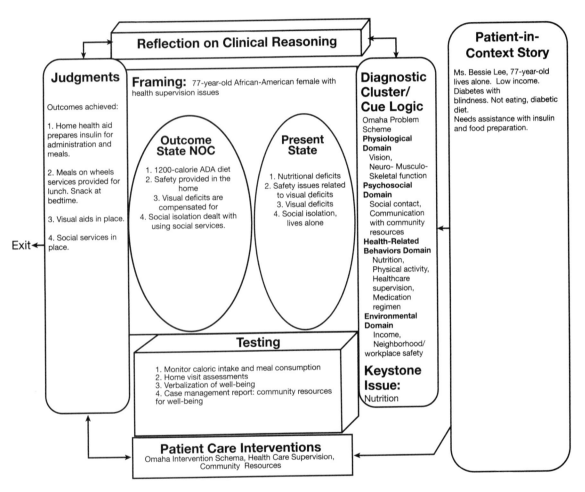

Figure 14.4   The OPT Model of Clinical Reasoning for a Community Health Patient Using the Omaha System.

Reframing

What if Ms. Lee did not meet and achieve her desired outcome-state criteria? Reframing would be a necessary sequel to this clinical judgment. Reframing is the thinking strategy of attributing a different meaning to the content or context of a situation given a set of cues, tests, decision-makings, or judgments. If new issues emerged or were not resolved, then reflection and decision-making would activate diagnostic cluster/cue logic to identify other issues as the nurse continues to reflect and reason about the story. For example, how long will Ms. Lee be able to maintain her independence?

Reflection Check

A reflection check pinpoints what has been done correctly, identifies errors, and provides insights and opportunities to identify and understand how to fix errors or reframe issues.

STOP AND THINK

1. If I were Ms. Lee's home health nurse, how would I reason differently about her story?

2. How do my past clinical experiences influence my reasoning about this case?

3. Given this case and the Omaha System, here are some instances of my own use of self-talk; schema search; prototype identification; hypothesizing; if-then, how-so thinking; comparative analysis; juxtaposing; reflexive comparison; reframing; and reflection checking.

4. How will experience with this case influence future clinical reasoning if I encounter a patient with a similar story?

SUMMARY

In this chapter, nursing care with a patient in a community context was discussed. The Omaha System provided the standardized nursing terminology for reasoning about problems, interventions, and outcomes given the community health contexts. The Omaha System was derived from a practice base and has been used and developed over a 20-year period. Advantages of the system include categories for problems, interventions, and outcomes. The system handles most types of problems that occur in community and home health situations. The Problem Rating Scale for Outcomes, although general, underscores the importance of focusing on outcomes in the areas of knowledge, behavior, and status. The OPT Model of Clinical Reasoning helps structure reasoning using Omaha System content given a patient's story. Thinking strategies that support clinical reasoning in general are also useful in the context of community care. Future developments and modification of the Omaha System in concert with other nursing knowledge development activities hold promise for future knowledge development in nursing and the development of clinical reasoning as art and science (Monsen et al., 2015).

KEY POINTS

- Healthcare is moving into the community. Some people suggest community care is the crux of professional nursing education and practice.

- The Omaha System is a practice-based classification system that consists of problem domains, interventions, and outcomes.

- Combining the Omaha System and the OPT Model provides structure for reasoning about patient care needs in community contexts.

STUDY QUESTIONS AND ACTIVITIES

1. Consider your own community health clinical experiences. What classification systems do the home health nurses in your community use? Why were these systems chosen? What are the advantages and disadvantages of these systems given the current state of classification system development?

2. Review Ms. Lee's case. How would you spin and weave a Clinical Reasoning Web for her if you had used another classification system and the standardized terminologies of NANDA-I, NIC, and NOC?

3. Pretend you are a nurse in a community health center that does not use the Omaha System. Create an argument for its adoption in your agency. Be sure to explain the value of a knowledge classification system for professional practice as well as quality patient care.

References

Bowles, K. H. (2000). Application of the Omaha System in acute care. *Research in Nursing & Health, 23*(2), 93–105.

Hitchcock, J. E., Schubert, P. E., & Thomas, S. A. (2003). *Community health nursing caring in action* (2nd ed.). Clifton Park, NY: Thomson Delmar Learning Inc.

Martin, K. S. (2005). *The Omaha System: A key to practice, documentation, and information management* (reprinted 2nd ed.). Omaha, NE: Health Connections Press.

Martin, K. S., Monsen, K. A., & Bowles, K. H. (2011). The Omaha System and meaningful use: Applications for practice, education, and research. *Computers Informatics Nursing, 29*(1), 52–58.

Martin, K. S., & Scheet, N. J. (Eds.). (1992). *The Omaha System: Applications for community health nursing.* Omaha, NE: WB Saunders Company.

Monsen, K. A., Banerjee, A., & Das, P. (2010). Discovering client and intervention patterns in home visiting data. *Western Journal of Nursing Research, 32*(8), 1031–1054.

Monsen, K. A., Holland, D. E., Fung-Houger, P. W., & Vanderboom, C. E. (2014). Seeing the whole person: Feasibility of using the Omaha System to describe strengths of older adults with chronic illness. *Research and Theory for Nursing Practice, 28*(4), 299–315.

Monsen, K. A., Peters, J., Schlesner, S., Vanderboom, C. E., & Holland, D. E. (2015). The gap in big data: Getting to wellbeing, strengths, and a whole person perspective. *Global Advances, 4*(3), 31–39.

Monsen, K. A., Schenk, E., Schleyer, R., & Schiavenato, M. (2015). Applicability of the Omaha System in acute care nursing for information interoperability in the era of accountable care. *American Journal of Accountable Care, 3*(3), 53–61.

Omaha System. Retrieved from http://www.omahasystem.org/

CHAPTER 15

USING THE OPT MODEL FOR CLINICAL SUPERVISION

LEARNING OUTCOMES

- Discuss the concept and purposes of clinical supervision.

- Explain how the OPT Model is used to promote reflection and organize the clinical supervision process.

- Describe how the OPT Model supports the development of critical, creative, systems, and complexity thinking skills.

- Discuss a set of questions that facilitate the supervision process and support the development and acquisition of reflective thinking skills to enhance the mastery of clinical reasoning.

As healthcare systems are restructured and redesigned, nurses have the opportunity to coach and supervise other nurses, protégés, and ancillary healthcare workers. Helping others reason about complex care situations is challenging. The purpose of this chapter is to explore the nature of clinical supervision using the OPT Model of Clinical Reasoning as a framework. Systematic use and application of the OPT Model of Clinical Reasoning with complex scenarios and patient stories supports the development of different types of intelligence including academic, practical, and successful thinking in nursing situations. The structure, strategies, and tactics that support the OPT Model of Clinical Reasoning can also be used to help people master the critical, creative, systems, and complexity thinking skills needed in many healthcare contexts (Kuiper, Pesut, & Arms, 2016; Pesut, 2008). Tools such as the Clinical Reasoning Web, OPT Model Worksheet, and Thinking Strategies Worksheet help organize thinking and reasoning about complex situations and can support the teaching-learning and supervisory processes (Kuiper, 2002; Kuiper, Pesut, & Kautz, 2009).

REFLECTIVE THINKING SKILLS AND NURSING INTELLIGENCE

Robert Sternberg (1985, 1988) makes distinctions between and among academic, practical, and successful intelligence. Academic intelligence is measured by Intelligence Quotient (IQ) tests. Academic intelligence is knowledge focused on what "should" work. Academic problems are well defined, formulated by others, and usually come with all the information that is necessary for problem solution. Generally, academic problems have only one correct answer and method for obtaining the answer. Often academic problems are unrelated to everyday experience. In contrast, practical intelligence (PI) is the ability to apply mental abilities to everyday situations. PI involves learning to manage oneself, others, and tasks. The street smarts of PI are tacit and embedded in experience.

Sternberg (1988) acknowledges that practical problems differ from academic problems in five ways:

- Practical problems are not well defined and are not formulated by others.

- Often one does not have all the information needed to solve the problem.

- There is rarely a single solution to practical problems.

- Everyday experience can be used to solve practical problems.

- Practical intelligence is knowledge focused on what does work.

Practical experiences gained through clinical dialogues, coaching, or supervision sessions combined with academic experiences (theory) build nursing knowledge and enhance individual and collective nursing intelligence. The combination of practical and academic intelligence when linked with experience and coaching helps one develop high Nursing IQ (NIQ).

For example, consider Patricia Benner's (1984) classic work related to the development of expertise over time. By talking with nurses, she "discovered" and made explicit the tacit knowledge or practical intelligences involved in the reality of nursing practice. Benner (1984) identified and defined the following practical domains of nursing:

- Helping role

- Teaching-coaching function

- Diagnostic and patient monitoring function

- Effective management of rapidly changing situations domain

- Administration and monitoring of therapeutic interventions and regimens

- Monitoring and ensuring the quality of healthcare practices

- Domain of organizational and work role competencies

Benner (1984) makes a distinction between "knowing that" and "knowing how." She suggests practical knowledge may elude scientific formulations. Benner (1984) believes knowledge development in an applied discipline consists of extending practical "know-how" through theory-based scientific investigations and through sharing the existent "know-how" developed through clinical experience. Today there is a call for radical transformation of nursing education and the development of a variety of thinking skills to support learning through unfolding of case studies (Benner, Sutphen, Leonard, & Day, 2009) and more intentional strategies to debrief clinical situations (Dreifuerst, 2009, 2012) and simulation (Kuiper, Heinrich, Matthias, Graham, & Bell-Kotwall, 2008).

Nursing Intelligence Quotient (NIQ) is a function of academic and practical intelligence modified by reflection-in-action. It is an ability to cope with demands created by novel nursing situations or new nursing problems. NIQ is the ability to apply what is learned from nursing care experiences and to use reasoning and inference effectively as a guide for the development of nursing care knowledge. NIQ is a function of knowing that, knowing how, and knowing why, as well as a function of a clinician's ability to maintain curiosity and a sense of surprise in his or her work. NIQ is enhanced every time nurses talk with themselves and others in a reflective way about patient care situations. The common denominator of NIQ is reflection-in-action.

Long ago, *reflection-in-action* was a term used by Donald Schön (1983) to describe the process by which professionals think and act. Reflection-in-action is the ability to consciously talk with yourself and others about a practice situation. Reflective practice is a valuable and important paradigm for nursing and provides a conceptual framework and model to support lifelong learning and the integration of knowledge across contexts (Sherwood & Horton-Deutsch, 2012, 2015).

The OPT Model of Clinical Reasoning thinking strategies of self-talk; prototype identification; schema search; hypothesizing; if-then, how-so thinking; comparative analysis; juxtaposing; reflexive comparison; reframing; and reflective check are the specific techniques of reflection-in-action. Reflective skills are central to the "art" by which practitioners deal with uncertain, unique situations. When someone reflects-in-action, he or she becomes a scientist-scholar in the practice context. As a scientist-scholar, the practitioner is concerned about what works but is also curious about what does not work. What doesn't work helps pinpoint the next target for inquiry.

Each clinical case, scenario, and vignette nurses encounter provides an opportunity for the development of NIQ through reflection-in-action. Coaching and clinical supervision are opportunities to help peers and colleagues reflect in order to develop prerequisite skills and the spirit of inquiry essential for professional practice.

STOP AND THINK

1. How can coaching and clinical supervision help develop the knowledge, intent, reflection, curiosity, tolerance for ambiguity, self-confidence, and professional motivation necessary for clinical reasoning?

CLINICAL SUPERVISION AND THE DEVELOPMENT OF SUCCESSFUL INTELLIGENCE

The purpose of clinical supervision is to promote an individual's success and therapeutic competence. Clinical supervision is an interpersonal process that helps people identify strengths, know weaknesses, capitalize on strengths, compensate for or correct their weaknesses, and contribute to their success. Loganbill, Hardy, and Delworth (1982) define *supervision* as an intensive, interpersonally focused, one-on-one relationship in which one person is facilitating the therapeutic competence in the other person. Webb (1997) notes that clinical supervision serves a number of purposes:

- It establishes a formal system for practitioners to explore, discover, and examine their practice in a safe and supportive environment.

- Clinical supervision allows individuals to develop their thoughts and actions in a way that leads to enhanced care delivery to the patient or patient group.

- Clinical supervision enables practitioners to accept accountability for their own practice and development.

- Clinical supervision serves the purpose of containing the stresses of working in a demanding environment within healthcare.

Clinical supervision enables people to learn, develop, and reflect on practice problems and gain insight, support, and guidance that enhance care and professional development (Pesut & Williams, 1990). Active use of clinical supervision is one way to sustain lifelong learning.

STOP AND THINK

1. What are my images, impressions, and associations with the term "clinical supervision"?

2. What are the differences in my mind between coaching and clinical supervision?

3. What qualities or characteristics of a clinical supervisor do I admire ?

4. To what degree has clinical supervision contributed to my personal or professional development and enhanced my NIQ?

Coaching and clinical supervision in nursing promote the development of successful intelligence. Sternberg (1996) defines and outlines what constitutes successful intelligence. Successfully intelligent people possess the following characteristics:

- They don't wait for problems to be apparent; rather they recognize the existence of the problems before they get out of hand and begin the process of solving them.

- They define problems correctly and thereby solve those problems that confront them, rather than solving extraneous problems. In this way, the same problems don't return. These individuals also make the effort initially to determine which problems are worth solving and which are not.

- They carefully formulate strategies for problem solving. In particular, they focus on long-range planning rather than rushing in and later having to rethink their strategies.

- They represent information about a problem as accurately as possible with a focus on how they can use that information effectively.

- They think carefully about allocating resources for both the short term and long term. They consider risk-reward ratios and then choose the options they believe will maximize their return.

- They do not always make the correct decisions, but they monitor and evaluate their decisions and then correct their errors as they discover them.

STOP AND THINK

1. As I review the characteristics of successfully intelligent people in regard to navigating complexity, what strengths and learning needs do I have?

2. Given the context of clinical supervision, how can I foster successful intelligence if I am the supervisor or if I am the supervisee?

Whether one is a supervisor or a supervisee, most supervision starts with a story. Sharing the elements of the story helps contextualize and frame the issues, problems, and learning challenges that need to be mastered. The authors believe the OPT Model of Clinical Reasoning provides strategies, tactics, and tools to organize and support the supervisory process and promote the acquisition of critical, creative, systems, and complexity thinking skills. Stories lead to framing and identification of present-state challenges. Creative thinking and contemplation of the complementary nature of problems and outcomes leads to insights about how to define and specify outcomes. After outcomes are determined, intervention decisions and action choices help resolve situations based on knowledge work and evidence. Finally, judgments about outcome achievement add to one's mental models and schemas about classes of patient care issues, challenges, and success. Supervisors help supervisees reflect, reason, and reframe facts when necessary. Because the word *supervision* means literally to "oversee," a supervisor oversees the work of another with the responsibility for the quality of that work (Leddick & Bernand, 1980).

The OPT Model of Clinical Reasoning is a useful way to think about and organize the oversight of a supervisee's thinking. The reflective clinical reasoning thinking skills for nursing practice depend on the cognitive and metacognitive processes of critical thinking, creative thinking, complexity thinking, and systems thinking (Kuiper & Pesut, 2004). Clinical expertise, clinical reasoning skills, and cognitive and metacognitive processes are needed to know when it is appropriate to deviate from evidence-based guidelines alongside the values and preferences of individual patients to deliver quality, patient-centered, safe care.

USING THE OPT MODEL OF CLINICAL REASONING FOR CLINICAL SUPERVISION

Thus far, we have used the OPT Model of Clinical Reasoning to help structure the reasoning about patient cases. Consider now how the OPT Model of Clinical Reasoning in Figure 15.1 can assist you in structuring a clinical supervision session. The elements and questions that support clinical supervision are contained within the OPT Model. We believe using the OPT Model of Clinical Reasoning to structure thinking and reasoning in clinical supervision sessions assists individuals in considering different types of thinking as well as the different levels of perspective one needs to consider given clinical reasoning challenges from patient care situations.

Students are most familiar with educational clinical supervision. These supervision experiences help students learn about nursing interventions for patient care. As students mature, they develop confidence and expertise. However, new situations emerge, and one might not have the experience to reason effectively about the situation. In these cases, it is wise to seek clinical supervision.

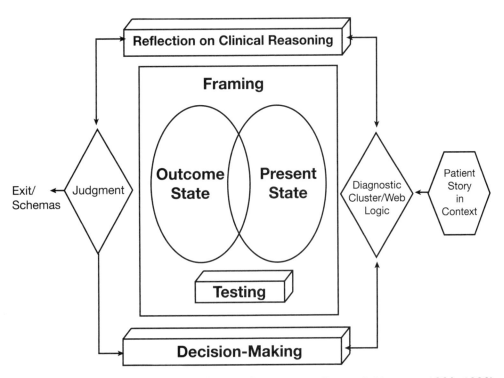

Figure 15.1 OPT Model of Clinical Reasoning (Pesut & Herman, 1998, 1999).

Clinical supervision is one mechanism to enhance the different types of thinking that support reflective clinical practice. Reflection is increased by talking with each other about situations encountered, responses observed, and care solutions that are effective. Case studies, patient care conferences, formal and informal consultations, and use of clinical exemplars or critical incidents increase reflection and dialogue among students and practitioners. Discussion of how cases are alike and how they are different is another way to encourage reflection and build clinical knowledge. The OPT Model of Clinical Reasoning coupled with the thinking strategies provide the structure and techniques for helping people think through complex situations. Given the OPT Model, clinical supervision is accomplished through a dialogue and set of questions that parallel the structure of the model.

There are several questions supervisors can use to help supervisees reason about specific situations with the OPT Model of Clinical Reasoning framework as a structure:

- Tell me the clinical situation-in-context story.

- How are you filtering, framing, and focusing the story/situation?

- What diagnoses have you generated for the clinical situation?

- What evidence supports those diagnoses?

- What outcomes do you have in mind given the diagnoses?

- How does a reasoning web reveal relationships between and among the diagnoses for the clinical situation?

- What keystone issue(s) (attractors) emerge?

- How are present states defined?

- What is/are desired outcomes?

- What is/are the gaps or complementary pairs (~) of outcomes and present states?

- What are the clinical indicators of the desired outcomes?

- On what scales/tests will the desired outcome be rated?

- How will you know when the desired targeted outcomes are achieved?

- What clinical decisions or interventions help to achieve the outcomes?

Most clinical supervision sessions begin with a discussion of a clinical problem. One of the key elements of a supervisory relationship is to help the supervisee reflect on the filtering, framing, and focus associated with the story. In fact, each part of the OPT Model of Clinical Reasoning can become the focus for a set of questions that encourage reflection. Asking supervisees how, specifically, they are *critically* thinking about each element enables the clinical supervisor to uncover hidden assumptions, values, beliefs, and ideas and hold them up for explicit analysis and understanding. Sometimes a clinical supervisor helps frame problems and issues in a new way. After a frame is established, outcomes are evident. Juxtaposing or making explicit the side-by-side comparison of specified outcome-state criteria with present-state data is also a clinical supervision opportunity. This juxtaposition creates a gap analysis and thus the conditions for a test. Because the goal of care management is bridging the gap between present state and desired outcome state, supervisors help supervisees make clinical decisions.

Decision-making is supported by *creative thinking* through the use and application of schema searches, prototype identification, and comparative analysis. The process of considering the strengths and weaknesses of competing alternatives is supported by if-then, how-so thinking and hypothesizing. Supervisors can explicitly ask questions that help supervisees recall facts and knowledge; think about prototypes; access schemas; and use if-then, how-so thinking, comparative analysis, and reflexive comparison in a systematic way. For example, a supervision question such as, "What are the facts?" and another that asks, "Have you had an experience like this one before?" facilitate recall and schema search. "What will happen if..." is a question that is likely to activate hypothesis generation and if-then, how-so thinking. "What were the baseline data associated with the patient's condition?" is a question that activates the thinking strategies of comparative analysis and reflexive comparison.

Clinical judgments are critical to achieve individual and system outcomes. Supervision questions that help thinking in this process are "Have you achieved your desired result?" "What is missing based on your desired outcome criteria?" and "Is there another explanation, frame, or way of looking at the problem that would account for facts at hand?" Certainly, other questions will arise during the course of this clinical supervision dialogue.

The OPT Model of Clinical Reasoning structures the clinical supervision process by organizing the elements of the story, frame, present state ~ outcome state, test, and judgment. The astute clinical supervisor knows what thinking strategies support clinical reasoning. Use of a Clinical Reasoning Web and OPT Model Worksheet helps make the thinking strategies explicit and relevant to the specific case under consideration. Fundamentally, supervising well requires learning how to manage clinical issues. It is important that supervisees perceive supervisors as role models. Use of the OPT tools and techniques may increase the effectiveness and efficiency of the clinical supervision process. The outcomes of such effectiveness will be an increase in the academic, practical, nursing, and successful intelligence that is a part of professional nursing practice. Figure 15.2 shows a blank OPT Model Worksheet. How might you use this structure to guide your thinking and interactions with the people whom you supervise?

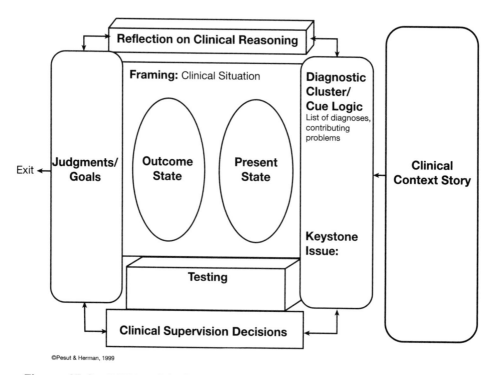

©Pesut & Herman, 1999

Figure 15.2 OPT Model of Clinical Reasoning Worksheet for Clinical Supervision.

In Figure 15.3, the essential cognitive and metacognitive thinking skills that support clinical reasoning are outlined.

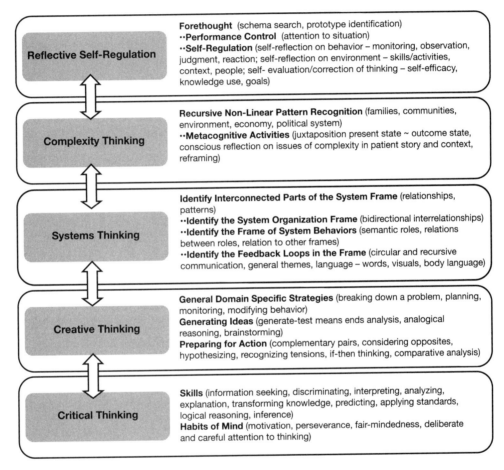

Figure 15.3 Thinking Skills That Support Clinical Reasoning.

SUMMARY

Academic intelligence alone is insufficient for successful performance in real-world settings. Successful *systems thinking* and practical intelligence are also needed. Nursing intelligence was defined as a function of a clinician's ability to maintain curiosity, and a sense of surprise in his or her work. Nursing intelligence develops when one appreciates strengths and recognizes barriers in understandings, skills, and abilities. Nursing intelligence is enhanced through clinical supervision and reflection as practitioners talk among themselves and make implicit knowledge explicit. Nursing intelligence grows when practitioners-scholars identify and discuss the multiple intelligences that exist in nursing and use insights gained to develop the practical and academic knowledge that is nursing science.

Use of the OPT Model of Clinical Reasoning structure can help guide clinical supervision because the thinking strategies used with the OPT Model are the techniques for reflection and clinical reasoning. The OPT Model of Clinical Reasoning encourages the use and application of the analytic, creative, practical, and successful intelligences that contribute to professional practice. Supervisors play a critical role in asking questions that stimulate reflection and the activation of the many thinking strategies that support clinical reasoning.

KEY POINTS

- Clinical supervision is both an art and science. As healthcare contexts experience restructuring and redesign, nurses are going to find themselves supervising a variety of ancillary healthcare workers. Clinical supervision is a skill that must be developed.

- Supervision as an intensive, interpersonally focused, one-to-one relationship in which one person is designated to facilitate the therapeutic competence in the other person. The word *supervision* means literally to "oversee." Thus, a supervisor is one who oversees the work of another with the responsibility for the quality of that work.

- Clinical supervision establishes formal systems for practitioners to explore, discover, and examine their practice in a safe and supportive environment. Clinical supervision allows individuals to develop their thoughts and actions in a way that leads to enhanced care delivery to the patient or patient group. Clinical supervision enables practitioners to accept accountability for their own practice and development. Clinical supervision serves the purpose of containing the stresses of working in a demanding environment within the workplace.

- The OPT Model of Clinical Reasoning can become the structure for guiding questions that encourage reflection. Asking supervisees how they are thinking about each element of the OPT Model of Clinical Reasoning enables the clinical supervisor to uncover hidden assumptions, values, beliefs, and ideas and hold them up for explicit analysis and understanding.

- The essence of clinical supervision is the conscious activation on the part of the supervisor to help the supervisee use the thinking strategies that support clinical reasoning.

STUDY QUESTIONS AND ACTIVITIES

1. What are the essential elements of clinical supervision in your mind? Write your own definition of clinical supervision and discuss it with a peer or colleague.

2. Develop a plan for how you will gain skill as a clinical supervisor.

3. Based on the OPT Model of Clinical Reasoning, develop a set of supervision questions that could be put on a card in your pocket. Make sure the questions raise the key issues for reflecting on clinical situations to achieve desired outcomes.

4. How is supervision of ancillary nursing personnel different from supervision with a peer or colleague? Can you adapt the OPT Model of Clinical Reasoning to accommodate for these differences?

5. What are some of the ethical and legal consequences of clinical supervision?

6. How might adherence to the OPT Model of Clinical Reasoning structure be useful as you consider the ethical and legal issues associated with clinical supervision?

References

Benner, P. (1984). *From novice to expert: Power and excellence in nursing practice.* Menlo Park, CA: Addison-Wesley.

Benner, P., Sutphen, M., Leonard, V., & Day, L. (2009). *Educating nurses: A call for radical transformation (Vol. 15).* Hoboken, NJ: John Wiley & Sons.

Benner, P. E., Tanner, C. A., & Chesla, C. A. (2009). *Expertise in nursing practice: Caring, clinical judgment, and ethics.* New York, NY: Springer Publishing Company.

Dreifuerst, K. T. (2009). The essentials of debriefing in simulation learning: A concept analysis. *Nursing Education Perspectives, 30*(2), 109–114.

Dreifuerst, K. T. (2012). Using debriefing for meaningful learning to foster development of clinical reasoning in simulation. *Journal of Nursing Education, 51*(6), 326–333.

Kuiper, R. (2002). Enhancing metacognition through the reflective use of self-regulated learning strategies. *The Journal of Continuing Education in Nursing, 33*(2), 78–87.

Kuiper, R., Heinrich, C., Matthias, A., Graham, M. J., & Bell-Kotwall, L. (2008). Debriefing with the OPT Model of Clinical Reasoning during high fidelity patient simulation. *International Journal of Nursing Education Scholarship, 5*(1), 1–14.

Kuiper, R. A., & Pesut, D. J. (2004). Promoting cognitive and metacognitive reflective reasoning skills in nursing practice: Self-regulated learning theory. *Journal of Advanced Nursing, 45*(4), 381–391.

Kuiper, R. A., Pesut, D. J., & Arms, T. (2016). *Clinical reasoning and care coordination in advanced practice nursing.* New York, NY: Springer Publishing Company.

Kuiper, R., Pesut, D., & Kautz, D. (2009). Promoting the self-regulation of clinical reasoning skills in nursing students. *The Open Nursing Journal, 3,* 76–85.

Leddick, G., & Bernard, J. (1980). The history of supervision: A critical review. *Counselor Education and Supervision, 19,* 186–196.

Loganbill, C., Hardy, E., & Delworth, U. (1982). Supervision: A conceptual model. *Counseling Psychologist, 10,* 3–42.

Pesut, D., & Herman, J. (1998). OPT: Transformation of the nursing process for contemporary practice. *Nursing Outlook, 46,* 29–36.

Pesut, D., & Herman, J. (1999). *Clinical reasoning: The art and science of critical and creative thinking.* New York, NY: Delmar Publishers.

Pesut, D., & Williams, C. (1990). The nature of clinical supervision in psychiatric nursing: A survey of clinical specialists. *Archives of Psychiatric Nursing, 4*(3), 188–194.

Schön, D. (1983). *The reflective practitioner.* New York, NY: Basic Books.

Sherwood, G., & Horton-Deutsch, S. (2012). *Reflective practice: Transforming education and improving outcomes.* Indianapolis, IN: Sigma Theta Tau International.

Sherwood, G., & Horton-Deutsch, S. (2015). *Reflective organizations: On the front lines of QSEN & reflective practice implementation.* Indianapolis, IN: Sigma Theta Tau International.

Sternberg, R. (1985). Implicit theories of intelligence, creativity, and wisdom. *Journal of Personality and Social Psychology, 49*(3), 607–627.

Sternberg, R. (1988). *The triarchic mind: A new theory of human intelligence.* New York, NY: Viking.

Sternberg, R. (1996). *Successful intelligence.* New York, NY: Simon & Schuster.

Sternberg, R. J. (1998). Metacognition, abilities, and developing expertise: What makes an expert student? *Instructional Science, 26*(1–2), 127–140.

Webb, B. (1997). Auditing a clinical supervision training program. *Nursing Standard, 11*(34), 34–39.

16

FUTURE TRENDS AND CHALLENGES

LEARNING OUTCOMES

- Explain how the OPT Model of Clinical Reasoning can be used to promote reflection and debriefing after a simulation experience.

- Discuss the use of the OPT Model of Clinical Reasoning as a conceptual framework that supports curriculum integration and learning clinical reasoning across a nursing education program.

- Discuss how the OPT Model of Clinical Reasoning provides a structure and model for teaching and learning in interprofessional health education and training contexts.

- Describe how to use the OPT Model of Clinical Reasoning to enhance thinking habits and advance competencies and skill sets to benefit patients, families, and communities that nurse cares for.

In Part I of this book, the OPT Model of Clinical Reasoning was introduced as a structure to emphasize content, process, and outcomes for patient and family care planning and targeted priority tests, interventions, and treatments. It's also used as an evaluative measure to determine the achievement of healthcare outcomes. We described reflective clinical reasoning and the thinking strategies associated with the process. In Part II, applications of the OPT Model of Clinical Reasoning were made explicit through a series of case studies and healthcare challenges and exemplars across the life span. In Part III, we propose and describe innovative applications of the model. For example, in Chapter 14 use of the OPT Model of Clinical Reasoning in conjunction with the Omaha System was illustrated in community health contexts.

The OPT Model provides structure, strategies, and tactics for clinical supervision. As development of the model evolves in the future, other applications of the model are likely to inspire readers to consider additional innovative uses and applications in clinical, education research, and theory development contexts. This chapter discusses use of the model for debriefing, curriculum development, and interprofessional health professions education and training.

THE OPT MODEL: SIMULATION DEBRIEFING

Simulation has been used as an experiential learning experience for many years to help students adapt to the clinical setting by refining practice skills and communication strategies (Foronda, Gattamorta, Snowden, & Bauman, 2014; Feingold, Calauce, & Kallen, 2004; Kovalsky & Swanson, 2004). Practice with simulated experience is important to scaffold the learning of clinical skills and activities. One innovative use of the OPT Model of Clinical Reasoning is as a debriefing tool following acute care, high-fidelity simulation experiences. Structuring debriefing with a teaching and learning strategy such as the OPT Model of Clinical Reasoning gives faculty and students direction for the discussion of clinical and scenario events. One of the most important activities surrounding simulation is debriefing; this reflection activity helps students recognize their actions and thinking to promote mastery and the development of clinical expertise (Feltovich, Prietula, & Ericsson, 2006; Sundler, Pettersson, & Berglund, 2015). The debriefing process extends the analysis of learning and helps students correct their thinking and develop advanced levels of cognition (Fanning & Gaba, 2007; Kuiper, Pesut, & Kautz, 2009; Rudolph, Simon, Dufresne, & Raemer, 2006).

Affective and behavioral learning occurs during simulations when debriefing is structured (Petranek, Corey, & Black, 1992). When debriefing is unstructured, the student responses may be at various levels of cognition and may be inappropriately transferred to future experiences (Petranek et al., 1992). In addition, Petranek et al. (1992) emphasize the importance of writing to develop analytic learning skills. The structure of the OPT Model Worksheet helps students organize their thoughts and serves as a writing outline for the presentation of essential elements of a case scenario. The kinds of thinking that support clinical reasoning defended in Chapter 3 of this text are useful for debriefing activities after simulation. Specifically, the cognitive critical thinking strategies of organization, comparison, classification, evaluation, summarization, and analysis (Petranek et al., 1992) can be described and explained as students work through the self-regulating reflection questions.

There is research evidence to suggest the OPT Model of Clinical Reasoning is an effective tool for debriefing after high-fidelity simulation (Kuiper, Heinrich, Matthias, Graham, & Bell-Kotwall, 2008). When the OPT Model Worksheet is used for debriefing as a scaffold for reflection and thinking, clinical reasoning following simulation experiences improves. Constructivist learning theory was used to organize and guide the project. Constructivist theory asserts that situated cognition occurs between a person and a situation (Schunk, 2015). This premise guided the hypothesis that problem-solving with high-fidelity simulation would be similar to authentic clinical experiences as measured by the analysis of the OPT Model Worksheets the students used for debriefing. A group of students who served as their own controls were compared on their use of the OPT Model Worksheet for debriefing before and after simulation, and then for debriefing after authentic clinical experiences.

The project involved 44 undergraduate senior-level baccalaureate nursing students who had no previous exposure to patient simulation apart from task trainer exercises in previous courses. OPT Model Worksheets were compared for a debriefing session after authentic clinical experiences (variety of critical care units) and simulation experiences (30 to 45 minutes with an acute care scenario). There were no significant differences on a measurement tool between the mean scores on the OPT Model Worksheets between the two groups ($t = -1.321$, $p = .194$). The inter-rater reliability was shown to be statistically significant on this tool in previous research studies [(Kendall's coefficient: $W = .703$, $X2 (24) = .573$, $p = .000$)] (Kautz et al., 2009).

The OPT Model Worksheet scores were higher after debriefing for simulation on the following measures: listing interventions, recording laboratory data, making judgments regarding tests, and connecting present-outcome states with NANDA-I diagnoses. Practicing thinking strategies, followed by feedback and monitoring, promotes higher-order cognitive skills and expertise to perform tasks efficiently and effectively (Feltovich et al., 2006; Kuiper & Pesut, 2004).

STOP AND THINK

1. How can debriefing with the OPT Model be used and combined with simulation and real-world practice to promote the development of clinical reasoning?

CURRICULUM INTEGRATION: USING THE OPT MODEL OF CLINICAL REASONING ACROSS THE CURRICULUM

Another innovative application of the OPT Model relates to curriculum development and integration in nursing education programs. The authors assert it is essential to assure that nurses have clinical reasoning skills to diagnose problems, initiate appropriate treatments, manage complications, and prevent adverse patient outcomes (Lapkin, Levett-Jones, Bellchambers, & Fernandez, 2010). Faculty in nursing education programs are challenged to help students learn and master these clinical reasoning skills despite the fact that there are limited teaching and learning strategies that promote and measure clinical reasoning outcomes (Boshuizen & Schmidt, 2000; Groves, O'Rourke, & Alexander, 2003; Hoben, Varley, & Cox, 2007; Kabanza, Bisson, Charneau, & Taek-Sueng, 2006; Liu, Chan, & Hui-Chan, 2000; McAllister & Rose, 2000; Norman & Eva, 2010; Rochmawati & Wiechula, 2010; Unsworth, 2001).

Some educators argue a paradigm shift is needed in healthcare education with a need to replace the hypothetical-deductive model of reasoning (Elstein, Shulman, & Sprafka, 1990) with narrative reasoning that supports contextually, socially constructed realities from multiple perspectives (Benner, Hughes, & Sutphen, 2008; Edwards & Richardson, 2008; Murphy, 2004). The educational and cognitive developmental research in nursing has not consistently shown a relationship between patient outcomes and critical thinking in clinical settings. Reflective thinking in practice contexts is promoted with the OPT Model structure, content, and process as individuals create meaning out of experiences and patient outcomes are achieved.

Expert reasoning has been shown to be complex and multidimensional in regard to knowledge and skills (Norman & Eva, 2010). Others suggest the key to promoting clinical reasoning is through practice in a variety of circumstances to formulate scripts or schema that build a bank of stored knowledge from case to case (Kabanza et al., 2006). The authors of this text assert that repetition with the OPT Model promotes the development of clinical reasoning in authentic situations to enhance intuition and insights, as well as influence and affect future patient interactions.

The OPT Model of Clinical Reasoning meets the standards for promoting clinical reasoning as it is context-dependent, domain-specific, and recursive in process (Gillespie, 2010). Clinical reasoning outcomes Tare derived from thinking strategies emerge from the relationship between and among domain-specific language, structure, and processes. The domain-specific language is *content* (clinical vocabulary) and knowledge represented by nursing language used to organize patient health issues for clinical reasoning. The organized use of standardized nursing terminologies is related to improvements in documented patient outcomes in some studies (Kautz, Kuiper, Pesut, & Williams, 2006; Müller-Staub, 2009). The OPT Model *structure* is used as a scaffold for thinking activities. The self-regulating reflective thinking *processes* pull experiences together to enhance efficiency reasoning. Figure 16.1 represents the relationship among *content, structure,* and *process* in a framework that services clinical reasoning outcomes.

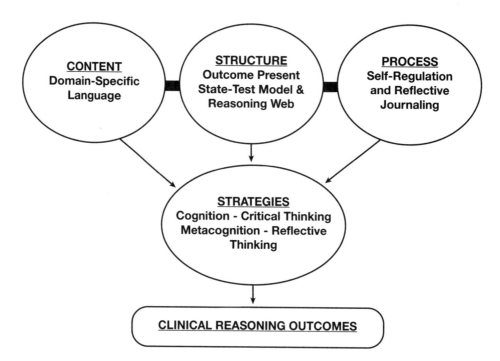

Figure 16.1 Content, Structure, Process Model.

Research with the OPT Model of Clinical Reasoning demonstrates that students increase their thinking to higher levels and refine their attention to patient problems (Kuiper et al., 2009). When students transition from traditional care plan formats, they are enthusiastic about using the OPT Model Worksheet and see the clinical assignment as more patient-focused.

Based on these findings, the undergraduate faculty at one school integrated the OPT Model of Clinical Reasoning across a curriculum as students progressed through different specialties, and advanced learning with more complex and acute patient assignments (Kuiper, 2013). The use of the OPT Model Worksheets varied by course while the students planned care specific to individual patients instead of copying prepublished plans from textbooks or articles. Faculty integrated the OPT Model of Clinical Reasoning into the following courses within the curriculum:

- *Clinical Reasoning and Scientific Inquiry:* Foundation course where the OPT Model Worksheets are introduced one section at a time and practiced in class.

- *Adult Health Nursing I:* OPT Model Worksheets are completed for seven clinical assignments.

- *Mental Health Nursing:* OPT Model Worksheets for inpatient and community experiences (Bland et al., 2009).

- *Maternal-Infant Nursing:* OPT Model Worksheets are completed for simulation debriefing and for three clinical assignments.

- *Gerontology/End-of-Life Care:* OPT Model reflection activity in long-term care for one assignment.

- *Pediatric Nursing:* OPT Model Worksheets completed four times.

- *Community Health Nursing:* OPT Model Worksheet for one comprehensive home care visit.

- *Adult Health Nursing II:* OPT Model Worksheet completed for three complex health problem patients in critical care.

The integration of the OPT Model Worksheets was not the same in every course because the clinical assignments and clinical contexts were different in each specialty area. However, the consistent use of the model and pedagogy throughout the program reinforced the structure, content, and process of clinical reasoning. Repetition and repeated application of the model contribute to the creation of habits of mind so that by the end of the curriculum, students have schemas and frameworks for thinking that are habitually embedded, so the scaffold of the worksheets are no longer needed.

The measurable outcomes for this integration are high licensure pass rates and employer satisfaction with new graduate performance. A recent graduate from a program with OPT Model integration commented that the OPT Model practice for problem-solving aided her in passing the licensure examination.

Successful integration of the OPT Model pedagogy requires annual orientation, supervision, and review of the ways new and experienced faculty understand and make use of the worksheets. Patient outcomes are similar for many healthcare educators as they strive to help students: a) understand patients and their issues in the context where they live, b) use procedural and content knowledge for concerns in the social and temporal situation, c) understand how patient conditions change and need to be managed, and d) consider patients' participation in their own care (Liu et al., 2000). Faculty guidance, mentoring, and expertise in the process of evaluating clinical reasoning are essential to promoting growth in student clinical reasoning ability and competence in solving patient problems.

To promote the adoption, application, and evaluation of the OPT Model in nursing curricula, the authors offer the following suggestions:

- Practice clinical reasoning in clinical situations.

- Use scaffolding methods to promote good habits of mind.

- Promote reflection to enhance the metacognition of clinical reasoning.

- Give ample feedback to promote growth in clinical reasoning skills.

- Practice with the thinking strategies promoted with the OPT Model to facilitate the transfer of these skills to new practice arenas.

STOP AND THINK

1. How does the structure, content, and process model incorporate the use of the OPT Model of Clinical Reasoning and relate to my current course work or learning experiences?

2. What specific faculty development, mentoring, and/or guidance is needed to assist faculty in helping students master thinking strategies and tactics associated with the OPT Model of Clinical Reasoning?

3. What might stop faculty or students from adopting the OPT Model of Clinical Reasoning?

THE OPT MODEL AND INTERPROFESSIONAL EDUCATION

The final example of an innovative application and use of the OPT Model relates to its adoption and use in interprofessional education. The future of healthcare delivery depends on the attention to interprofessional education and practice models. Nurses can educate their colleagues about the OPT Model of Clinical Reasoning and show how it promotes teamwork that is essential for coordinating care. Recently, statements put forth for competency-based education from the Institute of Medicine (IOM) report (2010) specify competencies that should be included in nursing and other healthcare provider education to prepare nurses for expert decision-making, quality-enhancement skills, systems thinking, and team leadership at all levels of preparation. These competencies include knowledge, skills, and abilities related to interprofessional teamwork, patient-centered care, using information technologies, promoting ethical standards, and developing leadership for health promotion and disease management. Interprofessional education ought to prepare new providers with the skills to keep up to date with knowledge development, evidence-based practice, and evidence-based teaching strategies.

Education mandates in the ANA Scope and Standards of Practice (ANA, 2015) include nurses' preparation for essential roles in care coordination in future healthcare contexts. Educational strategies are needed to teach clinical reasoning for care coordination in collaboration with others (ANA, 2015; Kuiper, Pesut, & Arms, 2016; Lamb, Zimring, Chuzi, & Dutcher, 2010), during didactic and clinical experiences to facilitate team-based, patient-centered care. Clinical reasoning for the coordination of care challenges nurses and all members of the interprofessional team to think and reflect about practice issues, interventions, and outcomes that support intervention plans of the interprofessional team. The knowledge, skills, and attitudes associated with interprofessional education provide the competencies and skill sets that are enhanced with the OPT Model of Clinical Reasoning.

Some of the pedagogical strategies to assist faculty in promoting clinical reasoning for interprofessional collaboration include creating situations where students work and interact together in teams in simulation or authentic clinical settings. Using the OPT Model of Clinical Reasoning with a group of provider students from different disciplines fosters systems thinking beyond the individual level. The complexity of clinical reasoning to coordinate care involves thinking about the individual patient while simultaneously considering the issues of working in an interprofessional team that must negotiate organizational and system issues. Clinical reasoning to coordinate care requires the simultaneous consideration of several levels of perspective: patient-centered, team-centered, and system-centered reasoning.

The literature also suggests an educational agenda surrounding interprofessional healthcare curricula with the goal of equipping students with interprofessional capabilities and the abilities to recognize professional boundaries, reflect on interprofessional relationships, and become aware of stereotypes that exist within self, others, and healthcare delivery teams (Thistlewaite, 2012). One reason to develop interprofessional curricula with embedded clinical reasoning strategies and tools is the fact that when students learn together in interprofessional clinical-learning experiences, confidence, competence, communication, and understanding of role clarity for teamwork improve patient care (Morphet et al., 2014). The meta-model structure that the OPT Model of Clinical Reasoning provides, combined with the filtering, framing, and focus from various healthcare disciplines, supports clinical reasoning, interprofessional understanding, and teamwork. The OPT Model of Clinical Reasoning for interprofessional teamwork provides a next-generation model of innovation and perspective taking in care coordination efforts that support team-based care, decision-making, and judgments about achieving patient outcomes from a shared plan of care.

STOP AND THINK

1. How are filtering, framing, focus, and the standardized terminologies and communication between interprofessional healthcare team members essential for clinical reasoning to coordinate care to address patient and family needs?

2. How can the structure, content, and process model enhance my interprofessional teamwork?

3. Given the current healthcare contexts, how can the OPT Model of Clinical Reasoning be used with interprofessional supervision?

SUMMARY

Three different and innovative uses of the OPT Model presented in this chapter are a) a debriefing tool following clinical simulations, b) a method of integrating reflective clinical reasoning pedagogy across a curriculum, and c) a tool to enhance interprofessional education and teamwork for the future of healthcare delivery. There are probably many more uses for the OPT Model that have yet to be described. The OPT Model is evolving as a valuable tool to enhance reasoning and thinking in healthcare settings. The flexibility of the tool to promote clinical reasoning in a variety of ways is based on its foundations in constructivist theory and situated cognition. The OPT Model can be used in a variety of clinical situations and contexts, with a variety of students and providers, and even in the education of patients and families to promote health and wellness.

KEY POINTS

• The OPT Model of Clinical Reasoning can be used as a debriefing tool following simulation experiences. Structuring debriefing with a teaching and learning strategy such as the OPT Model of Clinical Reasoning gives the faculty and students some direction for the discussion of thinking and clinical reasoning

• The OPT Model of Clinical Reasoning can be integrated throughout the curriculum of a nursing program. Promoting clinical reasoning over time enhances the student's ability to diagnose problems, initiate appropriate treatments, manage complications, and prevent adverse patient outcomes.

• The OPT Model of Clinical Reasoning can be incorporated into interprofessional education experiences. Nurses working with other disciplines can influence the coordination of care through appreciation and understanding of how those disciplines filter, frame, and focus care-planning activities.

STUDY QUESTIONS AND ACTIVITIES

1. Based on the OPT Model of Clinical Reasoning, develop a set of questions that you could ask yourself for the debriefing process following simulation. Make sure the questions raise key issues for reflecting on the simulation that did or did not achieve desired outcomes.

2. How is debriefing after simulation the same or different from debriefing following authentic clinical experiences? How does the OPT Model help to determine these differences?

3. Think about a nursing program and a particular curriculum. How would you integrate the OPT Model throughout to enhance reflective clinical reasoning in each course?

4. What are the essential elements of interprofessional education in your mind? Write your own definition of interprofessional education and share it with a peer or colleague.

5. Develop a plan for how you would introduce the OPT Model of Clinical Reasoning to an interprofessional team.

References

American Nurses Association (ANA). (2015). *Nursing: Scope and standards of practice* (3rd ed.). Silver Spring, MD: American Nurses Association.

Benner, P., Hughes, R. G., & Sutphen, M. (2008). Clinical reasoning, decision making, and action: Thinking critically and clinically. In R. G. Hughes (Ed.), *Patient safety and quality: An evidence-based handbook for nurses* (pp. 1–23). Washington, DC: Association for Healthcare Research and Quality. Retrieved from https://archive.ahrq.gov/professionals/clinicians-providers/resources/nursing/resources/nurseshdbk/nurseshdbk.pdf

Bland, A. R., Rossen, E. K., Bartlett, R., Kautz, D. D., Carnevale, T., & Benfield, S. (2009). Implementation and testing of the OPT Model as a teaching strategy in an undergraduate psychiatric nursing course. *Nursing Education Perspectives, 30*(1), 14–21.

Boshuizen, H. P. A., & Schmidt, H. G. (2000). The development of clinical reasoning expertise. In J. Higgs & M. Jones (Eds.), *Clinical reasoning in health professions* (pp. 15–22). Edinburgh, Scotland: Butterworth Heinemann.

Edwards, I., & Richardson, B. (2008). Clinical reasoning and population health: Decision making for an emerging paradigm of health care. *Physiotherapy Theory & Practice, 24*(3), 183–193. doi:10.1080/09593980701593797

Elstein, A. S., Schulman, L. S., & Sprafka, S. A. (1990). Medical problem solving: A ten-year retrospective. *Evaluation and the Health Professions, 13*(5), 5–36.

Fanning, R. M., & Gaba, D. M. (2007). The role of debriefing in simulation-based learning. *Simulation in Healthcare, 2*(2), 115–125.

Feingold, C. E., Calauce, M., & Kallen, M. A. (2004). Computerized patient model and simulated clinical experiences: Evaluation with baccalaureate nursing students. *Journal of Nursing Education, 43*(4), 156–163.

Feltovich, P. J., Prietula, M. J., & Ericsson, K. A. (2006). Studies of expertise from psychological perspectives. In K. A. Ericsson, N. Charness, P. J. Feltovich, & R. R. Hoffman (Eds.), *Cambridge handbook of expertise and expert performance,* pp. 41–67. New York, NY: Cambridge University Press.

Foronda, C., Gattamorta, K., Snowden K., & Bauman, E. B. (2014). Use of virtual clinical simulation to improve communication skills of baccalaureate nursing students: A pilot study. *Nurse Education Today, 34*(6), e53–e57.

Gillespie, M. (2010). Using the Situated Clinical Decision-Making framework to guide analysis of nurses' clinical decision-making. *Nurse Education in Practice, 10*(6), 333–340. doi:10.1016/j.nepr.2010.003

Groves, M., O'Rourke, P., & Alexander, H. (2003). The clinical reasoning characteristics of diagnostic experts. *Medical Teacher, 25*(3), 308–313. doi:10.1080/0142159031000100427

Hoben, K., Varley, R., & Cox, R. (2007). Clinical reasoning skills of speech and language therapy students. *International Journal of Language & Communication Disorders, 42*(1), 123–135. doi:10.1080/13682820601171530

Institute of Medicine (IOM). (2010). *The future of nursing: Leading change, advancing health.* Retrieved from http://www.nap.edu/catalog/12956.html

Kabanza, F., Bisson, G., Charneau, A., & Taek-Sueng, J. (2006). Implementing tutoring strategies into a patient simulator for clinical reasoning learning. *Artificial Intelligence in Medicine, 38*(1), 79–96. doi:10.1016/j.artmed.2006.01.003

Kautz, D., Kuiper, R., Bartlett, R., Buck, R., Williams, R., & Knight-Brown, P. (2009). Building evidence for the development of clinical reasoning using a rating tool with the Outcome-Present State-Test (OPT) Model. *Southern Online Journal of Nursing Research, 9*(1).

Kautz, D. D., Kuiper, R., Pesut, D. J., & Williams, R. L. (2006). Using NANDA, NIC, and NOC (NNN) language for clinical reasoning with the Outcome-Present State-Test (OPT) Model. *International Journal of Nursing Terminologies and Classifications, 17*(3), 129–138.

Kovalsky, A. A., & Swanson, R. (2004). Integration of patient care simulators into the nursing curriculum can enhance a student's ability to perform in the clinical setting. *Dean's Notes, 25*(5), 1–3.

Kuiper, R. (2013). Integration of innovative clinical reasoning pedagogies into a baccalaureate nursing curriculum. *Creative Nursing, 19*(3), 128–139. Retrieved from http://dx.doi.org/10.1891/1078-4535.19.3.128

Kuiper, R., Heinrich, C., Matthias, A., Graham, M. J., & Bell-Kotwall, L. (2008). Debriefing with the OPT Model of Clinical Reasoning during high fidelity patient simulation. *International Journal of Nursing Education Scholarship, 5*(1), 1–14.

Kuiper, R. A., & Pesut, D. J. (2004). Promoting cognitive and metacognitive reflective reasoning skills in nursing practice: Self-regulated learning theory. *Journal of Advanced Nursing, 45*(4), 381–391.

Kuiper, R. A., Pesut, D. J., & Arms, T. (2016). *Clinical reasoning and care coordination in advanced practice nursing.* New York, NY: Springer Publishing Company.

Kuiper, R., Pesut, D., & Kautz, D. (2009). Promoting the self-regulation of clinical reasoning skills in nursing students. *The Open Nursing Journal, 3,* 76–85. Retrieved from http://doi.org/10.2174/1874434600903010076

Lamb, G., Zimring, C., Chuzi, J., & Dutcher, D. (2010). Designing better healthcare environments: Interprofessional competencies in healthcare design. *Journal of Interprofessional Care, 24*(4), 422–435.

Lapkin, S., Levett-Jones, T., Bellchambers, H., & Fernandez, R. (2010). Effectiveness of patient simulation manikins in teaching clinical reasoning skills to undergraduate nursing students: A systemic review. *Clinical Simulation in Nursing, 6*(6), 207–222. doi:10.10116/j.ecns.2010.05.005

Liu, K. P. Y., Chan, C. C. H., & Hui-Chan, C. W. Y. (2000). Clinical reasoning and the occupational therapy curriculum. *Occupational Therapy International, 7*(3), 173–183.

McAllister, L., & Rose, M. (2000). Speech-language pathology students: Learning clinical reasoning. In J. Higgs & M. Jones (Eds.), *Clinical reasoning in health professions* (pp. 205–213). Edinburgh, Scotland: Butterworth Heinemann.

Morphet, J., Hood, K., Cant, R., Baulch, J., Gilbee, A., & Sandry, K. (2014). Teaching teamwork: An evaluation of an interprofessional training ward placement for health care students. *Advances in Medical Education and Practice, 5,* 197–204. Retrieved from http://dx.doi.org/10.2147/AMEP.S61189

Müller-Staub, M. (2009). Evaluation of the implementation of nursing diagnoses, interventions, and outcomes. *International Journal of Nursing Terminologies & Classifications, 20*(1), 9–15. doi:10.1111/j.1744-618X.2008.01108.x

Murphy, J. I. (2004). Using focused reflection and articulation to promote clinical reasoning: An evidence-based teaching strategy. *Nursing Education Perspectives, 25*(5), 226–231.

Norman, G. R., & Eva, K. W. (2010). Diagnostic error and clinical reasoning. *Medical Education, 44*(1), 94–100.

Petranek, C. F., Corey, S., & Black, R. (1992). Three levels of learning in simulations: Participating, debriefing and journal writing. *Simulation & Gaming, 23*(2), 174–185.

Rochmawati, E., & Wiechula, R. (2010). Education strategies to foster health professional students' clinical reasoning skills. *Nursing & Health Sciences, 12*(2), 244–250.

Schunk, D. (2015). *Learning theories: An educational perspective* (7th ed.). Upper Saddle River, NJ: Pearson Education Inc.

Sundler, A. J., Pettersson, A., & Berglund, M. (2015). Undergraduate nursing students' experiences when examining skills in clinical simulation laboratories with high-fidelity simulators: A phenomenological research study. *Nurse Education Today, 35*(12), 1257–1261.

Thistlewaite, J. (2012). Interprofessional education: A review of context, learning and the research agenda. *Medical Education, 46*(1), 58–70.

Unsworth, C. A. (2001). The clinical reasoning of novice and expert occupational therapists. *Scandinavian Journal of Occupational Therapy, 8*(4), 163–173.

GLOSSARY OF TERMS

A–B

Analogical Reasoning—Comparing a problem situation with one from experience that requires good domain knowledge and previous exposure.

Assessment—The collection of pertinent data and information related to the health of the patient, family, or community (Carpenito, 2017).

Brainstorming—Defining a problem, generating solutions, determining criteria to judge solutions, and then selecting the best solution for the outcome.

C

Care Coordination—The deliberate organization of patient care activities between two or more participants (including the patient) involved in a patient's care to facilitate the appropriate delivery of healthcare services (Agency for Healthcare Research and Quality [AHRQ], 2014).

Care Coordination Clinical Reasoning—The application of critical, creative, systems, and complexity thinking to determine the practice issues, interdependencies, and interconnections of role relationships for collaborative work in service of caring for people to address problems, interventions, and outcomes through time and across healthcare contexts and services.

Clinical Judgments—The meaning the provider attributes to the evidence derived from the test or gap analysis of the present state to the outcome state in the Outcome-Present State-Test (OPT) Model.

Clinical Reasoning—Reflective, concurrent, critical, creative, systems, and complexity thinking processes embedded in nursing practice that nurses use to filter, frame, focus, juxtapose, and test the match between a patient's present state and the desired outcome state.

Clinical Reasoning Web—A visual representation of the functional relationships between and among competing nursing care issues derived from systems and complexity thinking, which results in a convergence and identification of a central keystone issue that becomes the focus point for organizing nursing care.

Clinical Supervision—An interpersonal process designed to help people identify strengths, know weaknesses, capitalize on strengths, compensate for or correct their weaknesses, and contribute to their success.

Coaching—A collaborative relationship undertaken between a coach and a willing individual. It is time-limited and focused, and it uses conversation to help the clients achieve their goals (Donner & Wheeler, 2009).

Comparative Analysis—Process of considering the strengths and weaknesses of competing alternatives.

Competencies—Abilities to do something well (Merriam-Webster.com).

Complexity Thinking—Combining all types of thinking with an understanding of the complexity between relationships embedded in a particular patient story.

Concurrent Thinking—Simultaneous consideration of facts, concepts, and/or principles that support complexity thinking and reasoning.

Creative Thinking—A metacognitive process that supports clinical reasoning by generating associations, attributes, elements, images, and operations to solve problems (Pesut, 2008).

Critical Thinking—Purposeful self-regulatory judgment that results in interpretation, analysis, evaluation, and inference as well as the explanation of the evidential, conceptual, methodological, criteriological, or contextual considerations on which that judgment was based (Facione, 1990).

Critical Thinking Skills—Skills of interpretation, analysis, inference, explanation, evaluation, and self-regulation (Facione & Facione, 1996).

Cue—Sign, symptom, behavior, or characteristic displayed by a person that serves as data for clinical reasoning.

Cue Connection—The process of clustering two or more cues to form a pattern to guide framing, outcome specification, and establishment of a test.

Cue/Web Logic—Consideration of bio-psycho-social-spiritual facts, standardized terminologies system data, and functional relationships among diagnostic hypotheses. A reflective decision-making process that refers to inductive, deductive, and retroductive connection of cues and concepts in a Clinical Reasoning Web in order to establish an organizing frame for a clinical reasoning scenario.

D

Decision-Making—Considering and selecting interventions from a repertoire of actions that facilitate the achievement of a desired outcome state.

Deductive Reasoning—Reasoning from general to specific.

Diagnosis (as a component of the nursing process)—The analysis of data to determine actual or potential nursing diagnoses, issues, or problems (Carpenito, 2017).

Diagnostic Hypothesis—A guess; an explanation for circumstances intended to explain a situation and high-risk sequela.

Dialectic Thinking—An analytic thinking and reasoning strategy that involves appreciation of differences and multiple perspectives of contradictory positions, information, and stances. Dialectic thinking and reasoning attempts to synthesize the positions, stances, and/or phenomenon into a third integrative stance, position, or perspective. For example, the dialectic between the complementary pair of pain ~ comfort results in a synthesis perspective about pain control or comfort management.

E–F

EHR (Electronic Health Records)—The vehicle through which medical and nursing data derived from standardized terminologies is captured and stored.

Evaluation (as a component of the nursing process)—The determination of progress toward outcome achievement (Carpenito, 2017).

Filtering—The process of being conscious of the knowledge and perspectives one is using to gather data about a patient care scenario. Disciplines filter patient data differently. Sifting through and choosing significant disciplinary facts associated with a patient story.

Framing—Mental models that influence and guide our perception and behavior for the process of deriving the theme or meaning of a client-in-context situation. The frame then becomes the lens through which all thinking is viewed.

G–I

Generate-and-Test Strategy—Using knowledge to create a hierarchy of possible solutions and subsequent solution choice.

Hypocognition—Nonexistent or ineffective words or language to frame an idea that can lead to persuasive communication or orient a person for action (Lakoff, 2010; Mariotto, 2010).

Hypothesizing—Determining an explanation that accounts for a set of facts and that can be tested by further investigation.

If-Then, How-So Thinking—A thinking strategy that involves linking ideas and consequences in a logical sequence.

Implementation (as a component of the nursing process)—The execution of the developed plan of care that includes care coordination and activities related to teaching and health promotion (Carpenito, 2017).

Inductive Reasoning—Reasoning from specific to general.

Iterative Thinking—Repeated application of a rule, strategy, or tactic in service of concurrent thinking and reasoning.

J–K

Judgment—Conclusions drawn from a test of the comparison of present state to a specified outcome state. Judgments result in conclusions, clinical decisions, new tests, reframing, or exit from the reasoning task.

Juxtaposing—Side-by-side comparison of specified outcome state criteria with present state data.

Keystone Issue—Central supporting element of the client's story that guides reasoning and care planning based on an analysis and synthesis of concepts and diagnostic possibilities as represented in a Clinical Reasoning Web.

Knowledge Work—Active use of reading, memorizing, drilling, writing, and reviewing to learn clinical vocabulary (Kuiper, Pesut, & Arms, 2016).

M–N

Means-End Analysis—Comparing a problem situation with one from experience which requires good domain knowledge and previous exposure.

Metacognitive Check—The process one engages in to self-monitor, self-correct, self-reinforce, and self-evaluate one's thinking about a specific task or situation.

NANDA-I (North American Nursing Diagnosis Association)—An organization founded in 1973 with the purpose of providing a means to develop, organize, and test nursing diagnoses that are within the individual domain of nursing practice (Carpenito, 2017).

NIC (Nursing Interventions Classification)—A classification system of nursing treatments that is organized into three levels of taxonomy: domains, classes, and interventions.

NIQ (Nursing Intelligence Quotient)—The ability to apply what is learned from nursing care experiences and to use reasoning and inferences effectively as a guide for the development of nursing care knowledge.

NOC (Nursing Outcomes Classification)—System of nursing-sensitive patient outcomes that includes variable patient and family states, behaviors, or perceptions responsive to nursing interventions.

Nursing—The protection, promotion, and optimization of health and abilities; prevention of illness and injury; facilitation of healing; alleviation of suffering through the diagnosis and treatment of human response; and advocacy in the care of individuals, families, communities, and populations (American Nurses Association [ANA], 2015).

Nursing Analytics—Extensive use of data to describe, predict, prescribe, and compare data that drives decision-making with the goal of improving results surrounding patient/family care problems.

Nursing Art—Caring and respect of human dignity and a compassionate approach to patient care that embrace spirituality, health, empathy, mutual respect, and partnership (ANA, 2015).

Nursing Diagnosis—A clinical judgment about an individual, family, or community response to actual or potential health problems or life processes (NANDA-I, 2009).

Nursing Informatics—The science and practice that integrates nursing, its information, and knowledge with management of information and communication technologies to promote the health of people, families, and communities worldwide (American Medical Informatics Association [AMIA], 2015).

Nursing Minimum Data Set—A set of variables with uniform definitions and categories concerning the specific dimensions of nursing that meet the information needs of multiple data users in the macro healthcare system.

Nursing Process—A five-part systematic decision-making method focusing on identifying and treating responses of individuals or groups to actual or potential alterations in health. Includes assessment, nursing diagnosis, planning, implementation, and evaluation (MediLexicon International, 2016).

Nursing Science—Nursing using logic to understand and solve patient problems.

O

Omaha Nursing Classification System—A systematic means to classify and code problems and interventions relevant to community and home healthcare nursing practice.

OPT (Outcome-Present State-Test) Model—A concurrent iterative model of clinical reasoning that emphasizes reflective self-monitoring while filtering, framing, and focusing the context and content of clinical reasoning and juxtaposing outcome state with present state client data. Clinical decision-making in this model relates to choosing nursing actions. Clinical judgment in this model is attributing meaning to the results of a test or match between desired criteriological outcome state and present state.

Outcome Specification—Process of determining the desired end state of the client.

Outcome State—The desired condition of the client derived from the frame and initial present state data as well as criteria that define the desired condition.

Outcome-Focused Thinking—Thinking that emphasizes outcomes or end results.

P

Patient-Centered Thinking—Thinking about transforming problems through care-coordination activities and reflecting on the patient and family needs and issues to achieve success.

Patient-in-Context Story—The central issues of the patient's story which are derived from patient communications (both verbal and nonverbal), physical assessments, significant others and family interviews, and prior medical records.

Planning (as a component of the nursing process)—The design of strategies to achieve desired outcomes for the consumer or situation (Carpenito, 2017).

Present State—The initial condition of the patient derived from cue/web logic and defined by standardized terminologies that changes over time as a result of nursing actions and decisions as well as the current condition of the client at the time of the test.

Prototype Identification—Using a model or textbook case as a reference point for comparative analysis.

R

Reflection—The process of observing one's thinking while simultaneously thinking about the patient's situation, the goal of which is to achieve the best possible thought processes.

Reflection Check—The process of intentionally using self-regulation strategies of self-monitoring, self-correcting, self-reinforcing, and self-evaluating one's thinking about a specific task or situation (Herman, Pesut, & Conard, 1994; Kuiper & Pesut, 2004; Pesut & Herman, 1992; Worrell, 1990).

Reflective Thinking—Conscious application of the thinking strategies, functional relationships of self-talk; prototype identification; schema search; hypothesizing; if-then, how-so thinking; juxtaposing; comparative analysis; reflexive comparison; and reframing.

Reflexive Comparison—Making a judgment about the state of a situation after gauging the presence or absence of some quality against a standard using the current case as a reference criterion.

Reframing—Attributing a different meaning to the content or context of a situation given a set of cues, web logic, tests, decisions, or judgments.

S

Scenario—An outline of a hypothesized or projected chain of events.

Schema—Pattern imposed on complex reality or experience to assist in explaining it, mediating perception, or guiding a response.

Schema Search—Accessing general and/or specific patterns of past experiences that might apply to the current situation.

Scientific Method—Problem-solving approach where a problem is identified, possible solutions to the problem are hypothesized, and experiments are designed to test a solution to the problem.

Self-Regulation—Metacognitive process whereby individuals actively pursue and sustain behaviors, cognitions, and emotions, which are geared toward goal attainment (Zimmerman & Schunk, 2001).

Self-Talk—Expressing one's thoughts to one's self.

Spinning and Weaving a Web—The process of using thinking strategies to analyze and synthesize functional relationships among diagnostic hypotheses associated with a client's health status.

Standardized Terminology—Vocabularies and language commonly understood by those within a profession to provide a common means of communication.

Systems Thinking—Attention to distinctions (D), systems rules (S), relationship rules (R), and perspective rules (P) to make distinctions between and among ideas or things to split them into parts, lump them into a whole, or relate them to each other (Cabrera & Cabrera, 2015).

T–Z

Taxonomy—The classification or naming into ordered categories.

Test—The process of juxtaposing the present state and outcome state and evaluating the criteriological match between present-state data and the specified outcome.

Thinking Strategies—Specific cognitive and metacognitive techniques and strategies that nurses use when engaged in reflective clinical reasoning.

References

Agency for Healthcare Research and Quality (AHRQ). (2014). Chapter 2. What is care coordination? Care coordination measures atlas update. Rockville, MD: Agency for Healthcare Research and Quality. Retrieved from http://www.ahrq.gov/professionals/prevention-chronic-care/improve/coordination/atlas2014/chapter2.html

American Medical Informatics Association (AMIA). (2015). Retrieved from http://www.amia.org/about-amia/mission-and-history

American Nurses Association (ANA). (2015). *Nursing: Scope and standards of practice* (3rd ed.). Silver Spring, MD: American Nurses Association.

Cabrera, D., & Cabrera, L. (2015). *Systems thinking made simple: New hope for solving wicked problems.* New York, NY: Odyssean Press.

Carpenito, L. J. (2017). *Nursing diagnosis: Application to clinical practice* (15th ed.). Philadelphia, PA: Wolters Kluwer Health.

D'Amour, D., & Oandasan, I. (2005). Interprofessionality as the field of interprofessional practice and interprofessional education: An emerging concept. *Journal of Interprofessional Care (Supplement 1),* 8–20.

Donner, G., & Wheeler, M. M. (2009). *Coaching in nursing: An introduction* (p. 9). Switzerland: International Council of Nurses; Indianapolis, IN: Sigma Theta Tau International.

Facione, P. A. (1990). *The Delphi Report executive summary.* Montclair, NJ: Montclair State University Center for Critical Thinking, and Millbrae, CA: The California Academic Press. ERIC, ED 315423. 1–22.

Facione, N. C., & Facione, P. A. (1996). Externalizing the critical thinking in knowledge development and clinical judgment. *Nursing Outlook, 44*(3), 129–136.

Herman, J., Pesut. D., & Conard, L. (1994). Using metacognitive skills: The quality audit tool. *Nursing Diagnosis, 5*(2), 56–64.

Kuiper, R., & Pesut, D. J. (2004). Promoting cognitive and metacognitive reflective clinical reasoning skills in nursing practice: Self-regulated learning theory. *Journal of Advanced Nursing, 45*(4), 381–391.

Kuiper, R. A., Pesut, D. J., & Arms, T. (2016). *Clinical reasoning and care coordination in advanced practice nursing.* New York, NY: Springer Publishing Company.

Lakoff, G. (2010). Why it matters how we frame the environment. *Environmental Communication: A Journal of Nature and Culture, 4*(1), 70–81. doi: 10.1080/17524030903529749

Mariotto, A. (2010). Hypocognition and evidence-based medicine. *Internal Medicine Journal, 40*(1), 80–82. doi:10.1111/j.1445-5994.2009.02086.x

MediLexicon International Ltd. (2016). Nursing process. Retrieved from http://medical-dictionary.thefreedictionary.com/nursing+process

Merriam-Webster: Dictionary and Thesaurus. Retrieved from http://www.merriam-webster.com; http://www.learnersdictionary.com

National Library of Medicine. (2009). UMLS reference manual (2015). Retrieved from http://www.ncbi.nlm.nih.gov/books/NBK9676

North American Nursing Diagnosis Association (NANDA-I). (2009). *Nursing diagnoses: Definitions and classification 2009-2012.* Ames, IA: Wiley-Blackwell.

Nursing Working Group of the American Medical Informatics Association. (2015). Retrieved from http://www.amia.org/programs/working-groups/nursing-informatics

Pesut, D. (2008). Thoughts on thinking with complexity in mind. In C. Lindberg, S. Nash, & C. Lindberg (Eds.), *On the edge: Nursing in the age of complexity* (pp. 211–238). Bordentown, NJ: PlexusPress.

Pesut, D. J., & Herman, J. A. (1992). Reflection skills in diagnostic reasoning. *Nursing Diagnosis, 3*(4), 148–154.

Werley, H. H., Ryan, P., & Zorn, C. R. (1995). *The NMMDS: A framework for the organization of nursing language. An emerging framework: Data system advances for clinical nursing practice.* American Nurses' Association: American Nurses Publishing, #NP-94.

Worrell, P. (1990). Metacognition: Implications for instruction in nursing education. *Journal of Nursing Education, 29,* 170–175.

Zimmerman, B., & Schunk, D. S. (2001). *Self-regulated learning and academic thought.* Mahwah, NJ: Lawrence Erlbaum Associates.

INDEX

A

ABC (Alternative Billing Codes), 8, 36
academic versus practical intelligence/
    problems, 392–395
adolescent with traumatic injury case study
    background information, 177–179
    care plan, 179–180
    CRW (Clinical Reasoning Web), 181–190
    diagnostic cluster/cue logic, 191–192
    framing, 192
    interventions, 195–197
    judgments, 197–199
    nursing diagnoses/domains and
        connections, 182–189
    OPT Model, 200
    outcome-present state-tests, 192–193,
        198–199
    patient-in-context story, 190–191
    testing, 194–195
ADPIE (assess, diagnose, plan, intervene,
    and evaluate) model, 8–9
Alternative Billing Codes (ABC), 8, 36
ANA (American Nurses Association)
    NIDSEC (Nursing Information and Data
        Set Evaluation Center), 32
    Nursing: Scope and Standards of
        Practice, 3rd Edition, 4–6, 16–17
    standardized terminologies, 34–37
    Steering Committee on Classifications of
        Nursing Practice Data, 32–33
analogical reasoning, 54, 424
APIE (assess, plan, implement, and evaluate)
    model, 8–9
assessment domains, 126–132, 424

B

benign prostatic hyperplasia. See BPH
blindness and diabetes case study
    background information, 375–376
    comparative analysis, 382–383

CRW (Clinical Reasoning Web), Omaha
    System terminology, 376–377, 383–
    384
decision-making, 385
hypothesizing, 379
if-then, how-so thinking, 380–382
interventions, 385
juxtaposing, 384–385
OPT Model, 387
outcome-present state-tests, 373–375
prototype identification, 379
reflection checks, 388
reflexive comparison, 386
reframing, 388
schema searches, 379
self-talk, 378
BPH (benign prostatic hyperplasia) case
    study
    background information, 270–272
    care plan, 272
    CRW (Clinical Reasoning Web), 280–285
    diagnostic cluster/cue logic, 286–287
    framing, 287
    interventions, 290–293
    judgments, 293–296
    nursing diagnoses/domains and
        connections, 273–284
    OPT Model, 297
    outcome-present state-tests, 288–289,
        294–296
    patient-in-context story, 285–286
    testing, 289–290
brainstorming, 54, 424

C

Caregiver Role Strain case study
    background information, 207–209
    care plan, 209–210
    CRW (Clinical Reasoning Web), 211–220
    diagnostic cluster/cue logic, 221–222
    framing, 222

interventions, 225–227

judgments, 227–229

nursing diagnoses/domains and connections, 212–220

OPT Model, 230

outcome-present state-tests, 198–199, 223–224, 229

patient-in-context story, 221

testing, 224–225

care plans/coordination

case studies

adolescent with traumatic injury, 179–180

BPH (benign prostatic hyperplasia), 272

gerontology stroke patient, 308

middle-aged female with endometriosis and surgical intervention, 240–247

neonatal jaundice, 150–154

palliative care, 339

young adult and mental illness, 209–210

definition of, 424

case studies

adolescent with traumatic injury

background information, 177–179

care plans, 179–180

CRW (Clinical Reasoning Web), 181–190

diagnostic cluster/cue logic, 191–192

framing, 192

interventions, 195–197

judgments, 197–199

nursing diagnoses/domains and connections, 181–189

OPT Model, 200

outcome-present state-tests, 192–193, 198–199

patient-in-context stories, 190–191

testing, 194–195

BPH (benign prostatic hyperplasia)

background information, 270–272

care plans, 272

CRW (Clinical Reasoning Web), 280–285

diagnostic cluster/cue logic, 286–287

framing, 287

interventions, 290–293

judgments, 293–296

nursing diagnoses/domains and connections, 273–284

OPT Model, 297

outcome-present state-tests, 288–289, 294–296

patient-in-context stories, 285–286

testing, 289–290

elderly female with diabetes and blindness

background information, 375–376

comparative analysis, 382–383

CRW (Clinical Reasoning Web), 376–377, 383–384

decision-making, 385

hypothesizing, 379

if-then, how-so thinking, 380–382

interventions, 385

juxtaposing, 384–385

OPT Model, 387

outcome-present state-tests, 373–375

prototype identification, 379

reflection checks, 388

reflexive comparison, 386

reframing, 388

schema searches, 379

self-talk, 378

gerontology stroke patient

background information, 306–308

care plans, 308

CRW (Clinical Reasoning Web), 314–319

diagnostic cluster/cue logic, 320–321
framing, 321
interventions, 324–325
judgments, 326–328
nursing diagnoses/domains and
connections, 309–319
OPT Model, 328–329
outcome-present state-tests, 321–323,
327–328
patient-in-context stories, 319–320
testing, 323
middle-aged female with endometriosis
and surgical intervention
background information, 237–239
care plans, 240–247
CRW (Clinical Reasoning Web),
248–253
diagnostic cluster/cue logic, 254–255
framing, 255
interventions, 258–260
judgments, 261–262
nursing diagnoses/domains and
connections, 242–251
OPT Model, 264
outcome-present state-tests, 255–257,
262
patient-in-context stories, 253–254
testing, 257–258
neonatal jaundice
background information, 146–149
care plans, 150–154
CRW (Clinical Reasoning Web),
155–160
diagnostic cluster/cue logic, 161–162
framing, 162
interventions, 165–167
judgments, 167–169
nursing diagnoses/domains and
connections, 150–159
OPT Model, 169–170
outcome-present state-tests, 162–164,
168–169

patient-in-context stories, 160–161
testing, 164–165
palliative care
background information, 337–338
care plans, 339
CRW (Clinical Reasoning Web),
344–349
diagnostic cluster/cue logic, 350–351
framing, 351
interventions, 354–355, 357
judgments, 356–357
nursing diagnoses/domains and
connections, 339–349
OPT Model, 358
outcome-present state-tests, 351–353,
357
patient-in-context stories, 349–350
testing, 353
young adult and mental illness
background information, 207–209
care plans, 209–210
CRW (Clinical Reasoning Web),
211–220
diagnostic cluster/cue logic, 221–222
framing, 222
interventions, 225–227
judgments, 227–229
nursing diagnoses/domains and
connections, 211–220
OPT Model, 230
outcome-present state-tests, 223–224,
229
patient-in-context stories, 221
testing, 224–225
CCC (Clinical Care Classification), 8, 36
Center for Nursing Classification and
Clinical Effectiveness, 35
Clinical Care Classification (CCC), 8, 36
clinical decision-making
definition of, 426
Omaha System, 385

OPT Model, 116–118
thinking tactics, 64–65
clinical judgments
case studies
adolescent with traumatic injury, 197–199
BPH (benign prostatic hyperplasia), 293–296
gerontology stroke patient, 326–328
middle-aged female with endometriosis and surgical intervention, 261–262
neonatal jaundice, 167–169
palliative care, 356–357
young adult and mental illness, 227–229
definitions of, 133, 424, 427
OPT Model, 118–124
clinical reasoning. *See also* CRW; OPT Model of Clinical Reasoning
contemporary practice features, 15–17
definition of, 424
Omaha System terminologies, 367–375
clinical supervision
basics, 395–397
CRW (Clinical Reasoning Web), 402
definitions of, 395, 425
OPT Model/Worksheet, 395–403
cluster/cue logic. *See* diagnostic cluster/cue logic
coaching, 393, 425
comfort care. *See* palliative care/ovarian cancer case study
comparative analyses
basics, 62, 106, 382–383
definitions of, 61, 108, 425
compartment syndrome case study
background information, 177–179
care plan, 179–180
CRW (Clinical Reasoning Web), 181–190
diagnostic cluster/cue logic, 191–192
framing, 192
interventions, 195–197

judgments, 197–199
nursing diagnoses/domains and connections, 182–189
OPT Model, 200
outcome-present state-tests, 192–193, 198–199
patient-in-context story, 190–191
testing, 194–195
competencies, 425
complexity thinking
components of, 50, 57–58
CRW (Clinical Reasoning Web), 14
definitions of, 403, 425
concurrent thinking, 425
county nursing practice data level, 26–28
creative thinking
analogical reasoning, 54
brainstorming, 54
in clinical supervision, 401
components of, 50, 53–54
definitions of, 403, 425
critical thinking
components of, 50–52
definitions of, 403, 425
versus thinking strategies and reflective clinical reasoning, 136–139
CRW (Clinical Reasoning Web), 14, 424
case studies
adolescent with traumatic injury, 181–190
BPH (benign prostatic hyperplasia), 280–285
diabetes with blindness, 376–384
gerontology stroke patient, 314–319
middle-aged female with endometriosis and surgical intervention, 248–253
neonatal jaundice, 155–160
palliative care, 344–349
young adult and mental illness, 211–220
creating, 76–78
definition of, 14, 424

diagnostic cluster/cue logic questions, 78–83

framing and present-outcome state-tests, 102–104

keystone issues, 79–82

nursing domains and diagnoses connections, 79–80

outcome-present state-tests, 101–102

patient-in-context stories, 73–76

cue connections. *See* diagnostic cluster/cue logic

curriculum integration and OPT Model, 410–415

D

debriefing and OPT Model, 408–410

deductive reasoning, 74, 426

diabetes with blindness case study

background information, 375–376

comparative analysis, 382–383

CRW (Clinical Reasoning Web), Omaha System terminology, 376–377, 383–384

decision-making, 385

hypothesizing, 379

if-then, how-so thinking, 380–382

interventions, 385

juxtaposing, 384–385

OPT Model, 387

outcome-present state-tests, 373–375

prototype identification, 379

reflection checks, 388

reflexive comparison, 386

reframing, 388

schema searches, 379

self-talk, 378

diagnoses. *See* nursing diagnoses

diagnostic cluster/cue logic

case studies

adolescent with traumatic injury, 191–192

BPH (benign prostatic hyperplasia), 286–287

gerontology stroke patient, 320–321

middle-aged female with endometriosis and surgical intervention, 254–255

neonatal jaundice, 161–162

palliative care, 350–351

young adult and mental illness, 221–222

creating, 78–79

CRW (Clinical Reasoning Web), 76–83

definitions of, 425–426

filtering information, 94–95

keystone issues, 79–83

nursing domain and diagnoses connections, 79–80

patient-in-context stories, 74–76

types, 74

diagnostic hypotheses, 62, 426. *See also* hypothesizing

dialectic thinking, 74, 426

E

EHR (electronic health records), 31, 426

endometriosis in middle-aged female case study

background information, 237–239

care plan, 240–247

CRW (Clinical Reasoning Web), 248–253

diagnostic cluster/cue logic, 254–255

framing, 255

interventions, 258–260

judgments, 261–262

nursing diagnoses/domains and connections, 242–251

OPT Model, 264

outcome-present state-tests, 255–257, 262

patient-in-context story, 253–254

testing, 257–258

environmental practice domain
  case studies
    diabetes (type 2) with blindness, 378, 380–381, 383
    mental illness in young adult, 219
    neonatal jaundice, 153–154, 158
    palliative care, 347
  with diagnoses and web connections, 37–39, 79
  Omaha System, 367, 369, 377–378
evaluation, nursing process component, 426

F

The Fifth Discipline, 96
filtering
  definitions of, 108, 426–427
  with framing and focusing, 92–102
focusing, with filtering and framing, 92–102
framing
  case studies
    adolescent with traumatic injury, 192
    BPH (benign prostatic hyperplasia), 287
    gerontology stroke patient, 321
    middle-aged female with endometriosis and surgical intervention, 255
    neonatal jaundice, 162
    palliative care, 351
    young adult and mental illness, 222
  definitions of, 108, 427
  with filtering and focusing, 92–102
functional practice domain, 38–39
  case studies
    mental illness in young adult, 219
    neonatal jaundice, 151, 158
    palliative care, 347
  with diagnoses, outcomes, and interventions, 37–39, 79

G

generate-and-test strategy, 53, 427
gerontology stroke patient case study
  background information, 306–308
  care plan, 308
  CRW (Clinical Reasoning Web), 314–319
  diagnostic cluster/cue logic, 320–321
  framing, 321
  interventions, 324–325
  judgments, 326–328
  nursing diagnoses/domains and connections, 309–319
  OPT Model, 328–329
  outcome-present state-tests, 321–323, 327–328
  patient-in-context story, 319–320
  testing, 323

H

health-related behaviors practice domain
  diabetes (type 2) with blindness case study, 380–381, 383
  Omaha System, 369–370, 377
hospice care versus palliative care, 336–337
hypocognition, 49, 427
hypothesizing
  basics, 62, 105–106, 379
  definitions of, 60, 108, 427

I

ICNP (International Classification for Nursing Practice), 8, 19, 34
if-then, how-so thinking
  basics, 54, 62, 106, 380–382
  definitions of, 61, 108, 427
implementation, nursing process component, 427
individual nursing practice data level, 25–26

inductive reasoning, 74, 427
International Classification for Nursing
    Practice (ICNP), 8, 19, 34
interprofessional education and OPT Model,
    415–417
interventions, 114–116
    care planning/management worksheet,
        126–132
    case studies
        adolescent with traumatic injury,
            195–197
        BPH (benign prostatic hyperplasia),
            290–293
        diabetes with blindness, 385
        gerontology stroke patient, 324–325
        middle-aged female with endometriosis
            and surgical intervention, 258–260
        neonatal jaundice, 165–167
        palliative care, 354–355, 357
        young adult and mental illness, 225–
            227
    decision-making process, 116–118
    judgments, 118–124
    nursing practice domains, 37–39
    Omaha System, 370–372
Iowa Nursing Intervention project, 24
iterative thinking, 13, 92, 427

J

jaundice case study
    background information, 146–149
    care plan, 150–154
    CRW (Clinical Reasoning Web), 155–160
    diagnostic cluster/cue logic, 161–162
    framing, 162
    interventions, 165–167
    judgments, 167–169
    nursing diagnoses/domains and
        connections, 151–159
    OPT Model, 169–170
    outcome-present state-tests, 162–164,
        168–169
    patient-in-context story, 160–161
    testing, 164–165
judgments. See clinical judgments
juxtaposing
    basics, 63, 106–107, 384–385
    definitions of, 61, 108, 428

K–L

keystone issues
    CRW (Clinical Reasoning Web) and OPT
        Model Worksheet, 79–83
    definitions of, 14, 428
knowledge work
    basics, 58–59, 86
    definitions of, 60, 85, 428

Logical Observation Identifiers Names and
    Codes (LOINC), 8, 37
LOINC (Logical Observation Identifiers
    Names and Codes), 8, 37

M

means-ends analyses, 53–54, 428
mental illness in young adult case study
    background information, 207–209
    care plan, 209–210
    CRW (Clinical Reasoning Web), 211–220
    diagnostic cluster/cue logic, 221–222
    framing, 222
    interventions, 225–227
    judgments, 227–229
    nursing diagnoses/domains and
        connections, 212–220
    OPT Model, 230
    outcome-present state-tests, 198–199,
        223–224, 229
    patient-in-context story, 221
    testing, 224–225
metacognitive thinking/checks, 48–50, 403,
    428

middle-aged female with endometriosis and surgical intervention case study
  background information, 237–239
  care plan, 240–247
  CRW (Clinical Reasoning Web), 248–253
  diagnostic cluster/cue logic, 254–255
  framing, 255
  interventions, 258–260
  judgments, 261–262
  nursing diagnoses/domains and connections, 242–251
  OPT Model, 264
  outcome-present state-tests, 255–257, 262
  patient-in-context story, 253–254
  testing, 257–258

N

NANDA-I (North American Nursing Diagnosis Association) classifications
  ANA-recognized standardized terminologies, 7–8, 35
  case studies
    adolescent with traumatic injury, 183–186
    BPH (benign prostatic hyperplasia), 275–279
    gerontology stroke patient, 311–313
    middle-aged female with endometriosis and surgical intervention, 243–247
    neonatal jaundice, 151–154
    palliative care, 341–343
    young adult and mental illness, 213–215
  definition of, 428
  OPT Model Worksheet, 126–132
  purpose of, 40
National Hospice and Palliative Care Organization, 336
neonatal jaundice case study
  background information, 146–149
  care plan, 150–154
  CRW (Clinical Reasoning Web), 155–160
  diagnostic cluster/cue logic, 161–162
  framing, 162
  interventions, 165–167
  judgments, 167–169
  nursing diagnoses/domains and connections, 151–159
  OPT Model, 169–170
  outcome-present state-tests, 162–164, 168–169
  patient-in-context story, 160–161
  testing, 164–165
network nursing practice data level, 26–28
NIC (Nursing Intervention Classifications) system
  case studies
    adolescent with traumatic injury, 183–186
    BPH (benign prostatic hyperplasia), 275–279
    gerontology stroke patient, 311–313
    middle-aged female with endometriosis and surgical intervention, 243–247
    neonatal jaundice, 151–154
    palliative care, 341–343
    young adult and mental illness, 213–215
  nursing practice data levels, 31
  OPT Model Worksheet, 126–132
  standardized terminologies, 8, 35, 40
NIDSEC (Nursing Information and Data Set Evaluation Center), 32
NIQ (Nursing Intelligence Quotient), 393–395, 428
NMDS (Nursing Minimum Data Set), 34, 429
NMMDS (Nursing Management Minimum Data Set), 25, 27, 34. *See also* nursing practice data levels
NOC (Nursing Outcome Classification)
  basics, 40–41

case studies
  adolescent with traumatic injury, 183–186
  BPH (benign prostatic hyperplasia), 275–279
  gerontology stroke patient, 311–313
  middle-aged female with endometriosis and surgical intervention, 243–247
  neonatal jaundice, 151–154
  palliative care, 341–343
  young adult and mental illness, 213–215
definition of, 428
OPT Model Worksheet, 126–132
standardized terminologies, 8, 31, 35
North American Nursing Diagnosis Association classifications. See NANDA-I
nursing analytics, 429
nursing art, 16–17, 429
nursing diagnoses, 7
  case studies
    adolescent with traumatic injury, 182–189
    BPH (benign prostatic hyperplasia), 273–284
    gerontology stroke patient, 309–319
    middle-aged female with endometriosis and surgical intervention, 242–251
    neonatal jaundice, 151–159
    palliative care, 339–349
    young adult and mental illness, 212–220
  definitions of, 426, 429
  practice domains, 37–39
nursing informatics
  definition of, 429
  EHRs (electronic health records), 31, 426
  standardized terminologies, 29–37
    ANA recognition of, 32–37
    NIDSEC (Nursing Information and Data Set Evaluation Center), 32
    Steering Committee on Classifications of Nursing Practice Data, 32–33

Nursing Information and Data Set Evaluation Center (NIDSEC), 32
Nursing Intelligence Quotient (NIQ), 393–395, 428
Nursing Intervention Classifications system. See NIC
Nursing Management Minimum Data Set (NMMDS), 25, 27, 34. See also nursing practice data levels
Nursing Minimum Data Set (NMDS), 34, 429
Nursing Outcome Classification. See NOC
nursing practice data levels. See also NMMDS
  data elements, 27–28
  individual, 25–26
  network/state/country, 26–28
  overview, 24–26
  unit/organization, 26–27
nursing practice domains. See environmental, functional, health-related behaviors, physiological, and psychosocial practice domains
nursing process
  clinical reasoning, 15–17
  definition of, 429
  evolution of, 8–9
  history of, 6–12
  Omaha System, 8
  OPT Model, 9–15
  outcome specifications, 9
  planning component of, 430
  six-step process, 10–12
nursing profession
  definition of, 428–429
  interprofessional education, 415–417
  Nursing: Scope and Standards of Practice, 3rd Edition, 4–6
nursing science, 15–17, 429. See also nursing informatics
Nursing: Scope and Standards of Practice, 3rd Edition, 4–6, 16–17

O

Omaha System
  community care, 366
  definition of, 429
  interventions and targets, 370–371
  nursing practice domains/problems, 41–42, 367–370
  Problem Classification Scheme, 367–370
  Problem Rating Scale for Outcomes, 373–375
  standardized terminologies, 8, 35
OPT (Outcome-Present State-Test) Model of Clinical Reasoning, 9–15. *See also* CRW (Clinical Reasoning Web)
  case studies
    adolescent with traumatic injury, 200
    BPH (benign prostatic hyperplasia), 297
    diabetes with blindness, 387
    gerontology stroke patient, 328–329
    middle-aged female with endometriosis and surgical intervention, 264
    neonatal jaundice, 169–170
    palliative care, 358
    young adult and mental illness, 230
  definition of, 430
  Worksheet
    clinical judgments, 121
    diagnostic cluster/cue logic, 83
    framing, 98
    outcome-present state-tests, 99
    patient-in-context stories, 76
    reframing, 135
outcome-focused thinking, 100, 430
outcome-present state-tests, 93
  case studies
    adolescent with traumatic injury, 192–193, 198–199
    BPH (benign prostatic hyperplasia), 288–289, 294–296
    diabetes with blindness, 373–375

endometriosis, 255–257, 262
    gerontology stroke patient, 321–323, 327–328
    neonatal jaundice, 163–164, 168–169
    palliative care, 351–353, 357
    young adult and mental illness, 223–224, 229
  definition of, 430
  focusing, 99–102
  framing, 95–99, 102–104
  nursing practice domains, 37–39
  Problem Rating Scale for Outcomes, 373–375

P

palliative care/ovarian cancer case study
  background information, 337–338
  care plan, 339
  CRW (Clinical Reasoning Web), 344–349
  diagnostic cluster/cue logic, 350–351
  framing, 351
  versus hospice care, 336–337
  interventions, 354–355, 357
  judgments, 356–357
  nursing diagnoses/domains and connections, 339–349
  OPT Model, 358
  outcome-present state-tests, 351–353, 357
  palliative care versus hospice care, 336–337
  patient-in-context story, 349–350
  testing, 353
paradigmatic assumptions, 51
patient-centered thinking. *See* care plans/coordination
patient-in-context stories
  case studies
    adolescent with traumatic injury, 177–179, 190–191

BPH (benign prostatic hyperplasia), 285–286
  endometriosis, 253–254
  gerontology stroke patient, 319–320
  neonatal jaundice, 160–161
  palliative care, 349–350
  young adult and mental illness, 221
CRW Worksheet, 76
definition of, 430
Perioperative Nursing Data Set (PNDS), 8, 36
physiological practice domain, 38–39
  case studies
    diabetes (type 2) with blindness, 378, 380–381, 383
    mental illness in young adult, 219
    neonatal jaundice, 151–152, 158
    palliative care, 347
  with diagnoses, outcomes, and interventions, 37–39, 79
  Omaha System, 368–369, 377
planning nursing process component, 430
PNDS (Perioperative Nursing Data Set), 8, 36
practical versus academic intelligence/problems, 392–395
prescriptive assumptions, 51
present states. See outcome-present state-tests
Problem Rating Scale for Outcomes, Omaha System, 373–375
prototype identification
  basics, 61, 87, 379
  definitions of, 60, 85, 430
psychosocial practice domain, 38–39
  case studies
    diabetes (type 2) with blindness, 378, 380–381, 383
    mental illness in young adult, 219
    neonatal jaundice, 152–153, 158
    palliative care, 347

  with diagnoses, outcomes, and interventions, 37–39, 79
  Omaha System, 367, 369, 377

R

reflection checks
  basics, 64, 134–136, 388
  definitions of, 61, 431
reflection-in-action, 394–395
reflective clinical reasoning, 136–139
reflective self-regulation, 432
  components of, 50
  definition of, 403
  self-monitoring, 52–53
  Social Cognitive Theory, 52
reflective thinking skills, 392–395, 431
reflexive comparisons
  basics, 63, 107, 133, 386
  definitions of, 61, 109, 431
reframing
  basics, 63–64, 134–135, 388
  definitions of, 61, 133, 431

S

scenarios, 431
schema searches
  basics, 59–60, 87, 379
  definitions of, 60, 85, 431
Schön, Donald, 394
scientific methods, 431
Scope and Standards of Practice, 4–6, 16–17
self-monitoring. See reflective self-regulation
self-talk
  basics, 58–59, 86–87, 378
  definitions of, 60, 85, 432
Senge, Peter, 96
simulation debriefing, 408–410
SNOMED CT (Systematized Nomenclature of Medicine—Clinical Terms), 8, 37

Social Cognitive Theory, 52
spinning/weaving webs. *See* CRW (Clinical Reasoning Web)
standardized terminologies
    ANA-recognized, 32–37
    definition of, 432
    domains of practice/interest, 37–39
    future of, 42–43
    nursing data levels, 24–28
    nursing informatics, 29–32
    nursing process evolution, 8
state nursing practice data level, 26–28
Steering Committee on Classifications of Nursing Practice Data, 32
stroke patient case study
    background information, 306–308
    care plan, 308
    CRW (Clinical Reasoning Web), 314–319
    diagnostic cluster/cue logic, 320–321
    framing, 321
    interventions, 324–325
    judgments, 326–328
    nursing diagnoses/domains and connections, 309–319
    OPT Model, 328–329
    outcome-present state-tests, 321–323, 327–328
    patient-in-context story, 319–320
    testing, 323
supportive care. *See* palliative care/ovarian cancer case study
symptom management. *See* palliative care/ovarian cancer case study
Systematized Nomenclature of Medicine—Clinical Terms (SNOMED CT), 8, 37
systems thinking
    definitions of, 55, 403, 432
    filters and frames, 56
    key concepts of, 50, 54–55

T

taxonomies, 432. *See also* specific taxonomies
testing
    case studies
        adolescent with traumatic injury, 194–195
        BPH (benign prostatic hyperplasia), 289–290
        endometriosis, 257–258
        gerontology stroke patient, 323
        neonatal jaundice, 164
        palliative care, 353
        young adult and mental illness, 224–225
    definition of, 432
thinking strategies
    cognitive/metacognitive, 109
    versus critical thinking skills and reflective clinical reasoning, 136–139
traumatic injury of adolescent case study
    background information, 177–179
    care plan, 179–180
    CRW (Clinical Reasoning Web), 181–190
    diagnostic cluster/cue logic, 191–192
    framing, 192
    interventions, 195–197
    judgments, 197–199
    nursing diagnoses/domains and connections, 182–189
    OPT Model, 200
    outcome-present state-tests, 192–193, 198–199
    patient-in-context story, 190–191
    testing, 194–195

U–V

unit/organization nursing practice data level, 26–27

Visiting Nurses Association of Omaha, 41

W–X–Y–Z

young adult and mental illness case study
    background information, 207–209
    care plan, 209–210
    CRW (Clinical Reasoning Web), 211–220
    diagnostic cluster/cue logic, 221–222
    framing, 222
    interventions, 225–227
    judgments, 227–229
    nursing diagnoses/domains and
        connections, 212–220
    OPT Model, 230
    outcome-present state-tests, 198–199,
       223–224, 229
    patient-in-context story, 221
    testing, 224–225

Anatomy of Medical Errors:
The Patient in Room 2

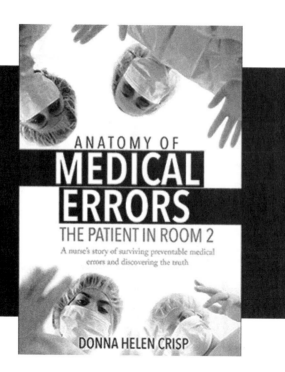

Donna Helen Crisp

To order, visit **www.nursingknowledge.org/sttibooks**.
Discounts are available for institutional purchases. Call **888.NKI.4YOU** for details.

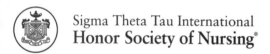
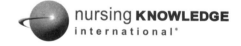

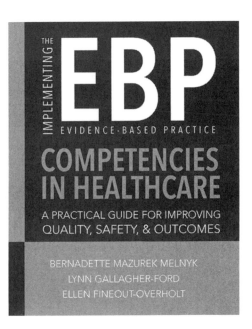

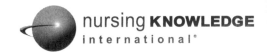

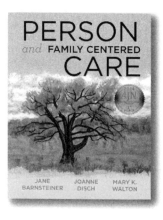
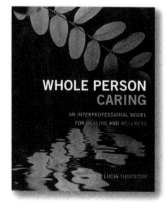
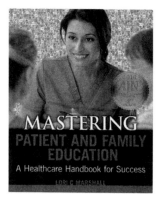
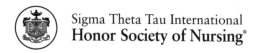
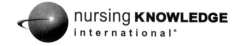

Reflection: A Valuable Tool for Change

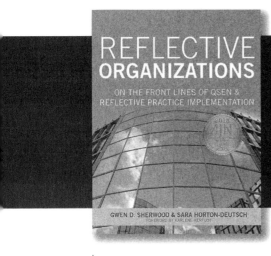

Reflective Organizations

Gwen D. Sherwood and
Sara Horton-Deutsch

Reflective Practice

Gwen D. Sherwood and
Sara Horton-Deutsch

To order, visit **www.nursingknowledge.org/sttibooks**.
Discounts are available for institutional purchases.
Call **888.NKI.4YOU** for details.

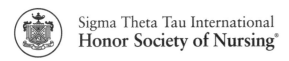
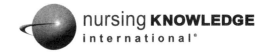

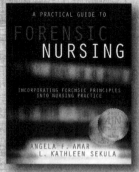
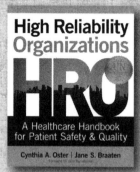
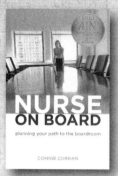
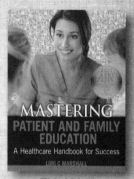
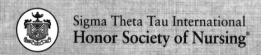
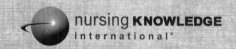